Improving Aid Effectiveness in Global Health

Elvira Beracochea

Editor

Improving Aid Effectiveness in Global Health

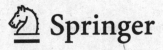 Springer

Editor
Elvira Beracochea
Realizing Global Health Inc.
Fairfax, VA, USA

ISBN 978-1-4939-4633-4   ISBN 978-1-4939-2721-0   (eBook)
DOI 10.1007/978-1-4939-2721-0

Springer New York Heidelberg Dordrecht London

Printed on acid-free paper

Springer Science+Business Media LLC New York is part of Springer Science+Business Media (www.springer.com)

Preface

I believe we are all destined to do big things. Sadly, some of us do not know it and never get to make the impact they were destined it to make. I believe reading this book you may not know it yet, but you can make a big impact on global health; in fact, you can make history. If you want to make a bigger impact and help save more lives, I think you are in good company. I think you can and in doing so you can make history in a small or big way, but you will make history anyway. I believe all global health professionals want to achieve big goals, not to boost our ego, but because it is the just thing we chose or were called to do. How? We work to prevent preventable deaths, fulfill the right to health and change injustice into justice, and inefficient health systems into self-reliant sustainable health systems that deliver quality health care to everyone, everywhere, every day.

Gandhi said, "Be the change you want to see in the world." I know it sounds cliche but I do believe that. Global Health professionals are being the change now more than ever after we learned how from almost 10 years of working hard to help achieve the Millennium Development Goals. We want to be the change in global health and we want our employers, clients, and partners to be the change too. We must all work together and make changes in a way that is reliable, faster, and sustainable. No excuses. Just results. Just lives saved. This book will show you how to be that change.

This book is for you if you ever woke up in the middle of the night because you wondered how you can help make a clinic, health center, or hospital serve more people or continue working after your project ended; or because you were worried about how to make sure that all the new global health and medical knowledge and technology be transferred faster to developing countries, or because again an epidemic is taking its toll uncontrolled, while you know how to stop it and deliver effective and sustainable aid. If you still remember the faces of the young woman that arrived too late or dead on arrival because she bled to death after an unsupervised delivery, or of the dead normal full-term baby that should not be dead if the mother had had a tetanus shot; or the disappointment and pain of the parent that left without the medicines his child needed. If you cannot sleep because you know that

v

the number of children that are not immunized is too high and you know the risk of an epidemic of vaccine preventable disease is imminent. If you are appalled by any of these ineffective results, this book will show there are others like you that cannot sleep well at night because of the millions of preventable deaths that must be prevented.

Don't get me wrong. I am not criticizing. I am taking responsibility because I have done these things myself and felt helpless at changing them for years. These deaths and many other ineffective things that should not happen in this century also kept me awake for years. What I do now is to get mad, but in a positive way and the energy of getting mad helps me figure out ways to change things. I believe I cannot complain about the things that I am not prepared to change. So I do not complain and I do not make excuses. I invite you to get mad and work together to figure out better and more effective ways to make things work. If you are also mad and want to make a bigger impact, you are in the right place. This book will show you how to change things.

I believe you found your way to this book because you are searching for a change, a solution, and a better way to practice global health. There must have been something in the circumstances you work in or the results you are getting that you want to change and the title of this book resonated with your mission in global health. You can make a bigger impact and you can contribute to realize global health goals; you can make global health really global for all. For the first time in history, we have the knowledge and the technology to improve health for everyone, everywhere, every day. Let's get it done. This book will show how others are doing it and you can too.

I believe it is time to make global health projects make health programs more effective and efficient and ensure health systems deliver quality health care to everyone, everywhere, every day starting from where you are now. Global health experts know how to do it; we have to make sure everyone knows it and does it too. It is now the time to change how we work in global health and prevent all preventable deaths. And as I always say: Now is always a good time.

So let's get started.

This book is going to take global health as it is in 2015 and reinvent it to make sure it is really global for everyone in every country by 2030.

We know that you have unique strengths, experience, and knowledge that will make you a global health leader. Our job is to help you through the chapters in this book to change how you see your role in global health and start to play much bigger. All you have to do is take action at a higher level than you are doing now and get others to support you. It is simple, not easy but simple.

Start by questioning everything you now take for granted in global health. Start asking yourself these and other challenging questions:

1. Do global health projects have to last several years? How about getting results in 1 year or in just 100 days?
2. Can we predict exactly the results a global health project will achieve? How much better will a country be as a result of a project? Can we guarantee results?
3. Do all global health projects have to have expensive mid-term and final evaluations? How about an ongoing system that monitors progress and evaluates results

in real time? Why is a global health project delivering ineffective or unsustainable solutions and nobody changes that? How about creating a system that delivers sustainable solutions every time? Is there a way to make sure donor and government's investments in health have a monthly measurable tangible return?

4. Does all training have to be expensive and take health providers out of their work? How about continuous training on the job that supports health providers to implement changes and improvements? Are there other ways for health professionals to stay up to date and keep learning and applying what they learn?

5. Do all projects have to focus on one disease or health problem? How about quality primary health care that meets the unique needs of every community? How about community-based approaches that deliver care for the most prevalent conditions in the communities or countries where we work?

6. Do global health projects always need to be followed by another project that does more of the same? How about designing projects that have an inbuilt successful exit strategy? What can we do to keep moving forward and take our work to higher level and make a bigger impact? How about projects that improve results in an upward and stepwise manner?

7. What must be the new effective role of development agencies and organizations in effectively delivering sustainable results in 2030? How will we get there?

Let's envision 2030 now in 2015. Imagine a health facility where there is a clean comfortable waiting room where patients arrive at the time of their appointment, are received by a friendly receptionist that checks their medical records are ready on the tablet of a smiling health provider that welcomes them after a short wait. Imagine every health provider has a consultation room to work in with the required equipment which is part of the facility's up-to-date inventory, a written job description, and an efficient work routine based on standard operating procedures. Now, imagine this healthcare provider is supervised and supported to improve themselves by a trained supervisor, and is accountable for serving a defined number of families in the community where the health center is. Imagine a well-organized pharmacy in that health center that has the right medicines that are needed in that facility, enough stock for the next 3 months and an inventory that is updated wirelessly daily to measure consumption of each product and automatically reorder next month's supply, and pharmacy staff that take time to ensure patients know how to use their medicines and ask them questions. Yes, this facility has electricity, running water, cleaning staff that ensure the hygiene of restrooms and patient care areas, and Internet access. This book will help you make good use of your imagination and make it come true. Global health is not science fiction. Global Health experts have the knowledge to transform health care and make sure that every health center and hospital works according to the above standards and does it efficiently. We cannot do it without you so keep reading and join the movement towards effective global health.

Realizing Global Health Inc.   Elvira Beracochea
Fairfax, VA, USA

Contents

Introduction

Imagine you are an adventurous space traveller and on one of your travels, you visit a planet where there is one species that dominates all other species and that lives in groups they call countries. This species has two main genders and you notice that one is significantly at higher risk of dying due to its reproductive role. You also notice that some groups of this species, depending mainly on where they are born, live shorter lives, and therefore contribute less to their countries, which in turn are less organized and poorer in relation to their share of the planet's resources. The shorter life span is mainly due the fact that the beings in these less organized countries have access to fewer resources, such as food, water, knowledge, technology and health services, and that they just do not know what the others that live longer do know about how to access proper nutrition, clean water, safety, and how to prevent disease, and provide enough for themselves and their offsprings. Some of those that live longer dedicate part of their resources, usually less than 1 % in most cases, to help those that live shorter lives. This help does save some lives, but it is not always designed to be effective and deliver lasting results and still millions of preventable deaths take place every year. Despite efforts to improve and prolong the life of those that live shorter lives, impact is limited and lasting changes and longer and equal life spans are still not achieved. In short, access to resources and services for survival on this planet is not fairly distributed among all and mortality rate is still dependent on where these beings are born and their gender.

On your visit to this planet, you also notice that some members of this species compensate for having been in the poor countries and for their lack of resources by moving from one part of the planet to another, others attempt to access resources by force and even kill others in an effort to gain access to more resources and impose their needs. Another group of these beings also work hard with various degrees of effectiveness and coordination to make sure that the aid that less than 1 % dedicated to improve services and save lives is increased and used effectively. You also notice that they particularly believe that health resources must be evenly distributed among all and in accordance to their individual need. These people have had some luck, but not been completely effective yet… but that is about to change.

Like you, the authors of this book live on such a planet and work to improve the effectiveness of aid programs in global health. We demonstrate through our individual work that effective and sustainable change is possible when designed to be in that way. Global health professionals must face the challenge and their responsibility of creating a fairer planet by working in ways that respect the human rights of all, by working in effective coordination with all stakeholders, and by sharing information within and across countries. Resigning to accept ineffective aid is not an option. I have been part of many projects and evaluated or just witnessed many projects. I have seen my reports gather dust and being forgotten. I now refuse to evaluate another project whose evaluation results were not carefully used to improve the country's programs and strengthen the health system. I encourage you to do the same. Also, I now advocate the use of evaluation results and scientific evidence to design effective projects and solutions that empower the host country and its health professionals to perform better. It is the job of global health professionals to transfer to the less developed country what we know and do and what the donors know and do. No, we won't lose our jobs. There is plenty of people to help and plenty of global health challenges to address. However, now is the time we must get out of the job of helping people survive preventable and treatable conditions and move on to improving quality of life. In 2015, it is not enough to help children survive beyond their fifth birthday; we must help them live healthy lives beyond their 85th birthday. Why save children from polio, and let them die of measles or malaria or even teen pregnancy a few years later. **The solution is simple, though not easy. It is time global health projects, organizations, and initiatives effectively help developing countries to manage their vertical programs so they can organize the delivery of horizontal packages of services to meet community-specific needs through efficiently managed health centers and hospitals. No excuses!**

This book has an agenda to truly realize the dream of global health for all by delivering quality health care to all by the year 2030 or sooner. It is time to care about others' well-being as much as ours. Health is a human right, not only because there are international treaties and conventions that say so, but because it is fair and the right thing to do. Yes, the skeptics will say "life is not fair" and they are right. It is up to us to make it fair. Now, for the first time in history we have the medical knowledge and technology to treat most conditions and prevent most of them too. The challenge is to apply that knowledge and deliver quality health care for all. The challenge is to achieve at least 10 % of that per year in the next 10 years and we will be ready to meet the next set of challenges.

I believe that on this planet, we are all human beings and all have the same human rights that are inalienable and universal. The authors of this book wrote it to set the baseline on what is done now and how and help develop a concerted effective approach to global health and development aid in general. Why measure and continuously strive for more effective aid in health? Because the right to health is a human right without which the other rights cannot be realized. There cannot be economic development when people are sick or go bankrupt due to health-related expenses. As Amartya Sen, the Nobel Prize Laurate said, development is freedom and there are many who are not free because they are sick or at increased risk of preventable disease or death unless we provide effective aid. Healthcare delivery must be developed to make sure that everyone's right to health is fulfilled.

In case you think all this is very idealistic and cannot happen in the "real" world, we suggest you prepare to change your mindset and accept that there is need for a new way, a more effective way to improve global health than we have been using for the last 15 years. Respecting the right to health of every human being by providing quality health care is possible. It is the main charge of our time and you can be part of the movement that is making it happen. Do not be left behind....

The most important part of this book is what you do with it: Take action every day to make a bigger impact. Choose wisely your daily actions. You will realize that every day you are presented with the choice to do things that will keep you busy and effective tasks that directly lead to a bigger impact. Choose the latter. Play big. The buck really stops with you. It is really up to you. Do not build your own medicine supply system in parallel and in isolation; instead, strengthen the country's medicine supply system. Do not implement a new vaccine campaign; strengthen the country's routine immunization program. Do not train health workers; strengthen the country's training institutions so they can continue training after you leave. Do not teach quality improvement; accompany health providers to deliver quality care every day. Do not donate equipment and leave; transfer and coach the local staff until you can ensure the new equipment is part of the facilities' inventory and someone's job description now includes its maintenance and repair. Do not implement HIV/AIDS counseling in facilities that do not have clean restrooms, a cleaning program or water for hand washing; help mobilize donor and local resources to ensure that restrooms are available for both men and women and janitorial staff are trained and supervised to maintain them clean. Do not just let local health staff work in rundown facilities, help the country develop a plan to refurbish, upgrade or replace at least 10 % of the country's facilities per year. Don't just let management work in disorganized offices, without computers, Internet access or filing systems, or standard operating procedures; help them improve how they work so they can work just as well as in any other donor, WHO or UN office.

If you read nothing else in this book but the introduction, I want you to at least know seven steps that I learned in my 30 year journey as a physician and from what it took to achieve part of the health targets of the MDGs:

1. Develop an accelerator health system strengthening (AHSS) plan and include in the plan how to coordinate and account for the contribution of every national and regional government, donor, stakeholder, and private provider and local civil society organizations.
2. Set up a human rights-based approach to implement the AHSS with annual targets that ensure every country's health system delivers vertical programs through horizontal services to all and everyone's right to health is fulfilled by the year 2030 or sooner.
3. Work to ensure donor-funded projects and initiatives demonstrate that their work effectively and efficiently contributes to improve the national public health programs and the quality and coverage of the healthcare delivery system.

4. Harmonize and ensure compliance with national policies and programs in quarterly donor meetings that report progress on national health targets.
5. Set the target to improve at least 10 % of the country's public health facilities every year and ensure they meet international quality healthcare delivery standards. In this way, our planet will have 100 % of the health facilities meeting quality standards in 10 years or sooner.
6. Report your work to the country's Ministry of Health so your work contributes to improve the country's health management and information and health surveillance systems. This will help track performance and track progress of the accelerated improvement plan as well as detect disease patterns and possible epidemics. Please no more Ebola epidemics uncontrolled and unmanaged for months!
7. Promote by modeling a professional service attitude among all local authorities, leaders, and health professionals working in the country and by recognizing achievements of health professionals that coordinate, collaborate, and play a unique role in the history of the country by ending preventable deaths in each community every quarter.

These are just a few of the ideas you will find in the book to improve the effectiveness of global health projects and initiatives. Keep reading. You are about to join a movement that will change how global health works.

Realizing Global Health Inc.   Elvira Beracochea
Fairfax, VA, USA
March 2, 2015

Part I
What Is Effectiveness
and How to Measure It

Chapter 1
Global Health and Aid Effectiveness: The MDGs and the Paris Declaration

Elvira Beracochea

It would be up to public health to find ways to bridge hatreds, bringing the world toward a sense of singular community in which the health of the each one member rises or falls with the health of all others. Laurie Garrett

> *Effective aid in global health must be by design. Short or long-term projects a donor funds must be designed to improve the quality and efficiency of the country's health programs so that the health system can deliver services that achieve the planned health outcomes and continue doing so.*

Introduction

What Is Effective Aid in Global Health?

Effective aid achieves global health goals. Ineffective aid achieves partial and/or incomplete or unsustainable results that create dependency on the donor aid, waste resources, and cost lives. Effective aid ensures that the country can sustain the improvements and becomes independent of that aid after the project ends. In this book, you will learn not only not to tolerate poor performance but ensure you, as a global health professional deliver effective performance.

E. Beracochea (✉)
Realizing Global Health Inc., Olley Lane 4710, Fairfax, VA 22032, USA
e-mail: elvira@realizingglobalhealth.com

© Springer Science+Business Media New York 2015
E. Beracochea (ed.), *Improving Aid Effectiveness in Global Health*,
DOI 10.1007/978-1-4939-2721-0_1

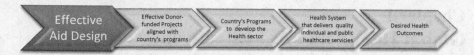

Fig. 1.1 The design of effective aid in global health

Aid effectiveness implies the existence and use of an also effective methodology to measure how well development aid projects and organizations work with developing nations to achieve economic and human development by progressively achieving and accounting for meeting development targets (Morra and Rist 2009). However, global health does not have a common measuring system or measurements that all use. Each global health organization has their own and does not contribute to the country's information system. The result is that information is fragmented, incomplete, and outdated most of the time.

It is simple, really. Effective global health aid is about getting the job done; **no excuses. Effective aid** is by design, not default. In global health, effective aid is that which delivers the required assistance for a country's health programs and facilities to work as part of an efficient, self-reliable, and sustainable health system that delivers quality health care consistently to every citizen anywhere in the country. Effectiveness is getting the planned and expected results and requires that there be a joint and common plan and results to be expected by all. The planned and expected results from aid-funded projects and organizations working in developing nations must be the result of providing the resources, knowledge, and skills to improve healthcare delivery and must facilitate the transfer of the new knowledge and expertise to the developing nation health workforce and institutions in the shortest time possible. In short, effective aid in global health must be designed so that short- or long-term **projects** a donor funds do improve the quality and efficiency of the country's health **programs** so that health **system** can deliver services that achieve the planned and expected health outcomes (Fig. 1.1). Just remember three words that need be in alignment: **Projects—Programs—System**. The existing evidence shows that a systems approach is accepted as the effective way to design, implement, and evaluate global health aid (40) (41). Why? Because we need a health system for healthcare providers to work and deliver health care to people the same way we need schools for teachers to teach students.

What Is an Effective Global Health Professional?

Global health professionals are professionals, usually a doctor, nurse or a professional with some other health-related degree, and with at least a master's degree and who practices in private donor foundations, government agencies, for profit consulting companies or assistance nonprofit organizations and the projects they fund and/or implement. The main goal of a global health professional is to help other human beings and save lives. An effective global health professional achieves results, does not make excuses and changes what needs to be changed to ensure that he or she does achieve results. That is professionalism.

Improving Aid Effectiveness in Global Health is a book about helping global health professionals and the organizations where they work to break with business as usual and practice global health in a different and more effective way using a different framework of reference, targeting the local health system, and using different intervention tools. I believe being a global health professional is the best job in the world because we have the honor and responsibility to participate in the development of humankind, serve others, and save lives. In my career that now spans over 30 years, I am humbled by the appreciation of my colleagues in developing countries where I provide assistance and can say I always feel I learn more about what works from them than I can teach or show them. My experience has taught me that nowadays health professionals in developing countries know their problems well and just need someone to help them uncover the options they have and help them decide their next step to address those problems. In many ways, our role as experts is playing as the midwife to the changes they make, but the change, like the newborn that stays with the parents, must be theirs if it is to last.

Lasting solutions cannot come from "outside" the health system; they have to come from those that are responsible for making it work. Consequently, I believe that it is the healthcare providers that I assist who deserve all the credit for the result of our joint work. The donor's contribution needs to be acknowledged as a catalyst of change and must share in the country's result in proportion to the contribution. The passion for service to others and to save lives I see in most health professionals everywhere is why I care about global health and effective aid. Who would not want to help the health professionals I met in rural Malawi a couple of years ago and that work so hard to treat acute malnutrition and save children's lives? Effective aid in global health must provide practical simple "real world" solutions that help local health professionals and their countries to succeed and deliver improved health services to their citizens at nationwide scale.

Effectiveness is a lifelong process. When I first became a doctor, I learned from peers and supervisors how to follow standard protocols and practices and operating procedures and became effective at serving one patient at a time. Then, I went into public health and by conducting sound epidemiological and health system research and learning to put procedures and checklists in place and being a good team player, I became effective at creating and managing programs that serve whole communities. Now, as a global health doctor, I ask questions and analyze existing information to help uncover gaps and create solutions that must contribute to the effective development of a whole country's health system. By doing that, I do my share and help make the world a better and more just place. I am really lucky to do this job. I believe you reading these pages will also want to impact the lives of one patient, one community, or one whole country. Wherever you are in this lifelong journey, this book will help you do so and become more effective at what you do and make a bigger impact.

The Foundation of Effective Global Health

The Universal Declaration of Human Rights is the foundation of all effective development aid programs (Universal Declaration of Human Rights 2007). A human rights foundation is the cornerstone of effective global health aid (Beracochea et al. 2011). The authors of this book are global health professionals who believe in justice, and believe their mission is to help protect and fulfill the right to health of all human beings. Aid is not effective if the right to health is not progressively fulfilled year in and out, and access to quality health care is not progressively available to reach everyone everywhere every day. Global health professionals must be committed to human rights as the legal framework for our work, to progressively fulfilling the right to health for all human beings by empowering all health professionals as equals, and ensuring access to quality health care as a birthright (Fig. 1.2). For that reason, the 2030 goals will only be achieved if we aim at 10 % annual improvement of the current global health indicators and at least 1/15 of the expansion required to meet population growth.

Human rights, equality, and quality healthcare delivery are the focus of an effective global health practice and why effectiveness is important. When you bring up these three values in all you do, you will inspire others around you and bring consensus on the topic of what is effective aid in global health. These values motivated me in 2007 to organize and moderate a panel on Aid Effectiveness in Global Health at the annual meetings of the American Public Health Association (APHA). Every year since then I invite like-minded speakers who also strive for the right to health and aid effectiveness to share their experience. This book collects most of those presentations and more. The simple chart in Fig. 1.2 is a symbol of our shared mission in global health and the mission of this book. I hope you make it your own. Your global health practice and career will never be the same. The fulfillment of human rights will fuel your work, and your mission will be to find those areas of inequality in access to quality health care, preventable deaths, and unfair circumstances which are not arbitrary and do something to end them. I believe we are at a unique time in which humankind has all the scientific knowledge and technology to deliver the highest standard of health care to all but have not yet implemented the

Fig. 1.2 The focus of effective global health

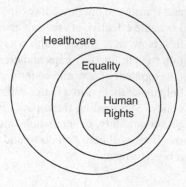

Healthcare

Equality

Human Rights

most effective ways to do it. Make aid effectiveness your mission so your work can effectively impact the present and future of global health.

One thing I learned from moderating the "Aid Effectiveness Panel" at APHA and working with the other coauthors of this book is that passion for your global health career mission is essential to success (Attwood and Attwood 2007) and the *only* solution to overcoming the inevitable complex challenges and drawbacks of working with multiple and different donors, stakeholders, and government systems. You will learn to trust your strengths (Buckingham 2007; Burchard 2007; Rath 2007; Rath and Conchie 2008), not to rest but build on successes and to perceive and share defeats as important valuable lessons (Tracy 2007). Throughout your journey towards effective global health results, you will need inspiration from colleagues, partners, and inspirational guides such as Mahatma Gandhi (Jack 1956) and Amartya Sen (Sen 1999a, b) who will guide you. Effective global health is a team sport. Don't do it alone. Surround yourself with effective colleagues and inspiring visionary leaders.

As Laurie Garrett said, it is up to you and me and all those who work in global health to look for ways to bridge hatred and create a sense of singular community to end the injustice of someone or his child dying because he is poor, was born in a country with a weak health system, where no one has yet figured out an effective way to prevent a preventable death. Become a global health revolutionary that does not accept that preventable deaths just happen. Become intolerant of preventable deaths and ineffectiveness. You are not alone. Together we have started a movement that will change how global health works and the results it achieves every year.

Now the question I ask you is: will you join the movement and commit to apply the effective global health aid principles and practices in this book? Let's get it started!

Human Rights and Effective Global Health Aid: A Historical Perspective to Show Where It All Began…

In the second half of the last century, several attempts were made to ensure universal access to quality effective health care. **Primary Health Care** (PHC) as defined in 1978 in the Alma-Ata (Alma-Ata Declaration 1978) conference of the then Soviet Union, marked a milestone in the development of a common global framework to aid in global health. However, in spite of several successful attempts to implement PHC, the approach was seen as a general and idealistic framework and did not spread worldwide due to a lack of concerted commitment by all stakeholders and lack of progressive coordinated action towards its realization. In spite of setting goals, aid was not effective enough, a commonly accepted way to achieve goals and deliver quality health care was not agreed upon, and the "**Health for All By the Year 2000**" goal was not met either.

In spite of lacking a universally accepted way to deliver quality health care in the year 2000, world leaders reached agreement on common global goals. Since the year 2000, development aid, by design or default, was mostly provided to achieve a number of goals known as **the Millennium Development Goals** (MDGs, see Box 1.1). Health dominated the MDG agenda, 3 out of 8 goals, because health was understood as a requirement of development and economic growth. These goals were chosen by the UN Assembly to address the differential mortality rates across developed and developing societies and nations, not the differential GDPs. The **Millennium Declaration (MD)** is a very important document that includes a lot more than the MDGs, it also sets values to guide our work in development, such as **Freedom, Equality, Solidarity, Tolerance, Respect for Nature and Shared Responsibility for Development**, and reaffirms the importance of good governance and human rights and protecting the vulnerable. These values are indeed the foundation of effective aid and of our collective global health practice. The MD was signed by 189 countries and gives us a basis for implementing effective aid projects in and with these countries. If you have not read it, please print a copy and keep it handy on your desk or briefcase and read it often. Every word counts.

The year 2000 was also important not only for the MD and the emphasis MDGs put into improving health care and reducing preventable mortality, but for "General Comment 14." As global health professionals, I believe that what is known as General Comment 14 is the **gold standard** against which we must measure our personal performance and organizational effectiveness. General Comment 14 (GC14) (see Box 1.2) defined the right to health as the right to the highest attainable standard of health care. "Health," as defined in article 12 of the International Covenant on Economic, Social and Cultural Rights (ICESCR), is **"an inclusive right extending not only to timely and appropriate health care but also to the underlying determinants of health, such as access to safe and potable water and adequate sanitation, an adequate supply of safe food, nutrition and housing, healthy occupational and environmental conditions, and access to health-related education and information, including on sexual and reproductive health."** GC14 further defined the right to health and emphasized the participation of the population in health-related decisions at community, national and international levels, as well as the role of the World Bank, the International Monetary Fund (IMF), and the UN family of organizations in their respective areas of expertise to provide effective assistance.

Box 1.1: <u>Millennium Development Goals</u>

1. Eradicating extreme poverty and hunger,
2. Achieving universal primary education,
3. Promoting gender equality and empowering women,
4. Reducing child mortality rates,
5. Improving maternal health,
6. Combating HIV/AIDS, malaria, and other diseases,
7. Ensuring environmental sustainability, and
8. Developing a global partnership for development.

Box 1.2: General Comment 14 Regarding (<u>Article 12 of the</u> <u>International Covenant on Economic, Social and Cultural Rights</u>)

Health is a fundamental human right indispensable for the exercise of other human rights. Every human being is entitled to the enjoyment of the highest attainable standard of health conducive to living a life in dignity. The realization of the right to health may be pursued through numerous, complementary approaches, such as the formulation of health policies, or the implementation of health programs developed by the World Health Organization (WHO), or the adoption of specific legal instruments. Moreover, the right to health includes certain components which are legally enforceable.

Box 1.3: <u>Core Obligations of States</u>

<u>Article 43</u>: Accordingly, in the Committee's view, these core obligations include at least the following obligations:

(a) To ensure the right of access to health facilities, goods and services on a nondiscriminatory basis, especially for vulnerable or marginalized groups;

(b) To ensure access to the minimum essential food which is nutritionally adequate and safe, to ensure freedom from hunger to everyone;

(c) To ensure access to basic shelter, housing, and sanitation, and an adequate supply of safe and potable water;

(d) To provide essential drugs, as from time to time defined under the WHO Action Programme on Essential Drugs;

(e) To ensure equitable distribution of all health facilities, goods, and services;

(f) To adopt and implement a national public health strategy and plan of action, on the basis of epidemiological evidence, addressing the health concerns of the whole population; the strategy and plan of action shall be devised, and periodically reviewed, on the basis of a participatory and transparent process; they shall include methods, such as right to health indicators and benchmarks, by which progress can be closely monitored; the process by which the strategy and plan of action are devised, as well as their content, shall give particular attention to all vulnerable or marginalized groups.

GC14 in its articles 43 and 44 (see Box 1.3) also states the core obligations of states to **respect, protect, and fulfill the right to health and five duties**:

(1) Ensure reproductive, maternal (pre-natal as well as post-natal) and child health care; (2) to provide immunization against the major infectious diseases occurring in the community; (3) to take measures to prevent, treat and control epidemic and endemic diseases; (4) to provide education and access to information concerning the main health problems in the community, including methods of preventing and controlling them; and (5) to provide appropriate training for health personnel, including education on health and human rights.

GC14 is important for effective aid in global health because focus on these five duties would help countries to allocate resources efficiently and effectively in those five programmatic priorities instead of diluting their efforts on focusing on controlling one or two diseases only at the expense of integrated health services for all. If the country you live in or work is a signatory of the MD and GC14, you have the legal foundation for improving programs and service delivery.

As for the duties of donors and other organizations providing assistance in global health, article 45 of GC14 says, that "For the avoidance of any doubt, the Committee wishes to emphasize that it is particularly incumbent on States parties and other actors in a position to assist, to provide "international assistance and cooperation, especially economic and technical" which **enable developing countries to fulfill their core and other obligations** indicated in paragraphs 43 and 44 above." Please note the emphasis added on enable countries to fulfill their duties.

In sum, the 2000 MD and GC14 are the foundation of twenty-first century effective aid in global health and must guide our professional work. In addition, two important documents produced in 2005 have helped define the implementation of the MD and GC14 and advance the work towards the MDGs, particularly the health goals: The **Millennium Project Report** (Earthscan 2005) and **Paris Declaration on Aid Effectiveness**. The Millennium Project Report to the UN Secretary-General gathered effective strategies and practical recommendations to achieve the MDGs that should have received the support and endorsement of all the UN family and global health leaders.

The **Paris Declaration on Aid Effectiveness** (PD) stated five principles and various strategies for effective aid to achieve lasting results. The PD five principles were agreed upon by over 90 nations and several aid organizations and include: ownership, harmonization, alignment, management by results, and accountability (Box 1.4). The beauty of the PD as a tool for increased effectiveness is in its simplicity. Just five powerful principles that put the ownership of the development process in the hands of its rightful owner, the developing nation and that calls for donors to harmonize their development assistance projects and align with the receiving country's development programs, to strengthen country's systems and institutions.

In addition, the PD emphasizes managing by results and mutual accountability, which are essential to have effective global health programs because despite good intentions, as you will see in the examples in the book, not all aid is good and effective, and not all development programs and projects deliver what they promise. By having accountability systems, timely corrective measures are possible. The accountability

---

Box 1.4: Principles of the Paris Declaration

1. Ownership
2. Harmonization
3. Alignment
4. Managing by Results
5. Mutual Accountability

systems are still under construction, though and as you will notice, not much attention is paid to them. Transparency and accountability will allow effective management and timely corrections which are essential to ensure effective results by the developing country and the donor or the grantees or contractor they hire. These have technical knowledge the receiving country needs; but the latter knows their situation and its own needs better than the donor for the simple reason that they are the ones running the health system, not the donor. So both sides of the aid partnership, the donor and the developing nation, (AKA the partners) need to commit to what each will do, do it and be accountable for their actions and the results they jointly committed to achieve. By working together in a coordinated and aligned manner, the partners can address many unanticipated challenges and benefit from opportunities when implementing development projects in the health sector, much like a pilot sets the flight course of an airplane and then needs to keep making corrections to stay on course. The application of the principles of the Paris Declaration helps make corrections and ensure global health projects stay on course towards the land of effective results.

The other important contribution of the Paris Declaration was to acknowledge the need of working at a country-wide scale when providing development aid. In addition to limiting the benefit to just a few groups or a geographic area, as opposed to all that need care and therefore violating their right to health, small-scale projects have very limited impact. In fact, investment in them may be questionable when they are not followed by a well-planned scaling up strategy and spread their interventions to the rest of the country does not take place.

Also, with the PD, it was the first time that elimination of duplication of efforts, high transaction costs, lack of integration, lack of performance standards, inefficiency, wastage, and corruption in development assistance were recognized and action was taken by a number of countries and donors. It became evident that we could not work any longer through an inefficient, fragmented, and unnecessarily complex donors' systems and procedures that become barriers to the development process itself. In sum, the Paris Declaration called for **scaling up Effective Aid and ending ineffective aid by setting targets, timetables, and measureable indicators and by making financial commitments anticipated and predictable. Progress has been slow, though and by 2010, few commitments had been kept, and no concerted effort is being made to continue monitoring its indicators. Global health professionals must bring the discussion of effectiveness monitoring of global health results back on the global health agenda**.

The Paris Declaration encompasses all areas of development aid, not only health, but it is in health where its impact is most important due to the urgent need to prevent deaths. It is unacceptable and a human rights violation, particularly the **Convention of the Rights of the Child** (UN 1989) that in this century children die or suffer due to vaccine-preventable diseases, dehydration due to diarrhea, malaria, and pneumonia. All these conditions are preventable and treatable. It is also unacceptable and a violation to the right to health and of the **Convention on Elimination of all Forms of Discrimination Against Women** (CEDAW, UN 1979), that there are not enough places for women to safely deliver their babies and get treatment for life-threatening pregnancy complications. No woman should be allowed to die during childbirth in this century when treatment for most conditions exists.

The challenge is to get consensus on how developed and developing countries allocate resources to prevent these deaths and to implement effective and sustainable programs making efficient use of those resources. **At the time of this writing approximately 300,000 women die every year due to preventable or treatable pregnancy-related conditions. We know where women die and why. We need to stop small uncoordinated projects and think globally: What about effectively coordinating the work of 3,000 organizations to create or improve 3,000 maternities that prevent 100 deaths each**?

The PD principles coupled with the existing knowledge to achieve the 2015 MDG targets are **the first global concerted attempt to fulfill the Declaration on the Right to Development (UN 1986)** (The Right to Development 2012). The Declaration on the Right to Development is different from other human rights declarations because it addresses a collective right to participate in the development process defined as "a **comprehensive economic**, **social**, **cultural and political process**, which aims at the **constant improvement** of the well-being of the **entire population** and of all individuals on the basis of their active, free and meaningful participation in development and in the **fair distribution of benefits** resulting therefrom."

The declaration of the Right to Development is really a visionary document that you must read too. It acknowledges the right to self-determination and sovereignty, the elimination of the violations to human rights and the role of disarmament to the progress of development, and that the person is central to that process and its main participant and beneficiary. Notice that it is not eradicating diseases the central subject, but the **progressive realization of the rights of every human**. The Declaration goes on to determine that "**States have the right and the duty of creating development plans and cooperating to ensure progress and eliminate obstacles to universal respect of human rights**." And finally, the declaration states that: "equal attention and urgent consideration should be given to the implementation, promotion and protection of civil, political, economic, social and cultural rights." In short, effective aid must help fulfill human rights and by using the principles of the Paris Declaration, we will be able to operationalize the cooperation between developed and developing nations to achieve global health goals.

This book will show you how you can improve your personal effectiveness, design effective projects, and improve the effectiveness of your existing projects and activities. The book will also help you focus aid projects in global health on achieving lasting impact by respecting, protecting, and fulfilling the right to health in accordance with human rights declarations and principles, and not only on controlling diseases such as polio, HIV/AIDS, Malaria, and TB. However, this book cannot not tell you what is best in your situation or how to adapt the approaches and tools in this book. That is why we invite you to engage the authors of this book in a dialog so you can find ways to apply what you will read and share your experience. Please find us on LinkedIn.

Leverage is the use of a resource in a manner that allows magnification, without practical limit, of the output realized from a given amount of input.

Improvements in global health will not come from global health only but from other sciences and fields that have figured out how to deliver results at global scale. Many of the innovative practices in this book come from the business sector and "sales" and marketing. Why? Because we must "sell" effective global approaches to governments and donors, and "market" new healthcare delivery practices to millions of health providers. Whatever problems we have in global health, I have realized that someone else has solved the same problem in another field or business sector. Do not doubt it: global health IS a business sector where competition for funding and market share is just as strong as in business. It is time we start looking at the bottom line of effectiveness in the number of lives saved and start making sound business decisions using reliable metrics and effective evidence-based practices. The main key to effectiveness and success is leverage. You must leverage your global health knowledge, time, technology and all resources, human and financial, tangible and intangible. Make the best of all you have and particularly all you learn in this book. Make leverage part of your everyday work (Pate 2004).

Summary

To create and implement effective aid programs and projects, you must start with a solid foundation which you will find in the following documents:

1. Declaration of Alma-Ata (1978)
2. Convention on the Elimination of Discrimination Against Women (1979)
3. Right to Development (1986)
4. Convention on the Rights of the Child (1989)
5. Millennium Declaration (2000)
6. General Comment 14 (2005)
7. Paris Declaration (2005)

These documents must be in your briefcase and night table and guide your work every day. Remember that effective aid is aid that is provided by human beings with human beings for human beings. It is not something you do to a group of beneficiaries or what you do to implement the scope of work of your project. You cannot just hope that the project will work out and after it ends, somehow the receiving country will adopt and/or scale up after you leave. You need to work together and make the health system the focus of your impact. You are responsible for implementing effective projects that improve the country's Ministry of Health programs and that will improve the procedures that make the health system work more efficiently **beyond the life of your health project**. If not, your project will be another project that will be forgotten after it is over. For example, if you are working on **a project** to help improve the nutrition outcomes of a certain country, you will aim at helping reduce the number of children with acute malnutrition and the number of stunted children so that every child's growth and development is according to their age. Your project must be part of **the country's nutrition program** along with other projects funded by other donors, agencies, and nongovernmental organizations, and must help improve how the country's nutrition program works so that the **country's health system** works better at delivering nutrition services. Your annual work plan must be part of the nutrition program annual work plan at national and local level to ensure your work contributes to the outcomes all are trying to achieve. Therefore, your project must also help improve the health system by improving staff's job descriptions, supervision checklists, performance reviews and career paths, annual procurement budgets, etc. that is what we mean by the effective impact sequence of **Project—Program—System**.

People tend to be able to find lots of explanations to explain why ineffective projects failed, but I want you to avoid that trap. These are not explanations; they are excuses. Instead of making excuses, think of how you can use the lessons in this book to make your **project** more effective, how it can be better aligned with the country's **program,** and how you can strengthen the health **system** so your project results are sustained after the project ended. Effective global health professionals do not explain, do not complain, and do not make excuses. They learn from mistakes and make programs work better to ensure the health system delivers quality health care through improved effective documented and streamlined processes and procedures. With the exception of testing the effectiveness of *new* health care delivery methods or interventions, effective aid must work at real life scale, so make sure that what your project does is part of and contributes to the respective national program that needs to cover everyone in the country. This is 2015 and best practices abound. It is time we effectively create projects that contribute for a country's programs and health system to ensure access to the highest attainable standard of health care to all. It is time to get started to make 2030 count as a milestone we will not miss. We invite you to start a dialog with us and join us in our mission to make aid in global health more effective.

What Is in This Book?

This book was designed to mark a point of departure for a new and more effective global health strategy, founded on international human rights legislation and on scientific evidence. This book gathers practical action-oriented strategies for global health professionals to use as a guide when planning and implementing developing projects, initiatives, and programs in global health.

The book is divided into four parts: the first part describes the main perspectives in regard to Aid Effectiveness and ways to measure and evaluate it. In Part I, Chap. 2, you will learn about the progress so far in global health, what works and what challenges donors, receiving countries and global health professionals face now. Chapter 3 presents how health systems work. Chapter 4 presents the experience of the OECD using health as tracer sector to measure effectiveness. Chapter 5 presents the perspective of the US government and the steps the Obama Administration is taking to ensure US taxpayers dollars are used effectively. Chapter 6 describes the results of an evaluation of the degree of implementation of the Paris Declaration by US agencies working in development.

Part II describes various ways the principles of the Paris Declaration are being applied by various global health stakeholders such a governments, international partnerships, NGOs, and the Private Sector. In Part II, Chap. 7 you will learn about the International Health Partnership and what it does to improve effectiveness. Chapter 8 will describe the role of the Global Fund and Civil Society in improving the effectiveness of healthcare programs. Chapter 9 presents practical recommendations for NGOs, the main providers of Aid to developing countries, to put the Paris Declaration to work. Chapter 10 describes how to work at countrywide scale, and Chap. 11, the important role of the private sector in effectively expanding access to quality health care and contribute to the advancement of local health programs. Chapter 12 describes the role of government and the people themselves in sustaining effective aid interventions in the case of Peru and the local health committees that are improving maternal health. Chapter 13 describes the role of academia in effective global health.

Part III presents three important challenges to effective aid: the challenge of charity without respect for dignity in Chap. 14 the challenge of respect of country ownership and accountability in the case of Rwanda in Chap. 15, and the challenge of having real partnerships in the experience of Peru with foreign aid in Chap. 16. Chapter 17 presents the challenge to effective food aid. Chapter 18 presents the work of the International Health Partnership in monitoring and keeping us all transparent and why you must be part of it.

Finally, Part IV presents approaches Global Health Professional can use now to maximize the effectiveness of aid in their global health programs, projects, organizations, or multi-partner initiatives and coalitions. Chapter 19 shows you ways to use social media to promote increased effectiveness. Chapter 20 shows you how one person can reach out to others who seem to be on the opposite side to work together and account for better results. Chapter 21 will show you why we must create, improve, and strengthen community-based health programs; and in Chap. 22 you will learn why you must learn to work in partnerships. Chapter 23 will show your story and yourself can be your most effective tools in global health, and Chap. 24 will show you do not need to know all the answers but you do need to learn to ask effective and powerful questions. Chapter 25 shows the link between effectiveness and sustainability and the lessons of a global health expert with over 50 years of experience, and Chap. 26 presents simple practical next steps for you to avoid the most common career traps and effectively apply what you learned in this book to make a bigger impact. Chapter 27 summarizes the conclusions the authors have identified to change and improve global health practice and make a bigger and more effective impact.

We wish you effective results and look forward to meeting you soon. Below are some questions to help you get the discussion on improving aid effectiveness in global health started in your place of work now. Organize a meeting in your organization or place of work and discuss these questions with your colleagues and partners.

Questions for Discussion

Select a country where you work or have visited and discuss:

1. How effective is aid in the health sector in this country?
2. Who are the main stakeholders of the development process in health in this country, what are they doing, and how are they coordinating their activities and sharing results and lessons learned?
3. How can you help apply the Right to Development in this country?
4. How can you help align global health programs with the principles of the Paris Declaration?
5. How will you work or career need to change to become more effective?
6. How effective is each and every global health project in improving the country's health system?
7. What is the exit and sustainability strategy of every donor?

References

(2007). *Universal Declaration of Human Rights: 60th anniversary special edition, 1948-2008.* New York: United Nations Department of Public Information.

Alma-Ata Declaration. (1978, September 6–12). *Report of the International Conference on Primary Health Care, Alma-Ata.* In: World Health Organization, "Health for All" Series, No. . Geneva, Switzerland: WHO. http://www.who.int/publications/almaata_declaration_en.pdf

Attwood, J. B., & Attwood, C. (2007). *The passion test: The effortless path to discovering your destiny.* New York: Hudson Street Press.

Beracochea, E., Weinstein, C., & Evans, D. P. (2011). *Rights-based approaches to public health.* New York: Springer.

Buckingham, M. (2007). *Go put your strengths to work: 6 powerful steps to achieve outstanding performance.* New York: Free Press.

Burchard, B. (2007). *Life's golden ticket: An inspirational novel.* San Francisco: Harper.

General Comment 14. Retrieved July 21, 2012, from http://www.unhchr.ch/tbs/doc.nsf/%28symbol%29/E.C.12.2000.4.En

Jack, H. A. (1956). *The Gandhi reader: A source book of his life and writings.* Bloomington, IN: Indiana University Press.

Morra, L. G., & Rist, R. C. (2009). *The road to results designing and conducting effective development evaluations.* Washington, DC: World Bank.

N/A. The Paris Declaration on Aid (2005) and The Accra Agenda for Action (2008), *1*, 21.

Pate, R. D. (2004). *Leverage: A key to success and wealth.* Rocky Mount, NC: VP Publisher.

Rath, T. (2007). *Strengths finder 2.0.* New York: Gallup Press.

Rath, T., & Conchie, B. (2008). *Strengths based leadership: Great leaders, teams, and why people follow.* New York: Gallup Press.

Sen, A. (1999a). *Development as freedom.* Oxford, NY: Oxford University Press.

Sen, A. (1999b). *Development as freedom.* New York: Knopf.

The Right to Development. Retrieved July 21, 2012, from http://www2.ohchr.org/english/law/rtd.htm

Tracy, B. (2007). *Eat that frog! 21 great ways to stop procrastinating and get more done in less time* (2nd ed.). San Francisco: Berrett-Koehler.

(2005). Investing in development: A practical plan to achieve the Millennium Development Goals, Earthscan. Retrieved from http://unmillenniumproject.org/reports/fullreport.htm

Further Reading

(2007). Draft summary of the 9th meeting. *DAC working party on Aid effectiveness, 1*, 10.

(2008). A joint commitment of principles and actions between the government and development partners. *Aid effectiveness in Papua New Guinea, 1*, 20.

(2008). Accra agenda for action. *3rd High Level Forum, 1*, 7.

(2014). Toward a world safe and secure from infectious disease threats. *The Global Health Security agenda, 1*, 2.

(2007). From Paris 2055 to Accra 2008: Will aid become more accountable and effective? *Draft for Discussion at Regional Consultation, 1*, 9.

High Level Forum on Aid Effectiveness, 4. (2011). Executive summary. *Aid effectiveness 2005–20: Progress in implementing the Paris declaration, 1*, 21.

Bliss, K. (2010). How Brazil, Russia, India, China, and South Africa. *The key players in global health, 1*, N/A.

Bliss, K. (2014). The transformation of the office of global affairs at HHS. *Global health within a domestic agency, 1*, 9.

Chandler, S. (2003). *The joy of selling: Breakthrough ideas that lead to success in sales.* San Francisco: R.D. Reed.

Chandler, S. (2012). *100 Ways to motivate yourself: Change your life forever* (3rd ed.). Pompton Plains, NJ: Career Press.

Dickinson, C. (2011). *Is aid effectiveness giving us better health results?* (Vol. 1, p. 10). London: HLSP Institute.

Dodd, R., Schieber, G., Cassels, A., Fliesher, L., & Gottret, P. (2007). Aid effectiveness and health. *Making Health Systems Work: Working Paper No. 9, 1*, 18.

Ehrenpreis, D. (2007). *Poverty in focus: Does aid work?-for the MDGs.* Brasilia, Brazil: International Poverty Centre.

Fee, D. (2012). *How to manage an aid exit strategy: The future of development aid.* London: Zed Books.

Garret, L. (2000). *Betrayal of trust: The collapse of global public health* (p. 2). New York: Hyperion.

Gladwell, M. (2000). *The tipping point: How little things can make a big difference.* Boston: Little, Brown.

Glennie, J. (2008). *The trouble with aid: Why less could mean more for Africa.* London: Zed Books in association with International African Institute, Royal African Society, Social Science Research Council.

IHP+. (2011). Outline. *The International Health Partnership, 1*, 29.

Jensen, B. (2000). *Simplicity: The new competitive advantage in a world of more, better, faster.* Cambridge, MA: Perseus Books.

Macrae, J. (2001). *Aiding recovery? The crisis of aid in chronic political emergencies.* London: Zed Books.

Millennium Declaration. Retrieved July 20, 2012, from http://www.un.org/millennium/declaration/ares552e.htm

Moyo, D. (2009). *Dead aid: Why aid is not working and how there is a better way for Africa.* New York: Farrar, Straus and Giroux.

N/A. (2007). Concept paper. *Civil Society and Aid Effectiveness, 1*, 22.

N/A. (2007). From Paris 2005 to Accra 2008: Will aid become more accountable and effective? A critical approach to the aid effectiveness agenda. *Draft for discussion at regional consultations, 1*, 9.

Partnership for Effective Development Co-operation, OECD, & UNDP. (2014). 2014 Progress Report. *Making Development Co-operation More Effective, 1*, 138.

(2008). *Global health watch 2: an alternative world health report.* Cairo: People's Health Movement. Print.

Prahalad, C. K. (2005). *The fortune at the bottom of the pyramid.* Upper Saddle River, NJ: Wharton School.

Progress Toward Enhanced Aid Effectiveness. (2005). Ownership, harmonization, alignment, results, and mutual accountability. *Paris Declaration on Aid Effectiveness, 1*, 12.

Rutigliano, T., & Brim, B. (2010). *Strengths based selling: Based on decades of Gallup's research into high-performing salespeople*. New York: Gallup Press.

Sanders, T. (2002). *Love is the killer app: How to win business and influence friends*. New York: Crown Business.

Shula, D., & Blanchard, K. H. (1995). *Everyone's a coach: You can inspire anyone to be a winner*. New York: Harper Business.

Smith, L. C. (2010). *The world in 2050: Four forces shaping civilization's northern future*. New York: Dutton.

Sogge, D. (2000). Aid chain analysis: Two models. *A pathological model, 1*, 2.

Tandon, Y., & Mkapa, B. W. (2008). *Ending aid dependence* (2nd ed.). Oxford, UK: Fahamu.

The Paris Declaration and the Accra Agenda for Action. OECD 2005–2008.

United Nations. (2000). Substantive issues arising in the implementation of the international covenant on economic, social and cultural rights. *Economic and Social Council, General comment no. 14*, 11.

USAID. (2012). USAID's global health strategic framework better health development. *USAID, 1*, 51.

World Bank, OECD, World Health Organization, (2008). Effective aid, better health. *3rd High Level Forum on Aid Effectiveness, 1*, 40.

Chapter 2
Aid Effectiveness in Global Health: Progress, Challenges, and Solutions

Elvira Beracochea

> *"If you can't **measure** it, you can't **manage** it."* Peter Drucker, *Management Leader*
> *"And if you measure what you do, you will manage to achieve effective results in global health."*
>
> Dr. Elvira Beracochea, Global Health Expert

Introduction

It is 8 a.m. in a health center in a rural area in a low income country; a nurse prepares for her day's work. Already, waiting outside, she can see over 20 patients with various illnesses, more or less the same number of mothers is also waiting for their antenatal checkup and an even larger number of mothers brought their children for their monthly growth monitoring and vaccination visit. The nurse opens the clinic's refrigerator and takes out enough vaccines for the day: tetanus vaccine for the pregnant mothers and polio, measles, and pentavalent vaccines for the infants. She looks at the temperature chart on the door of the refrigerator and realizes she has forgotten to record the temperature twice a day for the last couple of days. She will try to remember tomorrow; she is too busy today. She adds a couple of icepacks to the vaccine carrier, adds the vaccines, and closes the refrigerator door. She takes the carrier with her to the waiting area where all her patients, mothers, and children are waiting on long benches. She sits at her desk facing the patients in the benches, opens a large register, takes a pen out of her pocket, and calls the first person to come to sit at the chair next to her desk. She spends all morning delivering vaccines, weighing mothers and children, interviewing the sick and prescribing medicines she knows that are not available in the health center's pharmacy, and writing in the big register about each consultation until it is time for her lunch break. Patients will continue waiting until she comes back from her lunch break, then she will resume doing the same until they have all gone home. The nurse does not have a place nearby to wash

E. Beracochea (✉)
Realizing Global Health Inc., Olley Lane 4710, Fairfax, VA 22032, USA
e-mail: elvira@realizingglobalhealth.com

© Springer Science+Business Media New York 2015
E. Beracochea (ed.), *Improving Aid Effectiveness in Global Health*,
DOI 10.1007/978-1-4939-2721-0_2

her hands and although she knows she should get up and walk to the nearest hand basin to wash her hands between patients, she tells herself she is too busy to stop. She does not take the time to examine patients, take their temperature, pulse, or blood pressure because there is no privacy and she lacks the right equipment, time, and energy to do it. She could use one of the consultation rooms, but they are too dark without electricity. Her workload seems too much for her and she feels tired, frustrated, and trapped in a job that does not give her any motivation or satisfaction. Somehow she does not feel like smiling at her patients or take time to find out what other health problems they may have or other services they may need as she learned in school. The other staff in the health center work in more or less the same way. This type of healthcare is not what she was trained for, but she does not know how to change it.

Ownership of the Challenges to Deliver Quality Safe Healthcare

You and I know this story repeats every day in too many parts of the world. I am a doctor and have visited many facilities in over 40 countries. Most of the time I have surveyed, observed, and evaluated or interviewed health providers, I have found tired, overworked, frustrated, and unmotivated staff that lack clear job descriptions and performance standards, do not follow procedures they know they must follow and who have become indifferent to the chronic lack of supplies, equipment, and medicines. And worst of all, they also lack a supportive supervisor that would help them figure out ways to overcome these challenges. They do not have someone to help them figure out a different way to organize their work so the patients do not all come at the same time. The nurse and the staff in their health center in our story above need a new appointment system and a way to manage patient flow, do triage and prioritize the services patients need, and a simple and effective way to keep track of patients. Most providers often lack equipment and supplies but also, they do not know they have to fill out requests on time that will bring them at least a minimum of the supplies they need, or how to keep the inventory of the equipment and medicines to ensure they are accounted for.

Most health facilities are run down and the toilets are cleaned irregularly and rarely kept clean. Many do not have a local health committee including community leaders to leverage community resources to address basic facility maintenance and hygiene. The goal of effective aid is to put more efficient healthcare delivery processes in place that reduce errors like not monitoring vaccine temperature or not washing hands, and empower healthcare providers like the nurse in the story above to be proactive, take action, and overcome the challenges to deliver quality health services in the most efficient way consistently. If every health provider looked for ways to address a challenge every month instead of enduring them, they would have 12 fewer problems every year.

The main challenge is ownership of the problems that affect the quality of care and the lack of ability and support to do something about it. Clarity of the tasks to be performed to achieve measurable goals is the basis of an effective job description, performance evaluation, and supervision processes, which do not exist in most developing countries. Certainly, many problems are beyond the ability or resources of one person to solve, but there are opportunities for health providers to address many of the chronic problems that prevent them from delivering quality of care and sustaining improvements. I have seen donors creating "Rehydration Corners" but not changing work routines and job descriptions of staff and after a few months, the corners are abandoned. I have seen donors making improvements to allow for privacy of family planning visits and after a few months all goes back to the way it used to be in an open courtyard because the change was from outside and not self-started.

There are known solutions to many of these problems that can be implemented when all stakeholders and parties get involved. This chapter will show you how to find opportunities to take effective action making use of effective aid.

The Evitable Problem of the Complexities in Global Health

The increasing complexity in the global health field and international development field in general has two main causes and one important consequence. First, complexity is created by the large number of technical approaches and initiatives in global health without a coordinating mechanism that makes consensus about what brings about improvements confusing. Second, there is fragmentation in approaches because there is no effective technical leadership from WHO to guide the work of all these organizations, and consequently, there is duplication and more confusion about what each is doing and what countries need and want for improving the health of their people. Confusion does not lead to change, but to ineffectiveness. There are textbooks about cardiology or pediatrics that show what it takes to practice these specialties, but there is not a comprehensive textbook that shows how to practice global health in the current sea of organizations and initiatives. Until our book, there was not a global health book that gathers evidence-based knowledge about what is effective global health yet. Confusion supports the status quo.

Initiatives in global health emerge in waves of changing priorities that confuse the healthcare providers in the frontlines who have to deliver care every day. If we piled out all the manuals and guidelines donors and NGOs have developed and that a provider needs to have been trained in to deliver care, the pile would be several meters high. There was PHC (primary health care), Selective PHC, Health for all by the year 2000 (HFA 2000), GOBI (Growth monitoring, Oral rehydration, Breastfeeding, and Immunization) and GOBI-FFF (that added family planning, female education, and food supplementation), MNCH, FP/RH, IMCI (Integrated Management of Childhood Illnesses), then guidelines for diarrhea control, community management of malaria and pneumonia, home-based care guidelines and eradication efforts for various diseases, STOP TB, Rollback Malaria, and hundreds of tools and guidelines for improving for family planning and reproductive health. In the last 15 years, on the US side only, we have seen several initiatives such as PEPFAR (President's Emergency Plan for AIDS Relief), PMI (President's malaria initiative), GHI (global health initiative), along with UN's "Promised Renewed," just to name a few. The existence of so many of these initiatives raises many

questions about the effectiveness of these initiatives such as how does PMI complement the work of Rollback Malaria or improve the work of all the USG-funded
organizations that have malaria components in their projects that also contribute to
the GHI? The answer is not clear yet.

Technical fragmentation is due to the continuously increasing number of uncoordinated stakeholders and donors that choose to get involved in one or other health problem. There is WHO, UNICEF, GAVI for vaccines, Global Fund to improve malaria,
TB and AIDS programs along with so many other organizations. A recent evaluation
of Malawi's nutrition program (Social Impact 2013) showed that there were over 30
different organizations involved in the program and that although there were informal
coordination mechanisms, there was not an effective way to coordinating all their
inputs and plans, ensure their alignment the country's nutrition program, harmonize
their approaches or measure the effectiveness of each organization's contribution.
Their way of working would have been fine a few years ago when there were a few
stakeholders but now the number has increased and the complexity in fact, makes the
program hard to manage by three people at the MOH level who need to account for
the results and coordinate the work of all stakeholders and their collective impact. The
nutrition program is one of the most important services of Malawi's essential healthcare package due to the country's seasonal acute malnutrition and food insecurity and
high prevalence of stunting and of diseases such as HIV/AIDS. A national nutrition
program like this would require clearly defined roles and responsibilities, harmonized
and aligned work plans, and lines of reporting for each stakeholder.

The MOH of every developing nation and its partners must be able to oversee the
contribution of all involved in a simple and effective way to make the most of each
stakeholder's contribution without overwhelming the various levels of country leadership and causing high transactional costs. As complexity in aid increases, it is
impossible for the MOH to measure the progress of their health programs and keep
track of all the implementation activities unless a simple procedure for coordination,
collaboration, and communication between the MOH and its partners is in place. The
transactional costs of this type of aid may exceed their benefits. A new level of organization is required to ensure effective aid in global health. The five principles of the
Paris Declaration are not a choice but a must.

Clear Simple Goals Increase Effectiveness

The MDG agenda eventually brought simplicity and some degree of alignment for
all stakeholders as well as clear measures of accountability. At the time of this pub-
lication, there were less than 200 days to achieve the MDG targets and most of the
attention is not on what we have learned so far that can help accelerate achieving the
MDGs but on discussing the post- 2015 Agenda. Additional attention should be on
what needs to be done to achieve the targets that are most behind such as maternal
and child mortality rates because we know what to do and prevent those deaths. The
challenge is to change the global health aid industry to make it more effective in
delivering the much needed solutions (Bristol 2013). Table 2.1 below summarizes
the MDGs, the 2015 targets and the progress to date.

Table 2.1 Global health progress

MDG		2015 Target	1990	Progress
1.	Proportion of people living in extreme poverty	Reduce by 50 %	47 %	22% in 2010—700 million fewer poor. This target was met 5 years ahead and in spite of financial crises
	Hunger reduction	Reduce by 50 %	23.2 %	14.9 in 2010—within reach by 2015
2.	Universal primary education	100 %	80 %	90 % in 2011, although quality of education is unknown or uneven
3.	Gender parity in education	.97 to 1.03	.86	Not likely to be met, only two countries met the target
4.	Reduce child mortality	By 2/3	97/1,000 live births	57/1,000 live births, still 6.9 million children die every year, 19,000 a day, mostly in poor countries
5.	Reduce maternal mortality	By 3/4	440 deaths per 100,000 live births	240 deaths per 100,000 live births with wide disparity between rural and urban within country
6.	HIV/AIDS	Halt and reverse epidemic	0.09 infections per 100 people per year	0.06 new infections per 100 people per year
		Universal treatment	100 %	55 %
	Malaria	Halt and reverse	100 % net coverage of children	Range from 10 to 71, 660,00 deaths in 2010, 80 % of deaths are children
	TB	Halt and reverse	100 % diagnoses and treatment	In 2011, 8.7 million newly diagnosed, 2.2 % less in 2010, 13 % HIV+, 87 % successfully treated, 1.4 million deaths
7.	Environmental sustainability	Sustainability country policies and reverse loss of resources	CO_2 emission reduced	46 % increase
			Marine resources protected	1/3 marine resources overexploited
				Over 20,000 species risk extinction
			Water and land areas protected	Water 4.6–9.7 % and land 8.9–14.6 %
		Halve the population without safe drinking water	70 % with access to safe water in developing countries	87 % in developing countries
		75 % of the population without sanitation	49 %	67 %, another billion people need access to sanitation
		0 open defecation	24 %	15 %
		Improve living conditions of 100 million slum dwellers	100 million	200 million have access to safe water, sanitation, and durable housing. Target exceeded

(continued)

Table 2.1 (continued)

MDG		2015 Target	1990	Progress
8.	Global partnerships	ODA at 1 % of GDP		0.7 %
				Decrease of AID from DAC countries (Development Assistance Committee of the OECD)
				Increase of AID from Non-DAC countries
		Aid to least developed and landlocked countries		Decreased in favor of middle income countries
		Fair Trade	54 % of duty-free imports from least developed countries	80 % duty-free imports
		Debt	11.9 % debt ratio	3.1 % debt ratio in 2011
		Technology sharing		6.8 billion have mobile phones
				39 % of the population 2.7 billon are online

Table 2.1 is clear: **the job is not done yet**. We must stay on course and not change the goals. We have to change how we work and what we do to be effective and achieve the goals. I agree. We can be more ambitious, add more goals, and aim for continuous whole patient care goals so that a child that survives its fifth birthday does not die prematurely 10 years later due to a teen pregnancy or TB or gets infected with HIV due to unprotected sex. But let's not change the agenda! We must finish it. The rest of the chapter will discuss the unfinished agenda and what to do to finish it.

Challenges: The Unfinished Agenda by 2015

Global health experts have learned a lot about what works and what does not work by focusing on achieving the MDGs. However, there is no consensus yet and it is not clear as a profession what global health professionals accept as evidence-based best practices in the delivery of quality healthcare and public health programming. As mentioned above, increased number of actors, numerous, and conflicting information sources that lack consistent global health knowledge management (probably WHO's job), fragmentation in the architecture of technical assistance, and unharmonized implementation of interventions at country level reflect in the unfinished agenda of the MDGs (Box 2.1).

Box 2.1: The Unfinished Agenda of the Health MDGs

1. 970 million will still be living on $1.25 by 2015 and have higher risk of morbidity and mortality.
2. Measuring poverty to identify those that need healthcare and cannot afford it is still not effective and too many lack access.
3. Rural–urban gaps show rural communities bear higher mortality and morbidity.
4. There is a gender gap in employment in some regions more than others, and less secure jobs and fewer social benefits, women and youth suffer unemployment, poverty and higher morbidity and mortality.
5. Still 100 million children are underweight, and 1 in 4 are stunted.
6. Over 45 million people were refugees or displaced in 2012, the highest since 1994.
7. 1 in 4 of the children in school will leave before completing school. The reason: poverty. 250 million children do not know how to read and write and are at risk of higher morbidity and mortality.
8. Measles coverage 83 % in developing countries, 99 % in developed ones, the same gap applies to other essential vaccines in the global immunization program.
9. 50 million children are born without a skilled attendant, lack of access to antenatal care has gone from 37 to 51 %, that is about half of the pregnancies.
10. Contraceptive prevalence only 25 % in SSA, demand is increasing but the offer is not.
11. HIV treatment and access to ARV therapies, as with most treatments, is not universal: 8 million out of 14.4 million, still 45 % are not covered.
12. $5.1 billion are required to provide nets to all and more to keep the system supplying new nets as populations grow and replace old ones.
13. 768 million drew water from an unimproved source in 2011, 83 % in rural areas and are at risk of waterborne diseases.
14. Thousands of schools and health centers and hospitals are open despite not having water and sanitation or electricity.
15. The unfinished agenda does not include global health programs to respond to other highly prevalent conditions such as noncommunicable disease.

I know the reader will find many effective ways to address global health challenges in this book. It is essential that the lessons in this book and in other books, from global health projects and websites be coordinated and managed globally to be applied locally and global health donors stay focused on addressing this unfinished agenda. I do not think we should wait another millennium to end preventable deaths. I believe the MDGs can be achieved in the next decade with focused and coordinated strategies and effective monitoring and reporting. Now is time we make visible the invisible: the contribution each donor makes, the return on their investment, and their successes and failures to meet the MDG targets. Each project and donor must make visible how much is actually spent on direct assistance as opposed to headquarters overhead, travel, per diem and housing of consultants, and how much directly impacts health service delivery. More efficient and effective ways to improve healthcare will be found when we look at how we invest global health donations.

Measuring Progress in Global Health

Peter Drucker, the world's most influential management leader, made the point of why measurement is a must in business. He was not talking about managing development aid or global health projects but his business reference applies just as well to the nurse in our story, to the management of global health projects and organizations, and probably to just about everything we need to accomplish in life. Imagine tennis without knowing if the ball was in or out of the opponent's court or football without keeping score of the goals. How long do you think players would chase after the ball or you would watch the game on TV without knowing the score to know how well they are doing? Likewise, the nurse in the story is frustrated because she does not know if her work is recognized by anyone and if it is really making a difference. Likewise, donors and funding agencies responsible for projects are not sure daily if what their projects are doing is going to work or whether the results will last after the project ends. We should not accept providing aid or healthcare without keeping score or knowing if what is done has achieved lasting results, if the health services are provided with improved quality and efficiency, if the trained providers are applying what the donor-funded workshop taught, and if people that come to the health center every day are actually getting quality healthcare every day and really are better off.

Measuring Progress and Results, Not Just Inputs and Outputs But Outcomes

Measurement is essential to effective management, and effective measurement is essential to decide what activities or interventions to implement or change to achieve the desired results of global health projects. In short, there are two sciences you must master to deliver effective aid: **health measurement and health management**.

The science of "Health Measurement" includes several systems, starting with measuring patient or case health status and recording it in the "patient management information system" that includes medical records. It also includes the "health surveillance system" that monitors the incidence and prevalence of diseases and identifies epidemics and trends, so that policy makers and planners can develop or improve the management of health programs to address them. Next, is the measurement done in epidemiological and evaluation studies that study the risk factors, causes of diseases and health status of population, and the effectiveness of health services. Finally, there is the "health management information system" that measures how well a country's health system and its programs are doing, and it should also include how well global health projects doing, and if aid delivers lasting results. Every organization, health program, and health facility teams must have a health scorecard that measures how well they are doing and inform their actions (Table 2.2). In this way, the index case of Ebola or some other priority disease would not be disregarded for months.

Table 2.2 Sample health facility scorecard

Month:_____		Facility:_____		
Clinic no. 1 Annual target/ objective indicator	Monthly average score or result	Score/result this month	Progress to date	Action
1. Immunize 900 infants and children	75	85	785	No action required
2. Antenatal care to 300 mothers	25	32	216	No action required
3. Maternal deaths	0	0	0	No action required
4. Infant deaths	0	1	1	Traffic accident. Completed home visit and audit report
5. New malaria cases	12	**34**	137	Planning for bednet re-impregnation month
6. New tuberculosis cases	2	3	27	All patients are on treatment
7. New HIV infections	3	2	23	All patients are in support program and referred to the PLWHA Association
8. Percentage of supervised deliveries	80 %	82 %	81 %	201 births in the district this month
9. Low birth weight babies	0	3	19	All from rural areas; working to improve referrals from and antenatal care at Aid Posts
10. Adult deaths	3	1	17	One AIDS death; orphans are in family custody and are visited every week
11. Number of home visit	80	78	632	All patients defaulting treatment or antenatal visit were visited this month
Total indicators: 12	Coverage Area: all 14 villages in coverage area have met their monthly targets	Indictors on target: 11	Progress: on track to meet annual objectives	Number of actions to be taken: none. All issues resolved
	Responsible:_____			
		Signature		

The science of "Health Management" is the science of <u>planning and implementation of effective processes</u>, <u>procedures, and controls to ensure the consistent delivery of health services to achieve a desired health outcome</u>. Health management helps us make changes and improve the processes and procedures that do not achieve the desired results. The goal of health management is to design and implement the minimum number of effective processes required to deliver quality health services. Therefore, more than what is effective is not better but a waste of resources and may even be detrimental to healthcare quality.

<u>Quality</u>, <u>efficiency, and consistency</u> (QEC) are the main principles of effective health management and require health staff to manage effective health processes and procedures to ensure quality efficient and consistent healthcare delivery. These processes and standard procedures are included in the country's health program or facility "<u>operations manual</u>." Management of development aid also must follow the QEC principles and use operations manuals. Management requires effective measurement to monitor and evaluate the effectiveness of global health interventions. However, management and measurement of global health aid are not well-studied, standardized, and documented sciences **yet**. Much of the development aid started 60 or 70 years ago as part of humanitarian assistance. Then, charity was not perceived as a science and effectiveness was not measured consistently. In the twentieth century, having the good intentions to help was enough, even if one did not deliver what was planned and it was not sustainable. Even USAID did not start to systematically evaluate its projects until 20 years ago and it did not have an M&E policy until 2011 and still lacks an ongoing monitoring system in global health that coordinates the work of its offices in Washington and overseas. Much of the measurement is still related to inputs such as how many people were trained, babies delivered, or how many condoms were distributed but not about how many countries assisted have a better performing HIV/AIDS or malaria program or are able to deliver quality child survival services in an increasing number of facilities are at any time given.

Now, that is, in 2015, having good intentions to help improve the health of others is **no longer enough**. We need to demonstrate effectiveness and a return on every dollar invested in global health. Since the MDGs were set in 2000 and particularly since 2005 when people started to really focus on the MDG agenda, what is clear is that in global health we must set shared goals, plan, and coordinate how to achieve them at global scale, measure how well we are doing in real time, and account for country results not outputs. I believe the WHO must effectively lead this coordination effort in accordance with its constitution.

Progress in global health must be a continuous process that involves choosing the **minimum cost-effective interventions** in the right sequence in a way that strengthens the country's programs and health system so that they work better and keep doing so after the project ends. Deciding how and where to best implement interventions is also a continuous joint process that requires measuring the results we get on an ongoing basis. In conclusion, measurement is essential in global health. If you work in global health, you must measure what you do so you manage your project, facility, or organization and account for the resources used and the results achieved because they contribute to the overall global results. **Remember more aid is not better aid. The minimum required aid in the right sequence and place that delivers the desired lasting result is better aid**.

Effective Project and Program Planning and Monitoring

Having managed several projects and now managing a global health professional and consulting business, I have learned that planning is important to achieve progress in business as it is an important activity to achieve progress in global health projects. The maxim "If you fail to plan you plan to fail" still holds. Having plans is not important only because donors want to approve plans before releasing funds, but because having a plan is the only way to ensure that the right activities take place to achieve the desired results and to make corrections when necessary. Monitoring the implementation of the plan to ensure that the intermediate results are achieved is part of the planning process as plans should not be carved in stone but be flexible management tools.

Progress in global health projects is sometimes unknown or unpredictable because planning is usually based on assumptions and not an informed process making use of monitoring data from the country's health measurement systems. Work plans then become unrealistic and planning is a very time-consuming process that sometimes takes months and prevents staff from focusing on the real work that is implementing the project so that the country's programs work better and better services are delivered.

Health planning is one of the governance functions of a country's health system. Health planning is usually not a very productive activity in most countries where governance structures are not well defined or clearly managed. Many countries have national health plans, provincial or state plans that are used to produce the annual budget but are not used as daily management tools to achieve results. Plans are written annually and are usually set in stone despite the fact that the budget is usually insufficient to implement all that is included in the plan. In addition, these plans do not usually include the contribution of donors and partners so it gives the impression that the MOH is doing it all. Moreover, health plans are not continuously monitored to make corrections as challenges and opportunities arise and planning assumptions change.

Planning in global health projects is determined by the original project design that defined the project's framework. Design errors that were not perceived at the start of a project become apparent as implementation starts but most projects stay constrained by the original framework. Most importantly, opportunities to make a bigger impact also emerge that sometimes were not there when the global health aid project started such a Global Fund grant is awarded and then an HIV/AIDS project has the opportunity to contribute to the country's HIV/AIDS program in a different way. These errors and missed opportunities are usually not discovered until an evaluation takes place 2 or 3 years later, when it is too late to take effective corrective action. The important thing is not the plan but the results. **A Plan is a tool not an**

end. We must stick to a plan as long as it is delivering effective results. Plans must not be carved in stone; the desired end results in the form of improved quality and quantity of healthcare must be carved in stone. Plans must be flexible implementation tools and not constrict innovation and informed problem solving. Why? Because in global health results mean lives saved. We cannot afford to fail.

Planning is a continuous process. We must review annual plans monthly, and monthly plans must be reviewed weekly and weekly plans must be reviewed daily to ensure we are working on the right priorities. That is how I aim at getting done at least three important tasks every day. By important, I mean those that contribute to our shared goals and results.

Global Health Progress and Impact

Progress in global health is the result of the progress of the development plan of each country and of the effective aid that assisted them. Health status impacts the overall development plan because countries need a healthy workforce and investments in health must deliver the expected results. The development process of a country also impacts health because it increases people's choices and better livelihoods, better security, roads, and water and sanitation lead to better life quality and longer life expectancy (Box 2.2).

The adoption of the MDGs and the principles of the Paris Declaration and easy access to technology and information through the Internet have also led to progress in global health. An important factor in the recent progress in global health, as measured by the annual reports on progress towards the Millennium Development Goals (MDGs) (UN 2005–2014), is having measurable global goals and targets and the technology to measure and account for results towards those targets. It is clear from the international legislation discussed in Chap. 1 that the right to development is a right and a responsibility of all nations, developed and developing ones. The MDGs allowed nations to measure how they perform and create programs to meet the targets. What was missing at the time of Alma-Ata and therefore, the Health for All by

---

Box 2.2: *Development and Health*
The basic purpose of development is to enlarge people's choices. In principle, these choices can be infinite and can change over time. People often value achievements that do not show up at all, or not immediately, in income or growth figures: greater access to knowledge, better nutrition and health services, more secure livelihoods, security against crime and physical violence, satisfying leisure hours, political and cultural freedoms and sense of participation in community activities. The objective of development is to create an enabling environment for people to enjoy long, healthy, and creative lives.

Mahbub ul Haq (1934–1998)
Founder of the Human Development Report

the Year 2000[1] strategy was not measured in the same way the MDGs are. WHO must continue the global health monitoring in every country in a way that helps inform all stakeholders.

There has been progress as shown by the "Human Development Index" (HDI). Health as measured by the life expectancy at birth is part of the HDI (HDR 2013) and along with education and per capita gross national income, they constitute the HDI, which helps measure how well we are doing as a whole as a species. The 2013 HDI report shows important improvements. More nations are raising the quality of life of their citizens. Countries such as Mexico, Turkey, Thailand, and Indonesia are joining Brazil, Russia, India, China, and South Africa, now known as the "BRICS." Countries that used to receive aid are now providing it such as Turkey, Poland, Korea, and Russia are now global leaders and provide more opportunities for aid and innovation (Mawdsley 2012). However, having more development partners means that developing countries are at risk of costly unnecessary complexity that limits progress, and need to put more effort to keep things simple and ensure efficient use of all the resources. There are two options so far: either to limit aid or to create coordinating mechanisms. Mozambique, Rwanda, and Liberia have had to put a limit to uncoordinated aid projects that are not aligned with the countries' development agenda, a trend that must be supported and respected. The Global Fund Against AIDS, Malaria, and TB requires countries to create "country coordinating mechanisms" (CCM). The CCMs have democratic representation of government, donors, civil society, and the populations affected by these diseases. The CCM helps plan and measure progress of control and healthcare delivery activities for these diseases as well as with the effective and efficient management of performance-based grant funds.

Not all progress is good, effective, or even helpful due to lack of communication, collaboration, and coordination among all stakeholders at global and country levels (Dickinson 2011). For example, aid delivered by some international NGOs focuses only on achieving "their project objectives" and do not effectively collaborate with the government staff to help them do their work better. Instead, it is the project staff that do the work and the government staff are not empowered to get better results with the help of the project. In addition, even when each project does communicate with the authorities and other partners regularly, they sometimes use different approaches to provide services such as a different diagnostic process or treatment protocol which can cause confusion among health providers that do not know what the standard procedure is. That is why you may see an organization using one approach to promote child health in one province and another project or organization using another in another part of the same country, and this not because they are coordinating and comparing which is more effective.

Lack of coordination is also seen in donor-driven campaigns that drain human and financial resources from routine service delivery. Donor-funded projects that drain health professionals from the health sector must also be stopped. Instead, donors should use funds to support the local health facilities and the local training institutions to increase output, strengthen human resource management and support

---

[1] http://undp.by/en/who/healthforall/

to existing health staff to help them do their job, and supplement or hire more staff and second experts to the MOH and its facilities while new staff is being trained.

The MDGs set the agenda about what to do, what to achieve. The MDGs, however, did not state how to do it in spite of the fact that we have the knowledge and technology. There has been significant progress in the use of evidence-based practices about how to achieve the MDGs and since the Millennium Project report that listed the "Quick Wins,[2]" a list of the effective ways to achieve the MDGs that include effective interventions that would benefit mostly health programs. Unfortunately, donors and governments did not place much emphasis on the "Quick Wins," many of which are still valid today. There is no doubt that we know how to prevent a large number of deaths in developing countries because we do it in developed nations. Progress is now limited by our limited collective ability to implement improvements in public health and healthcare service delivery in a coordinated, effective, and efficient way. Below is a discussion of why and what to do about it to improve the effectiveness of global health aid and help contribute to the post2015 agenda.

Factors That Determine Progress to Effective Global Health Aid

Factor 1. The global health agenda must set clear desired goals and results to be achieved in every country and set annual targets. Progress is a function of effective management, which is a function of effective measurement, which is a function of having clear goals and targets. In short, we must plan and manage to achieve clear outcomes, not outputs, and the outcome must be focused on providing continuous whole patient care not on implementing disease control programs. These programs are not the end but the means to deliver continuous whole patient care services which must be the objective of most development projects. Now, most projects are usually output focused and focus on objectives such as numbers of mosquito nets distributed, without ensuring that these nets are part of a national program that ensures that every child and pregnant mother gets a net from their health provider and that this service needs to continue after the project end. Projects sometimes focus on numbers of health providers trained without measuring or ensuring if these trained providers have the supplies or the ability to change their work environment to actually implement what they were trained to do; or the number of supervised deliveries without ensuring the postpartum care and services for spacing of the next birth were also received satisfactorily, or the baby is breastfed exclusively and both mother and child survived. The disease and output focus of donor-driven approaches has resulted in fragmentation of the continuous healthcare delivery process and weakened the health system in many countries by creating parallel structures. You, as a global health professional, must work with all stakeholders and choose clear results to be achieved so you can "**Manage by Results**," a

---

[2] http://www.unmillenniumproject.org/resources/quickwins.htm

principle of the Paris Declaration (PD). When managing by results, the whole patient, not one disease, must be the focus and population-based well-being rates the ultimate result. The MOH of the country must coordinate the implementation of a countrywide health plan with targets so that each donor or stakeholder will have their share of those targets and contribute by taking responsibility for a number of activities and/or for a geographic area or by supplying funding or a number of inputs and/or supplies that are distributed through the country's strengthened logistics system. In this way, the 2030 results will be shared by all and contributions by each party will be accounted for and acknowledged.

Factor 2. The global health agenda must stay on course. When goals and results are agreed, all parties must stay focused on achieving these goals. The MDGs had targets for the year 2015. However, these targets were not achieved by all countries and even then, these targets do not get all the work done. For example, MDG4 calls for reducing child mortality by 50 %. Even if all countries achieved this target, there remain the other 50 % of preventable deaths that must be prevented, as well. The job is also not done yet when reducing maternal deaths, malaria, TB, or HIV/AIDS deaths either, but the UN is already thinking of changing the goals in the post 2015 era. There are "fads and fashions" in global health that change the course and limit our collective progress must be stopped. We must stay focused on the health MDGs. **The job is not done yet.** I agree there is the need to add other goals that address new knowledge, evidence, and prevalent development and health issues, such as mental health that affects millions of people, or tobacco-related deaths that are estimated to be one billion in the next 10 years, the threat of Ebola, and the prevention of neglected tropical diseases and noncommunicable diseases such as diabetes and cancer. However, it is not responsible to change course and reduce the momentum that took several years to gain in improving gender equality, and maternal and child health. This stop-and-go approach is not effective use of aid. The solution is for WHO to lead and keep the focus on the set goals that address all priority health problems (Annex) and on helping coordinate the improvement of the health system in its member countries.

Factor 3. The global health agenda must include consensus on measuring results to monitor progress and take corrective action. Measurement in global health is usually a complex process. The information for results and productivity measurement comes from various sources: a country's weak and incomplete health information system (HIS) or local disease surveillance system, or from national or local demographic and health surveys (DHS) that are conducted every 5 years or so, or from specific surveys funded by donors such as Knowledge, Practices, and Coverage Surveys (KPC). Most projects are not required to collect management information, and therefore, the management data they collect are limited, which prevents them from making timely corrections. The lack of comprehensive up-to-date information is compounded by the fact that most projects have monitoring and evaluation (M&E) systems that are designed to show output indicators and good results and do not report to the country's HIS or other MOH information systems. Projects do not measure errors or negative performance outcome information that can be used to make timely corrections. For example, health facilities measure number of children vaccinated, but they do not measure the number of children missed and therefore vaccines that still need to be given. Or projects and facilities do not measure which child misses which vaccines or does not have a mosquito net to sleep under so that the health workers can do home visits and reach the missed child. Also, few countries do actual immunization studies to measure the effectiveness of the vaccination in terms of the antibodies actually developed due to an effective vaccine, and consequently measure "injected" children as opposed to actually immunized children.

Factor 4. Global health results must be measured as a fraction or percentage of the total number of people that need the service. A fraction requires a numerator, that is, the number of people that actually got the service such as vaccines; and a denominator, that is, the total number of people that needed to receive the service. For example, in the case of children's vaccines, the denominator is the number of children born in the coverage area of the project or facility. Numerator data such as the number of children that were actually vaccinated are usually available and quite reliable and can be triangulated with the number of doses of vaccines reported to have been used to check for accuracy. However, the lack of "denominator" data is a limiting factor in measuring how effective the project or the facility is in achieving the expected result of vaccinating 100 % of the children born in their coverage area. Most facilities and projects do not have reliable numbers or data of their coverage population and therefore do not know their catchment population, that is, the actual number of people they need to serve so they can plan services accordingly. We must ensure that every facility regularly conducts a local census, works with the local government to have access to local vital statistics (births and deaths), and has accurate coverage area population figures, that is, denominator data, and use the data to measure their effectiveness in serving population needs.

Factor 5. Global health projects and country programs must reduce the number of errors that cost lives and human suffering. Zero error tolerance must be the new policy. Like the nurse in our story at the start of this chapter, every day somewhere a child misses a vaccine dose that would prevent a serious and even deadly disease such as polio or measles; a mother does not get her prenatal checkup, and another dies of childbirth complications; a person living with AIDS cannot have his or her medication because the local health center has run out of medicines. These are errors that can be prevented and anticipated. We know what interventions would save lives and have the technology to make it happen. We need to put "operations manuals" with the right processes and controls in place that we use in developed countries to ensure these errors do not happen again. These errors are human errors that can be prevented if measured and identified and corrected. We can do it by providing effective aid; global health projects must put the right standard operating procedures into place to deliver services in a way that errors are prevented and achieve the planned number of effective results. Global Health Six Sigma processes, that is, those processes that deliver results within less than six standard deviations of the norm must be used to ensure that errors are less than 3.4. per million opportunities.

Factor 6. Global health professionals must have a code of ethics that includes demonstrating accountability, and that they are responsible for effective results. The effectiveness of each person depends on whether they have performance goals and targets and are able to measure their performance and that performance in linked to the results to be achieved in the geographic area of the project of the facilities. Global health results usually depend on the effectiveness of the professionals responsible for them. Staff working on global health projects must have up-to-date job descriptions, performance goals, and short-term targets to deliver and have supervisors that ensure they are on track. Project evaluation must include evaluation of the effectiveness of the human resources responsible for the project activities. Join us in our online community as we develop the 2030 code of ethics.

Factor 7. Global health organizations and donor agencies must consider effectiveness and sustainability in the life cycle of a global health project when designing new projects. Most projects funded by the United States Government (USG) are designed to be implemented over a 5-year period, which is the budget cycle of the USG. In a 5-year project, year 1 must be the year when advisors and counterparts work together to develop a health development plan if there isn't one or align with the existing one and create a joint implementation plan that includes the roles and activities each party will play in the life of the project. Coordination and harmonization mechanisms with other donors and lines and frequency of communications and reporting as well as results and measures of success are agreed upon in alignment with the country's national health plan. Then, years 1–3 are usually "effectiveness years" in which the project delivers results through intense intervention testing, training, and implementation to ensure maximum coverage, and harmonization with other stakeholders. By year 3, the project must be ready to start the transition to structures that will sustain the achievements of the previous years by institutionalizing and systematizing the interventions of the previous years.

The goal of the fourth year of the project is usually to let go and sustain the capacity built in previous years so eventually activities become part of the country's budget and programs and can continue being implemented by project counterparts without assistance. Years 3–4 must be "sustainability years," in which project staff work to assist counterparts to seamlessly include the new interventions in their daily routines, work plans, and annual budgets. The project team must assist to include new interventions and activities in the next year's health plan and budget or they won't be funded or sustained.

For example, in years 1–3, it is expected that project staff would train trainers in the MOH and the country's nursing and medical schools, as well as supervisors of health providers to implement the new state-of-the-art health delivery interventions, reorganize patient flow and facility operational procedures, create or revise policies, job descriptions, and operations manuals, and procedure checklists to ensure the services are delivered according to the new quality standards the project introduced. The project staff at this time also helps identify and sort out problems, bottlenecks, and gaps that prevent sustainable efficient implementation.

Results in the first 3 years of a project are measured by the actual number of people served according to the new procedures. For instance, if the goal is to improve child health, the result would the number of health providers observed to deliver child health services according to the new child health quality standards and the number of children actually served according to the new standards as measured by patient records; these result indicators would be an indicator expected to progressively increase from 0 to 100 % as the months and the project's work progresses.

In years 3–4, it is usually the time when project staff work with counterparts to assume a more effective management role and effectively perform as managers, trainers, supervisors, and problem solvers. At this time is when the project staff start to get themselves out of their jobs as "doers" and move on to play the role of mentors and consultants. Local counterparts are now becoming able to manage the training and supervision on their own and measure their results indicators. For example, in the case of a project designed to improve child health, the result indicators would include in addition to the indicators mentioned above, the increasing number of facilities that now deliver services according to operating standards, and the number of local program managers that now manage the program with less support from the project.

Finally, year 5 is the year of effective transfer of the implementation capacity to the counterparts and in which project staff accompany the work of counterparts to monitor effectiveness and efficiency, tie any loose ends, and assist in problem solving, playing the role of consultant and sounding board.

WHO must lead general consensus about the life cycle of an effective project and make the description above or similar the standard in global health. If each project progresses in a different way without standardization, regular monitoring of the effectiveness of their work is hard if not impossible to measure. We encourage the systematic design and planning of aid programs to ensure their effectiveness and their alignment with the principles of the Paris Declaration.

Conclusion

Every year, millions of children, men, and women die of preventable and treatable conditions, some of which they would have never even acquired had they known how to prevent them. Our civilization as a whole has the knowledge and the technology to prevent these deaths. It is simply unprofessional, a human right violation and morally unacceptable to keep this situation going on year in and year out. Resourcefulness is the ultimate resource, the ability to make the best of whatever resources we have. We must apply resourcefulness to the global health agenda and deliver better aid (Trafton 2013). More resources without first creating the ability to use them efficiently will just lead to more waste. This chapter presented a number of factors towards the development of a framework of effective global health aid, the prevention of wastage of resources, and rapid and effective transfer of knowledge and skills for effective country owners which is required to prevent millions of deaths.

Effectiveness is getting the expected results (Riddell 2007). Effective aid is getting the expected results when aid is provided by those that have the knowledge and skills to improve healthcare and transfer that to those that do not. In development, we usually cite the Chinese proverb of teaching people to fish and not just giving fish. In the case of natural or man-made disaster, humanitarian assistance is essential and providing "fish," that is, water, food, and medical care is essential as communities are unable to sustain basic services and normal life has been disrupted. However, in the case of development aid, effectiveness is about teaching people to fish and motivating the want to fish, i.e., deliver quality healthcare and to be proactive, resilient, and competent no matter what.

The keywords in development assistance are "effective transfer" and that means the complete transfer of knowledge and expertise from experts to the local health authorities and program managers. In other words, it is not about giving "fish," and it is about just teaching others to fish. It is about transferring the ability to fish, ensuring they have the right equipment and supplies to fish, knowing where and how to find the fish, the ability to develop new fishing strategies and train future generations of fishers, and of manufacturing simple fishing rods for all fishermen and fisherwomen, as well as developing and sustaining the infrastructure to process the fish and distribute it. Without that, the cycle of dependence on foreign aid will not be broken, countries will not be able to provide quality health services on their own and continue improving them, and most importantly the general feeling that "quality healthcare for all" cannot be achieved in countries such as Haiti or Nigeria or India will continue permeating throughout. Health for all can be achieved by 2030. I got into the global health field because I wanted to end deaths of malaria, diarrhea, and pneumonia, and stop women from dying delivering their babies. We have the knowledge and technology to do it, but we must break with business as usual. Will you?

In global health, there is widespread inequity in the distribution of knowledge and skills. There are countries with more significant knowledge and skills to provide public health and healthcare services, and at least a minimum of quality healthcare to its citizens while others are not. Those with the knowledge and expertise are in general willing to share it but have not been able to do it very effectively yet. Until recently, most of the aid projects were designed by the donor funding the project, with limited and sometimes without the participation of the country that is about to receive the aid. Things are changing, but still most US-funded projects are designed and implemented by US experts and/or contractors, who are well trained and have lots of knowledge and many useful skills but who sometimes do not take into consideration that the solutions they design must be simple enough and work at countrywide scale within the constraints of the country's health system and resources not within the small scale and resources of the donor. For example, a project would train health workers on how to assess their pharmaceutical system that procures, stores, and distributes medicines to the government health facilities, but would not help them conduct the assessment. Or when a project is designed to improve the delivery of medical supplies and does actually get the supplies to the facilities, but through a parallel system that weakens the country's logistics system and does not help or support those in charge of the country's supply chain to use the project's lessons learned to fully plan their annual work plan and budget and identify areas for continuous improvement every year.

The "three C's" of communication, collaboration, and coordination must be practiced at all times by all aid projects. Aid projects must be designed, implemented, and evaluated in terms of how successfully they have been in effectively transferring the knowledge and skills.

The Development Assistance Committee (DAC) of the Organization for Economic Cooperation and Development (OECD) is working to expand their definition of "overseas development assistance" (ODA), which must keep measuring ODA in health in development. We cannot have economic development without health. OECD used health as a tracer measure of economic development because they thought that when economies get better, people will invest in health, which is true but not the whole truth. In fact, it is the other way around, when people are healthy they are able to contribute to economic development. The Right to Health as defined in General Comment 14 of the ICESCR must be part of the ODA definition and the way to work in global health.

Now as for the 2030 agenda, remember it is good to expand the MDG agenda but not to change it until we really achieve the targets. Many of the targets of the MDGs, particularly related to women's and children's health, have not been achieved yet and need more time. Let's stay on course and implement effective ODA projects to meet and exceed the MDG targets (See Annex).

Annex: Integrated Global Health Goals and Targets by 2030

MDG 3: Promote gender equality and empower women

4: Eliminate gender disparity in primary and secondary education preferably by 2005, and at all levels by 2015

NEW! Goal 3: Increase the number of nations that implement legislation making 18 years of age as the legal age of marriage and that implement nationwide gender equalization programs

1. *100 % of the countries have legislation and enforce 18 as the legal age of marriage.*
2. *Increase by at least 10 % per year the number of women that participate in Government.*
3. *Increase by at least 10 % per year the number of women that own businesses.*
4. *Increase by at least 10 % per year the number of women and men that have access to family planning and birth spacing education and services.*
5. *100 % of countries prosecute 100 % cases of rape, trafficking, pedophilia, and domestic and gender-based violence.*
6. *Increase by at least 10 % per year the number of victims of rape, trafficking, pedophilia and domestic and gender-based violence that receive support and rehabilitation.*
7. *Increase by at least 10 % per year the number of women that are paid the same as men for the same job.*
8. *Increase by at least 10 % per year the number of women that are not circumcised against their will.*

MDG 4: Reduce child mortality

5: Reduce by two thirds the mortality rate among children under five

NEW! Goal 4: Increase the number of children that survive their 18th birthday

9. *Increase by at least 10% per year the number of health facilities that implement IMCI and provide comprehensive preventive health services (vaccines, growth monitoring, etc.).*
10. *Increase by at least 10% per year the number of newborns that are born assisted by a trained attendant, breastfeed immediately and kept warm.*
11. *Increase by at least 10% per year the number of infants that are fully immunized, breastfed exclusively for at least 6 months, receive Vitamin A and Iron, and that sleep under a long-lasting impregnated mosquito net.*
12. *Increase by at least 10% per year the number of children that are well nourished and receive appropriate treatment for anemia, pneumonia, diarrhea, malaria, and prevalent children's illnesses at home and at a health facility by their fifth birthday.*
13. *Increase by at least 10% per year the number of pre-teens (6 top 12) and teens (13–18) that receive relevant immunizations, preventive health education, including reproductive education, and age-appropriate health services.*
14. *Increase by at least 10% per year the number of orphans that live in safe family-like settings and receive the same education and services as other children.*

MDG 5: Improve maternal health

6: Reduce by three quarters the maternal mortality ratio

NEW! Goal 5: Increase the number of women that survive pregnancy and delivery.

15. *Increase by at least 10% per year the number of health facilities that can provide quality antenatal, delivery, and postpartum health services.*
16. *Increase by 10% per year the number of women that have wanted pregnancies.*
17. *Increase by 10% per year the number of women that receive antenatal care.*
18. *Increase by 10% per year the number of pregnant women that have a supervised delivery.*
19. *Increase by 10% per year the number of pregnant women that have access to emergency obstetric care within 6 h.*
20. *Increase by 10% per year the number of pregnant and breastfeeding mothers that sleep under a long-lasting impregnated mosquito net.*
21. *Increase by 10% per year the number of women that have appropriate nutrition and work load during pregnancy and postpartum.*

MDG 6: Combat HIV/AIDS, Malaria, and other diseases

7: Halt and begin to reverse the spread of HIV/AIDS
8: Halt and begin to reverse the incidence of malaria and other major diseases

NEW! Goal 6: Increase the number of people that prevent or recover from the conditions responsible for 80 % of the mortality in each country

22. *Increase by at least 10 % per year the number of people that know how to prevent HIV/AIDS, Malaria, Trachoma, Fistula, obesity, cardiovascular disease, diabetes, cervical cancer, and other prevalent conditions.*
23. *Increase by at least 10 % per the number of people that have healthy lifestyles and protect themselves from HIV/AIDS, Malaria, Trachoma, Fistula, obesity, cardiovascular disease, diabetes, cervical cancer, and other prevalent conditions.*
24. *Increase by at least 10 % per year the number of people that receive integrated care and treatment for HIV/AIDS, TB, Malaria, Trachoma, Fistula, obesity, cardiovascular disease, diabetes, cervical cancer, and other prevalent conditions.*
25. *Pass legislation to ban smoking in public places and reduce by at least 10 % per year the number of people that smoke.*

MDG 7: Ensure environmental sustainability

9: Integrate the principles of sustainable development into country policies and programs; reverse loss of environmental resources
10: Reduce by half the proportion of people without sustainable access to safe drinking water
11: Achieve significant improvement in lives of at least 100 million slum dwellers, by 2030

New Goal 7: Increase the number of communities that have healthy environment programs and therefore have clean air, safe water, safe waste disposal, and limited carbon footprint

26. *Increase by at least 10 % per year the number of people that have clean indoor air.*
27. *Increase by at least 10 % per year the number of cities that manage their watershed systems.*
28. *Increase by at least 10 % per year the number of schools that have running water and safe clean bathrooms by gender.*
29. *Increase by at least 10 % per year the number of clinics, health centers and hospitals that have electricity, running water and safe clean bathrooms by gender.*
30. *Increase by at least 10 % per year the number of people that have access to clean drinking water and safe waste disposal.*
31. *Increase by at least 10 % per year the number of people that recycle and contribute to their community's Recycle and Garbage Management Program.*
32. *Increase by at least 10 % per year the number of cities and towns that know their Carbon footprint and have programs to reduce it by 10 % per year.*
33. *Increase by at least 10 % the number of trees in cities, rural areas, and deforested areas.*
34. *Increase by at least 10 % per year the number of households that have the seven elements of a healthy environment: clean air, clean water, toilets and sanitation, electricity, garbage disposal, live in forested areas and that recycle.*

References

(2006). International human solidarity day. *United Nations, 1*, 2.

(2007). An introduction to the World Health Organization. *Working for health, 1*, 21.

(2011). Eliminating health inequities every woman and every child counts. *International Federation of Red Cross and Red Crescent Societies, 1*, 42.

(2011). Join up, scale up: How integration can defeat disease and poverty. *n/a, 1*, 12.

(2011). Progress and challenges in aid effectiveness. *Fourth high level forum on aid effectiveness, 1*, 55.

(2012). Making a real difference—delivering real results. *An effective aid program for Australia, 1*, 66.

(2013). Annual letter. *USAID, 1*, 27.

(2013). Building relationships in development cooperation: Traditional donors and the rising powers. *IDS Policy Breifing, 1*(36), 6.

(2013). The millennium development goals report. *United Nations, 1*, 60.

(2006). Aid effectiveness 2006 survey on monitoring the Paris declaration overview of the results. *OECD, 1*, 130.

Bristol, N. (2013). *Do UN global development goals matter to the United States?* Washington, DC: CSIS.

Dickinson, C. (2011). Is aid effectiveness giving us better health results? *HLSP Institute, 1*, 10.

Human Development Report (HDR). (2013). Retrieved from http://hdr.undp.org/en/media/HDR2013_EN_Summary.pdf

Mawdsley, E. (2012). *From recipients to donors: Emerging powers and changing development landscape*. London: Zed Books.

Riddell, R. C. (2007). *Does foreign aid really work?* New York: Oxford University Press.

Social Impact. (2013). Final evaluation of the community-based therapeutic care institutionalization in Malawi (CTCIM). Retrieved from https://dec.usaid.gov/dec/content/Detail.aspx?ctID=ODVhZjk4NWQtM2YyMi00YjRmLTkxNjktZTcxMjM2NDBmY2Uy&rID=MzM5MjI5&inr=VHJ1ZQ==&dc=YWRk&bckToL

(2013). The Millennium Development Goals Report. Retrieved from http://www.un.org/millenniumgoals/pdf/report-2013/mdg-report-2013-english.pdf

Trafton, A. (2013). MIT's Institute for Medical Engineering and Science brings many tools to the quest for new disease treatments and diagnostic devices. *New approach to global health challenges, 1*, 2.

Chapter 3
Realizing Global Health: Effective Health Systems

Elvira Beracochea

Introduction

The Director of Health Services and the Directors of the Nutrition, Child Health, Maternal Health, Non-communicable diseases, HIV/AIDS, and TB programs in the Ministry of Health of a country somewhere in South America or sub-Saharan Africa or Asia are meeting to discuss their plan for the following year. Each of them has an average of 30 or more donors and donor-funded organizations and projects that work in their field and in some part of the country. However, they do not have real ownership ("Capacity Development and Country Ownership" 2014) of their programs and lack a unified plan that shows where each donor, project, or organization makes an effective contribution to their national programs or even where these partners work and what results they commit to achieve on behalf of the government in the next year. Each of them has 30 or more annual project reports and cannot make sense of all of them. Most partners do not work at national scale, which is what the directors do; they only work in some part of the country and influence part of the programs the directors are responsible for. For example, there is a donor working to improve the Prevention of Mother to Child Transmission of AIDS, but that project is not part of the country's child health program or even the HIV/AIDS, neither is there a plan by the donor to make it so. The directors need rapid scale up ("A Guide for Fostering Change" 2007) and know the partners are willing to help, but they do not know where or how much or how to scale up their many interventions or whether they are effective. The program directors also want to have tangible results and to know where most sick people are and where they need to focus their programs, but the national health information system is not effective in providing timely, complete, or accurate information for them to plan effectively. If only they could have

E. Beracochea, M.D., M.P.H. (✉)
Realizing Global Health Inc., Olley Lane 4710, Fairfax, VA 22032, USA
e-mail: elvira@realizingglobalhealth.com

© Springer Science+Business Media New York 2015
E. Beracochea (ed.), *Improving Aid Effectiveness in Global Health*,
DOI 10.1007/978-1-4939-2721-0_3

donors strengthen their health information and surveillance system, they could create a common plan with common goals and divide the responsibility and accountability for results among all the partners and pool the resources to target the unserved or areas with poor access (Ruger 2007). In addition to the numerous and unmanageable donor-funded projects, vertical programming without horizontal service delivery integration has made their jobs more ineffective and fragmented. The Director of the Nutrition program would like to coordinate with the Directors of the Child Health and Maternal Health programs and with the Directors of the other disease control programs, so they include nutrition services. After all, they serve the same people. If only they could integrate their work and take care of the whole person and not just part of them… The Director of Child Health would like to work with the other directors too. After all, she knows that children grow and become mothers and fathers and what is the use of saving them from childhood illnesses to see them die in childbirth, of AIDS, TB, or smoking-related conditions as young adults. If only they could have a life cycle approach to serve their people and not just fragmented periods of people's lives… you, the reader, must be wondering… If only they knew about how global health works, how programs translate into integrated packages of services that meet every person's needs and according to their needs, and if only they knew about how effective health centers can be for providing continuous healthcare along the human lifecycle to the communities in their coverage area… If only they had common effectiveness principles for all to put into practice and improve global health… The meeting adjourns without a plan and the directors agree to meet again next week to continue looking for a solution.

Frustrating and unproductive meetings like the one described above take place in every country in one way or another, but the story does not end there. In the meantime, in one of the many schools of public health in a North American or European country, every year over 200 graduates are getting their Master's degree in global health and are eager to get a job at one of the UN or donor organizations or foundations and start helping to improve global health. However, these graduates do not know about the effectiveness principles of global health, about ineffective projects, how countries have ineffective health systems that implement ineffective programs that deliver fragmented and discontinuous services, or how a new global health MPH can really contribute in effective ways, without reinventing the wheel. These graduates are passionate and want to help but they often are unaware of the operational aspects of ensuring quality Primary Health Care (PHC) and how global health works to implement PHC through facility and community-based programs. The idea of PHC was accepted in 1978, but its diffusion like most intangible ideas is slow (Gawande 2013). These new professionals as well as the more experienced ones need and want to be effective and really add value from the start and see tangible results. Unfortunately, most of these global health professionals have learned old-fashioned humanitarian or expert-consulting models and have rarely been introduced to how health systems work or really been involved in the design, management, and phase-out/handover of a project. Most find it very hard to find entry level jobs after graduation that would help them get a start in their profession and at the same time pay their student loans. And now you wonder if only they knew how Effective Global Health works and learned to be team players that ask the right questions to coach and contribute to teams that manage programs or deliver services. They would make an effective contribution to problem solving and help spread all the new knowledge they have.

But wait, the story does not end there either. Back in the developing country, healthcare professionals and all kinds of healthcare workers are being trained in outdated ways in the country's nursing and medical schools. These professionals are very resourceful after having been trained and worked in facilities with very limited resources. Most of the time, their training is clinical and they know little about managing vertical programs, community-based programs, or how health systems work to help them deliver services, ignoring basic operating procedures of the supply chain or the national health information system. Unfortunately, in spite of their reduced numbers, students are not actively recruited from their places of origin or helped to return to them after graduation. Production of new professionals is slow and in deficient numbers, their expertise is not leveraged, and they are not supported with up to date information that helps them solve the challenges they face every day (Perry 2013). So, now you wonder if only they could have access to the latest medical information and existing standard treatment protocols (Olmedo et al. 2013) and procedures (Joulaei et al. 2010) and could relate personally with their counterparts who graduated from European and North American Universities... Their schools' curricula have not been updated to include new knowledge and lessons learned from most of the country's donor-funded projects which use the "done for you" model and do not systematically transfer their knowledge to local health providers in training or in practice. In addition to not having access to up-to-date medical and nursing textbooks, health professionals in most developing countries have learned old-fashioned healthcare delivery models that are impersonal and unsatisfactory and do not allow them to measure their performance and see the results of their work for all the effort they make. If only they knew about different healthcare delivery models ("Tackling Pneumonia and Diarrhea Together" 2013) and had the right support to implement the required changes, they would be able to lead innovation and transform healthcare delivery process and its outcomes where they work, a much more rewarding professional experience compared to being trapped without visible solutions or a way out besides emigration.

But thanks to this chapter and the whole book, the current uncoordinated, unaccountable, and fragmented way of working in global health will start changing (we hope) and wherever you are, you will be able to start making a bigger impact because health professionals will start using the same principles and the same global health language with professionals worldwide. Please start now applying and sharing what you are about to learn today.

In this chapter you will learn how to apply the Principles of the Paris Declaration and about technical principles that ensure the effectiveness and sustainability of global health projects. You will also learn how health systems work, so the three groups of professionals described above finally converge and you can help them. You will learn about healthcare delivery models and how to effectively assist and implement change. With these principles and the tools presented in this chapter, global health professionals and healthcare providers will be able to coordinate their work, make a much bigger impact and save more lives, and know how much impact has been achieved and how many lives have been saved. It is that simple. After all, the goal of global health is to realize the right to health and progressively reach equity worldwide and improve quality in the provision of health services. Let's get started.

Three Questions

The first step to improve the effectiveness of a country's health system is to assess the effectiveness of all existing projects and organizations working in the health sector. There are usually several projects and NGOs and FBOs as well as private organizations working to improve some aspect of the health system through training and various reforms. A large number of these organizations also provide healthcare services as well. The first step is to make sure their participation and contribution is documented and part of the country's programs. The "Three Effectiveness Questions" (Box 1) are not the only questions to inquire about effectiveness, but are the first ones every global health professional should ask other partners and ask themselves on a regular basis to ensure they remain effective.

Question 1 is to determine whether the project or organization is effectively aligned with the country's programs. Thus, any HIV/AIDS project is expected to clearly contribute to improve how well the country's HIV/AIDS program works as well as the delivery of healthcare serves to people with HIV/AIDS.

Question 2 is to determine whether the project or organization has effectively harmonized its work with the country's health information system and is able to account for results and lessons learned, thus effectively contributing to one complete information system and working as a team player with others in the same field. The Three C's, that is, communication, collaboration, and coordination, is an approach that every project and global health organization must have in place. It consists of an effective strategy to communicate with the MOH and all partners and stakeholders to benefit all citizens in the country; an effective strategy to collaborate with the country's authorities and partners and prevent competitive strategies; and an effective effort to coordinate its daily activities to avoid duplication and wastage of resources. Thus, a malaria project or FBO providing malaria services must report to the country's health information and malaria program to ensure that the country's program objectives and strategies are informed and the coverage of services is comprehensive. Sometimes, you will find projects that do not document who they trained in a treat-

---

Box 1. Three Effectiveness Questions

1. Is my/your project or organization improving the country's programs and the delivery of health services?
2. Does my/your project or organization report to the country's health information system, account for results, and share lessons learned?
3. Does my/your project or organization have an exit strategy to move on to another region or a higher level of work?

Fig. 3.1 Stepwise
improvement approach

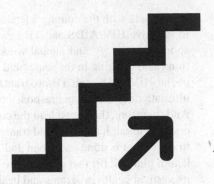

ment protocol for malaria for example, or the number of patients receiving the new treatment is not known and the country and its partners are unable to monitor the effectiveness of the new treatment. This is not an acceptable practice.

Finally, Question 3 is to determine whether the project or organization has anticipated how the country will sustain the innovations or new interventions introduced or how these will be scaled up to the rest of the country. Scaling up will be discussed in detail in the corresponding chapter. So here I will just say that you have to think of global health projects and the work global health organizations do as part of a *stepwise improvement process* (Fig. 3.1) that is measurable and moves up every quarter until plateauing when all the population has been covered. Therefore, one would expect the follow-on project or type of work of that organization to be at a higher supervisory and supportive level or in another region in the country, thus increasing the impact and coverage of its work.

At the end of the project, the country's program and its services should be able to work better and the project's results have been included in the country's corresponding policy; the project or organization must have moved its operations to another area in the country to continue the scale up; and/or the new interventions or services have been made part of at least two annual health plans and budget cycles and implemented routinely across the country.

Paris Declaration Principles and Effectiveness Global Health Indicators

The next step is to ensure that all those involved in the health sector follow the principles of the Paris Declaration (PD), and like the Department of Health of Papua New Guinea, they use the PD indicators to ensure all stakeholders do too as well. The principles are: ownership, alignment, harmonization, management by results and mutual accountability. Below are the questions you should ask to find out if the principles are followed:

1. **Ownership** does the country have ownership? Does the country have a 5–10 year health plan and an annual health work plan and budget that include the contribution of each partner or organization? Does this project or organization follow, ignore,

or compete with the country's leadership? For instance, an organization working to improve HIV/AIDS and TB treatment should be part of the country's corresponding strategy and annual work plan so that other resources and organizations also working in the same field may complement their work. The ownership of the HIV/AIDS and TB programs remains with the government, which is the ultimate duty bearer and responsible for the well-being of the country's people. And therefore, they must lead the corresponding program. There cannot be ownership without leadership and transparent collaboration of all involved. The tool to own what is done and when and by whom in the health sector is the national health plan (NHP) that includes the country's policies and objectives for each of its vertical health programs and health facilities that deliver horizontal services.

2. **Alignment** is this project or organization in alignment with the country's policies and plans (Wiggins et al. 2012)? If the answer to the questions above is yes, then you will be able to determine whether what projects or other NGOs do is in alignment with the country's policies, strategies, and plans. For example, an NGO working in nutrition must be included in the country's nutrition plan and its activities be aligned with the country's nutrition policy. If the policy is outdated, the organization must share the new information and assist the government to update its policy in collaboration with all other organizations working in nutrition before doing anything else.

3. **Harmonization** is this project or organization using harmonized strategies or approaches? Or is it creating parallel systems? If the country's systems are weak, the project or organization should look for ways to strengthen them in a top-down or bottom-up way and look for ways to minimize inefficiencies caused by temporary alternate solutions.

4. **Managing by Results** is the project or organization managing its activities to deliver results? By results, I mean outcomes not outputs. Thus, it is not enough to be training health workers in a new malaria treatment if they cannot apply it because their work routines and job descriptions have not changed, or the new malaria medicines are not available or there are frequent stock-outs. The result or outcome must always be improved quality of the services and/or improved coverage in global health, that is, patients get better and are satisfied or more people are served. All other activities are intermediary towards achieving those results. It is not acceptable to see incomplete processes that do not lead to results. In our example about malaria training, training would be preceded by improvements in the country's malaria policy, improvements in the supply chain to ensure continuous supply of diagnostic supplies and medicines, and supportive coaching to ensure the trained staff actually implement the new treatment when they go back to their jobs. Monitoring of patient outcomes through the statistics of each facility by a strengthened health information system and onsite supervision and patient interviews must be included as well.

5. **Mutual Accountability** are country and donor-funded projects and organizations mutually accountable? Monitoring must be an ongoing process in which all parties report on whether they fulfilled their commitments. The more involved, the greater the transparency. For example, if a project was to deliver 100,000 long-lasting impregnated nets (LLIN) to prevent malaria, how many have been distributed so far? How many are actually used? And how many are being replaced per year? Are there any "leaks"? LLINs or mosquito nets do not last forever and need to be

replaced and also, new people are born that need nets, therefore a continuous replacement system must be in place as well. It is not acceptable to distribute LLINs without a replacement system in place. I am talking about a countrywide health program to control and prevent malaria, not about the distribution of nets to the victims of a natural disaster or displaced persons, which may be a one-time effort. Every monthly monitoring report and annual evaluation must be a mutual assessment of the participation of each of the parties and an opportunity to improve processes, simplify procedures, and improve results in the next cycle.

In 2008, there was a meeting in Accra, Ghana; a document known as the Accra Agenda for Action (AAA) was produced, and 12 indicators were chosen to monitor the progress of the application of the PD principles. Global health projects and initiatives as well as donors and organizations must ensure that these indicators are monitored and reported and related procedures are enforced to ensure the effectiveness and sustainability of their work (Accra Agenda for Action 2008). The indicators are adapted to the health sector in the table below and must be monitored annually to set targets and discuss performance findings and make decisions (Table 3.1).

Table 3.1 Global health effectiveness indicators (Adapted from the AAA indicators)

Principles		Indicators
1	Ownership	The country has an operational development strategy for the health sector (and my project and organization contribute to it)
2	Alignment	The country moves up in the "Country Policy and Institutional Assessment Scale" (CPIA) and that applies to the MOH too
3		% of Global health aid that is reported in the country's health budget and that is increased annually
4		% of Global health technical assistance that is provided through a coordinated program consistent with the country's health development strategy and health plan
5a		% of Global health aid is provided through the MOH technical, managerial, information and financial systems and demonstrates improvement of their performance yearly
5b		% of Global health aid in the form of supplies that is provided through the country's procurement system and technical assistance is provided to improve the performance of the procurement system for commodities, medical supplies, and medicines
6		No parallel project implementation units
7		% of global health aid that is disbursed in the year it was scheduled
8		Global health aid is untied
9	Harmonization	Global health aid is part of a program-based approach and is reported as part of the corresponded program
10		Assessments, fact finding missions, studies and evaluations are conducted jointly by the MOH authorities and donor agencies
11	Managing for results	All global health projects and organizations in country are part of a national transparent and monitorable performance system and contribute to the national health information system through the district or local authorities
12	Mutual accountability	All global health donors participate in a mutual assessment review of the progress by health sector objective with the MOH annually and produce an annual report that informs the planning cycle for the following 2 years

Global Health Effectiveness Principles

In addition to the overall PD principles and indicators, there is need for principles of effectiveness to meet the unique global health challenges of quality healthcare, efficiency, countrywide scale, continuous healthcare, consistent whole patient care delivery, and sustainability. These principles are simple and clear, but not easy to put into practice unless all partners understand how healthcare delivery works and practice the "Three C's," that is, communication, collaboration, and coordination. The goal of these principles is to take the PD principles and indicators a step further to ensure that all global health aid effectively improves healthcare delivery and patient outcomes. These principles will help you understand the impact global health projects and initiatives that usually focus on one disease or aspect of the health sector have on the rest of the health system of a country and that the rest of the system has on the sustainability of the work they do.

1. *All global health projects must contribute to improve the performance of the country's health system.* Every country has a more or less effective health system. In the US, we have a mixed public-private healthcare delivery system that provides care to all insured according to the standards defined by the Health Insurance companies or health maintenance organizations about what is reimbursable. Although Canada and the UK have private providers, they also have a national health service (NHS) that ensures access to healthcare in accordance to services that meet standard quality criteria to all. Health reform is the continuous process that analyzes the performance of the health system and looks for ways to improve the quality, efficiency, and coverage of the health system. The Patient Protection and Affordable Care Act (ACA), is a new policy developed by the Obama Administration that is part of a number of health reform efforts in the last 25 years to improve the equity in the US system. Several health reforms have been implemented to improve delays in these centralized systems and quality of care has improved recently.

   Countries in SSA have health systems inherited from colonial times and health reform efforts are usually part of the work of a small team in the Policy and Planning Unit of the MOH and donor-driven and funded. Improving the effectiveness of how the health system works is the goal of every health reform effort and of every global health project or program or initiative. It is your job, the job of every health professional, and the job of every global health project and organization to understand how the health system and health reform works, its strengths and weaknesses. Yes, most ministries of health appear to be bureaucratic and need improvement and support to become more efficient and need to conduct research and develop and implement health reforms. That is why, they need global health professionals' advice to uncover the options they have to change and improve the system that was most likely designed to meet the needs of a much smaller population with a very different epidemiological profile in the colonial days. By getting to know the structure and function as well as the dysfunctions, the MOH and you can ensure that what you do will help build on and sustain strengths and overcome weaknesses. Remember weaknesses cost lives and money.

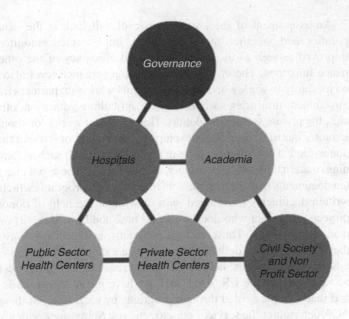

Fig. 3.2 The anatomy of a health system

2. *All global health aid must be based on the assessment of the performance of the health system of the country, which is a pyramid that includes three functional levels* (see Fig. 3.2): (1) governance level, (2) leadership level, and (3) PHC delivery level. All global health projects and aid must be designed on the basis of a joint assessment of the strengths and weaknesses of each level and designed to build on the strengths and correct weaknesses.

   (a) *The governance level is at the top of the pyramid and guides the performance and development of the health system through health reforms* (Fig. 3.2). The governance level includes national, state, or provincial and district or county governance levels. Governance includes the ten basic functions: policy and health reform, planning, budgeting and financing (Hughes et al. 2012), monitoring, evaluation, health surveillance, regulation, accreditation, partnerships, and donor–grantee coordination and management. The governance level is represented by the MOH and the provincial and district health offices in most countries. In the US, the Department of Health and Human Services with its operating divisions and agencies and regional offices is the federal governance level as well as the Departments of Health in each state and county are the state and county governance levels. Governance governs the health sector and works through policies that are implemented through vertical programs that then are "translated" into horizontal services to the citizens of their country. The ability of the governance level to enforce policies and implement programs depends on its structure, capacity, and effectiveness of staff in charge of the various agencies and programs, and their efficient management of resources.

An assessment of the governance level will look at the existence of policies and whether these are being implemented, monitored, and improved as well as the effectiveness and efficiency of the other governance functions. The effectiveness of the governance level also depends on its ability to work with and coordinate its work with partners from other government ministries such as finance, agriculture education, other agencies, the private sector, and donors. Here is how it works (or should work) in most countries: the MOH develops policies (with or without the help of donor-funded consultant experts in the technical field, such as family planning, maternal health, HIV, cancer, diabetes, etc.). These policies are written documents that are then implemented through programs which are also written documents (developed with or without the help of donor-funded projects) that state who does what and how and how to report on performance and results. These vertical programs, called in this way because they rule top-down, define what services are delivered and how in hospitals and health centers and clinics. So the sequence is Policy >>> Program >>> Services. In the US, since 2010 we have the ACA, which is a policy and that is implemented through programs by each state. In this way, the ACA determines the services our citizens get. Sometimes policies encompass several government agencies such as in Malawi, the government has a nutrition policy that is implemented through various programs by the MOH, the Ministry of Gender, the Ministry of Agriculture, and the Ministry of Education ("Final Evaluation of the Community" 2014). In South Africa, the Department of Health (similar to MOH) has based management of acute malnutrition project various policies in place that govern how the country provides health services to its citizens (http://www.health.gov.za/policies.php).

(b) *The mid level of the pyramid is the "leadership level" which provides Specialty Care, Education, and Research and includes hospitals, universities, and research or specialized medical centers* (Fig. 3.2). This level is called the leadership level because it provides medical care leadership to the PHC level and determines the indications for when a patient needs a referral to hospitals, as well as scientific and educational leadership to future health professionals in the country through universities and schools and research centers. This level includes more complex organizations that sometimes provide at least one, two or all three of the specialized care, education, and research functions and includes organizations such as hospitals, where most specialists such as oncologists, endocrinologists, and cardiologists, and specialized surgeons are; medical and nursing schools and teaching hospitals and other training institutions where doctors, nurses, and allied health sciences professionals are trained; and institutes of health where research and education usually take place (Macagba 2010). In global health, it is our job to assess how well this level performs and improve how hospitals deliver services and support their referring facilities, that is, the health centers and clinics in their coverage area.

(c) *The base of the pyramid is the PHC delivery level where the impact of global health aid is measured* (Fig. 3.2). Since the 1978 Alma-Ata declaration (Declaration of Alma-Ata 1978), the PHC concept has been well-defined and known (Joulaei et al. 2010). Now it is the time to put it to work at global scale. There are many resources on PHC in the WHO website (http://www.who.int/topics/primary_health_care/en). An in-depth description of PHC is beyond this book, so here I will just say that PHC has demonstrated to be an effective approach to provide healthcare particularly at the community level, which is where the majority of the public and private (for and nonprofit) health facilities are ("Direct Sales Agent Models in Health" 2013; Herzlinger 2012). Health centers and clinics are the real center of the health system because they provide "public health" and clinical care services, that is, health promotion and preventive health services to keep all people healthy and diagnose and treat those that get sick in the communities where they live and work. Thanks to WHO, most countries have adopted PHC to deliver health services as a policy. Community-based PHC (CBPHC), Community-oriented PHC (COPC) (Kark 1981) and Community-based participatory research (CBPR) are widely accepted approaches to ensure the design, provision, and access to PHC services that meet the needs of the facilities serve (Fleischman & Kramer 2013; Gaynor 2006; Wallerstein & Minkler 2008). A joint assessment of the effectiveness and efficiency of performance of the PHC level will determine if the facilities are providing quality healthcare and whether the facility and community-based services they provide and manage are run effectively and efficiently (Wennberg et al. 2010). For example, there may be a number of private facilities that have not been accredited, do not meet national quality standards, and their staff do not have the credentials to deliver care. This must be corrected. Also, an assessment may show that a number of facilities are overcrowded, while others are underused and some lack equipment and cannot account for the equipment provided by donors in their facility inventory.

3. *The PHC level must include a number of organizations that deliver healthcare services, both facility- and community-based services in their area of coverage.* In the absence of an effective health information system, an assessment of the PHC level is essential for the MOH and its partners to develop an operational development strategy of the health sector, AKA a national health plan for the next 5–10 years. The assessment must include the assessment of quality of the services provided as well as the knowledge, practices, and coverage (aka, KPC surveys) of the services provided. The assessment will help PHC level improve the deficient health information system afterwards and must include a sample of public or government-run facilities; private sector clinics and diagnostic centers such as radiology or medical laboratories; and non-profit, civil, and faith-based organizations providing various services that respond to needs in the communities they serve, such as, free home care to AIDS patients, bed-ridden elderly, disabled or terminal patients, screening and counseling, education, food supplementation, daycare for disabled persons, elderly or young children, etc. These

Fig. 3.3 Map of the
coverage area of a health post
in Peru

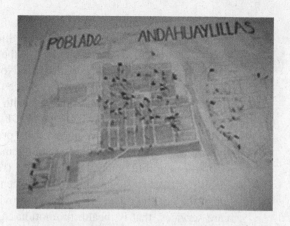

facilities provide healthcare services that implement various promotion, prevention, and treatment programs that are governed by the policies and plans of
the MOH in the country.

Each facility must have a defined coverage area and a known population that
serves as the denominator for the facility indicators. You will find that most
facilities have a map with the households (Fig. 3.3) with color-coded pins indicating where there is pregnant mother, a child under 1 or 5, and patients with
special needs. As mentioned above, most facilities do not have accurate census
data and must also conduct their own census and have a reliable denominator to
plan their services. For example, knowing the number of births allows the facility to plan the number of vaccines to be provided, the number of weighing sessions and nutrition, growth and child development education sessions that will
be required to meet their needs. Many facilities also manage a number of paid
or volunteer community health workers (CHW) that provide services under the
supervision of the facility nurse in charge of community services. CHW are
essential in most developing and developed countries because of the lack of
health professionals and due to the fact that most communities need basic
health promotion services that can be delivered through trained volunteers. The
US has several programs that make use of paid CHW such as the doulas that
provide a number of services to pregnant mothers, children, and elderly. Other
countries such as El Salvador, Israel, the UK and France have public health
nurses that do similar work in the community.

4. *The health center is the center of the health system.* Each health center (HC)
must deliver a horizontal integrated package of quality healthcare services efficiently and consistently ("Capacity Development and Country Ownership"
2014). Improving the effectiveness of every health center to deliver quality
healthcare to the population in their coverage area is the goal of every project,
program, or assistance organization working in their coverage area. The global
health target must be to improve or sustain the performance of at least 10 % of
the country's health centers per year, and with population growth, more centers
will have to be built.

The importance of effective leadership and managing an effective health team at every health center cannot be underestimated. The motivation of the Officer in Charge or HC Director is essential for every member of the health team to consistently follow standards operating procedures (SOP), process checklists, and proactively solve problems and address challenges. An assessment of the performance of a health center usually includes interviews with the health team, all of them preferably, or at least a sample of those at work at the time of the assessment. If there are several shifts; observations of consultations to assess whether they meet quality standards; and assessment of the condition of the facility and its assets, including hygiene, signage, and crowd control, inventory control and maintenance must be done at all shifts if possible. Health centers should have a clean waiting areas and separate bathrooms by gender in the sick and well patient areas. Health centers also must have individual consultation rooms for each healthcare provider and an effective appointment system that manages the time of each healthcare provider efficiently. Each healthcare provider must be responsible for a well-defined population and program. For example, one healthcare provider is responsible for all newborn and infants identified in the local census of the coverage area and the newborn and infant health programs; and another for all pregnant mothers and the antenatal and family planning programs. In this way, each health provider has a "denominator" to plan their services and that they can monitor and report on the facility scorecard.

Health centers usually have a laboratory for simple diagnostic tests; a medical records and information room and a storage room to store resources not in use, and a pharmacy with a preparation and dispensing areas and with its safe storage room for medicines, products and equipment. There must be well-defined organizational units in a HC and staff assigned to each area need to follow SOPs and meet productivity goals. For example, the staff in charge of the infant healthcare program are responsible for meeting at least 95 % vaccination coverage and preventing malnutrition by monitoring the growth of all newborns in the coverage area in accordance with the country's policies and program guidelines.

"*Global health Six Sigma*" (GH6δ) (Beracochea 2013) is an approach used to reduce medical errors and stop leaks in the management of health facilities. "Zero" error and leaks policies must be developed. In every clinic and HC, we see errors for action or omission, such as not washing hands before vaccinating a child, or giving the wrong dose of wrong medicine, or not checking the date of expiration of a medicine or not consistently providing family planning counseling to every pregnant mother to space the birth of the next baby, or not cleaning the labor room before the next delivery. Most HC do not have an assigned cleaner with clear duties to clean particularly toilets and patient areas every hour. Many donors as well as program managers are concerned about leaks. However, most health facilities do not have an updated SOPs or an inventory of the supplies and equipment they have received. Consequently things "disappear" because no one is responsible. The HC team along with members of the community must routinely conduct an inventory or form a local health committee including local members of the community that among other things can do quarterly and random inventory checks. The more people watching the inventory, the better as it is become easier to identify the leaks and the responsible party.

5. *Hospitals are the second line of care for patients* whose conditions cannot be diagnosed or treated in a health center due to the type of condition, its stage of progress, or urgency. It is not efficient for patients to bypass the HC for services that can be provided at the HC because it costs more to provide the same service at a hospital than at a HC. Patients do that when they perceive the quality of the health center services is not up to standard or they were treated rudely by staff. Hospitals are sometimes overlooked by global health programs that tend to focus on improving the delivery of services at the base of the health systems pyramid. However, without efficient and effective hospital services, it is impossible to sustain quality healthcare delivery in PHC facilities after the donor funding and their projects end. Hospitals are complex organizations with several diagnostic and treatment departments, clinical departments (emergency, internal medicine, cardiology, etc.), diagnostic departments (diagnostic imaging and radiology, microbiology lab, etc.), treatment departments (occupational therapy, physical therapy, nuclear medicine, oncology, etc.), and management departments, such as nursing, pharmacy, nutrition and dietetics, medical records and statistics, housekeeping, engineering, transportation, etc. Hospital resources should not be used to provide HC services. An effective referral system is managed by hospitals that support and supervise the quality of healthcare delivered at HCs.

   Managing a hospital requires special training and skills because it means managing a "hotel" as well as "restaurant" services and the delivery of a very specialized "menu" of services to out-patients and outpatients (Macagba 2010). Most hospitals have directors that have been promoted to that job without the proper training and support (Arthur 2011). It is essential that the director of the hospital as well as the heads of each department receive hospital management training, are able to interact with peers, and stay up to date with new management and organizational development practices, and the hospital meet accreditation standards. The "Global Health Six Sigma" (GH6δ) approach must also be used to ensure every hospital department meets quality standards and reduces error to the desired level of less than 3.4 errors per one million opportunities. An assessment of hospitals must include a number of assessments, one for each department. Hospitals also have a "denominator" because every hospital in the country must have a multi-year development plan and monitor the impact it has on the PHC facilities it supports and the communities served.

6. *Vertical programs must follow the national policy and have clear objectives, standards procedures, and performance measures as well as one manager or responsible person for its performance.* Programs define the objectives to be achieved in four services areas: health education and promotion of health behaviors, prevention, treatment, and rehabilitation. Programs are by definition "vertical" because they address one age group, one gender, or one disease that has specific health needs such as children, women, or people with malaria, TB, or HIV/AIDS top-down. Services are delivered by doctors and nurses and other health professionals who follow the program guidelines. Services are by definition

"horizontal" because they integrate the various programs at the point of delivery, i.e., clinic or hospital to provide "whole patient care." For example, the integration of programs for service delivery would work like this: an HIV (+) woman just had a baby and both need their HIV/AIDS treatment, in addition to the usual child health services HIV (−) newborns also get and the postnatal care and family planning HIV (−) women also get. Therefore, the mother would also get the following services: education about breastfeeding, malaria prevention and when to bring the baby for vaccination as well as advice to plan the birth of the next child or prevent future pregnancies, she would be screened for domestic violence and mental health disorders such as postpartum depression, and she would be asked about the health needs of other older children or members of her household. As mentioned above, global health projects, organizations, and initiatives must align their work with the country's program and help improve its performance by delivering effective horizontal health services.

7. *Projects must be effective and deliver the planned results. No excuses.* At least once a week, I repeat that projects must deliver results not outputs. Projects can make programs work well or make excuses, but not both. So I will say it again here: effectiveness is achieved by design. Many projects are designed based on unrealistic assumptions such as there are going to be enough medicines or commodities to implement a child health or family planning project. On the contrary, projects must be designed based on an assessment of the corresponding country program and to address the most important and debilitating weaknesses found in the program. A global health project must achieve and demonstrate improvement in the country's program and the delivery of its respective program in a defined area of the country, preferably countrywide, and manage the risks that would prevent it from succeeding. Risk management is usually not included in the scope of work and results framework of most projects. Therefore, there are projects that fail because they did not look for a way to address medicine stock outs by working in coordination with other projects addressing logistics and supply chains or the shortage of healthcare workers. This is why I call risk management putting the pieces of the healthcare delivery puzzle together. A family planning project does not have to address all aspects of healthcare delivery system, but must coordinate with others to ensure that problems or inefficiencies in other parts of the system do not prevent it from achieving its results. Consequently, from day 1, the project staff need to work with MOH and MOF partners to ensure the next year's budget includes enough supplies and with the training institutions to help look for ways improve production of health workers. Without a design based on the assessment of the country's corresponding program and risk management, projects are not effective. It is that simple.

8. *The "Three C's" must be included in the operations of every global health project, initiative, and organization: Communication, Collaboration, and Coordination.* As you know, there are many "Initiatives" and organizations in global health. However, many are not as effective as they could be because they do not communicate their plans, collaborate with others in the same geographic or technical area, do not coordinate their work with other existing efforts, and are

not evaluated for the actual value they provide to advance the development of the country's health system and global health goals. Before starting a new initiative, we must really ensure we are making the best of the existing ones and ending those efforts that are not giving the maximum return on the investment. Next, those working for the global health organization or initiative in question must work with the country program manager and other local authorities and identify their "effectiveness partners," that is, with whom they must communicate, collaborate, and coordinate. For example, an initiative to improve family planning, vaccination, or child health or access to TB treatment, must identify at global and country levels all the organizations in the same topic and communicate with them to ensure that their plan will complement what others are doing. They must also meet and communicate regularly, quarterly is the most effective interval in my experience, to report progress, share lessons learned, and communicate next quarter's objectives. They must look for ways to collaborate to implement SOPs and simplify work by doing things jointly or dividing the work among others to cover more people and not reinvent the wheel due to lack of prior knowledge of the institutional memory.

Coordination of activities simplifies implementation and increases efficiencies. For example, coordinating trainings with local training institutions and other organizations ensures that all healthcare providers receive training and this training is included in the curricula of future providers; and prevents including the same providers in a workshop about malaria one month and then family planning the next. Uncoordinated training makes it impossible for the provider to apply what they learn and wastes valuable time the providers must use to care for patients. Another example is the coordination of the use of vehicles, which must be part of a coordinated pool, so we do not have three project-funded vehicles going to the same facility and the country's supervisor not having the opportunity to accompany any of them or use the opportunity to deliver supplies. In general, pooling resources is a good idea (Hughes et al. 2012).

9. *Campaigns, pilots, and demonstration projects and scaling-up must be planned, implemented, and evaluated as part of a harmonized strategy to improve the performance of country programs and the quality and coverage of the delivery of services.* Campaigns are by definition short efforts to rapidly reach a large number of people or group. They do not substitute routine program activities but complement them. For example, a vaccination campaign must not be a substitute for the improvement of the "Routine Immunization Program." Hence, mop-up vaccination campaigns are used to rapidly protect a group of children or people that for some reason (migration or displacement, usually) were not reached by the routine program, and in this way, mop-up those that are susceptible to the disease in question. Sometimes, multi-year campaigns are designed. These campaigns should not exist and must be terminated because they drain resources from the country's programs.

Pilot AKA demonstration projects are used to test new approaches and procedures and must be part of a long-term strategy to improve a country's program and to scale up if proven cost-effective. Their design and implementation must be part of the 3C's process and their evaluation a multi-partner effort to ensure objectivity and transparency. Pilots must also demonstrate that the new or proposed procedure or practice is more cost-effective or efficient than the current one. Isolated pilots that are not evaluated or costed or whose lessons learned are not shared to contribute to the country's knowledge management capital should not have taken place and is a waste of resources.

Scaling-up is unfortunately an after-thought in many global health projects. It is very frustrating to see successful projects end and the team with capacity required to scale up disbanded because there is no expansion or scale-up plan. In fact, scale-up must be anticipated in the design of the project. What is the use of demonstrating something works if it does not benefit everyone? Please see the chapter on scaling-up to avoid this very expensive mistake.

10. *For every global health intervention to be effective, it must also be sustainable. Here are the "Five Keys to the Sustainability" in global health to effectively and sustainably achieve global health goals: (1) the health system, (2) the health programs, (3) the health center, (4) the healthcare provider, and (5) the Country's ownership.* These five keys must guide the work of every global health professional and organization to be effective:

Key 1. *The Health System.* Everything a global health project or organization does must improve how the country's health system works, that is, its three levels: governance, leadership, and delivery.

Key 2. *The Health Center.* The health center is the center of the health system. Global health projects must increase the number of well-functioning health centers that deliver quality healthcare services, manage community-based programs that meet the needs of communities it serves, and refer patients to hospitals when appropriate.

Key 3. *The Health Program.* Global health projects must improve how the country's health programs work, that is, a TB project must improve how the country's TB program works, a MCH project must leave a better performing MCH program in the host country, etc.

Key 4. *The Health Worker.* Global health projects must improve how the country's health professionals and workers perform and how their training institutions train them.

Key 5. *The Country's Ownership.* Global health projects must align their activities with the country's health policies and national health plan and assist to include their activities in the next year's national health plan and budget.

Conclusion

Bilateral donors such as USAID, DfID Irish Aid, the Bretton Woods institutions (IMF, WB), and other multilateral donors such as WHO, UNICEF, and others as well as private donors such as the Gates and Clinton Foundations must strive for effectiveness and pay for it. They must strive and pay for the "Three C's," ask their teams the "three questions" often, and enforce the PD principles.

The Millennium Development Goals showed us that the PD principles are essential to achieve success and that country ownership and leadership ensure sustainability of their investments.

Health is essential to development because a healthy workforce is good to the economy. In addition, most countries are signatories of international human rights treaties and therefore have endorsed the right to health, that is, the right to the highest attainable standard of care. Approaches based on human rights and on economic development goals make sense in every country. Human rights imply the government is the duty bearer and has to ensure access to the highest attainable standard of care. They do not have to provide services themselves, but they do have to protect the vulnerable and help fulfill the right of all citizens, particularly those that cannot afford it.

The issue of resources is important too, and many times used to justify poor results. However, I have not found evidence that shows that existing resources have been or are being used by donor-funded projects in the most effective and efficient manner. The most important conclusion is that global health professional must use what they have well and efficiently. Health is a human resource intensive sector because we need people to take care of people. In a school, one teacher can teach 30 or 40 or even more students. In healthcare, we need one on one care time as well as group care time. The health workforce must be managed effectively and the supervision and support of those in hard rural posts must be sustained. Effectiveness is a professional responsibility of all those working in global health.

References

A Guide for Fostering Change to Scale Up Effective Health Services. (2007). *Implementing Best Practices in Reproductive Health, 1*, 45.

Accra Agenda for Action. (2008). Paris: OECD.

Arthur, J. (2011). *Lean six sigma for hospitals: Simple steps to fast, affordable, and flawless healthcare*. McGraw-Hill.

Beracochea, E. (2013). *Health for All NOW* (2nd ed.). Fairfax, VA: MIDEGO.

Capacity Development and Country Ownership: Thinking Globally, Leading Locally. (2014). *USAID, 1*, 8.

Declaration of Alma Ata. (1978). Geneva, Switzerland: World Health Organization.

Direct Sales Agent Models in Health. (2013). *USAID, 1*, 32.

Final Evaluation of the Community-Based Therapeutic Care Institutionalization. (n.d.). USAID. gov. Retrieved September 1, 2014, from http://pdf.usaid.gov/pdf_docs/pdacy084.pdf

Fleischman, J., & Kramer, A. (2013). A trip report of the CSIS delegation to Zambia. *Strengthening U.S. Investments in Women's Global Health, 1*, 15.

Gawande, A. (2013, July 29). Annals of medicine, slow ideas. *The New Yorker*, p. 8.

Gaynor, C. (2006). Paris Declaration commitments and implications for gender equality and women's empowerment. *1*, 14.

Herzlinger, R. E. (2012). Let's put consumers in charge of health care. *Harvard Business Review, 1*, 11.

Hughes, J., Glassman, A., & Gwenigale, W. (2012). Innovative financing in early recovery: The Liberia health sector pool fund. *Center for Global Development, 1*, 30.

Joulaei, H., Honarvar, B., Zamiri, N., Moghadami, M., & Lankarani, K. (2010). Introduction of a pyramidal model based on primary health care: A paradigm for management of 2009 H1N1 flu pandemic. *Iranian Red Crescent Medical Journal, 12*, 7.

Kark, S. L. (1981). The Practice of Community-oriented Primary Health Care. New York: Appleton-Century-Crofts. Print.

Macagba, R. L. (2010). *Innovations in hospital management: Success with limited resources.* Santee, CA: Author.

Olmedo, B., Miranda, E., Cordon, O., Pettker, C. M., & Funai, E. F. (2013). Improving maternal health and safety through adherence to postpartum hemorrhage protocol in Latin America. *International Journal of Gynecology and Obstetrics, 1*, 4.

Perry, H. B. (2013). *Primary health care: A redefinition, history, trends, controversies and challenges. 1*, 31.

Ruger, J. (2007). Rethinking equal access: Agency, quality, and norms. *Global Public Health, 1*, 18.

Tackling Pneumonia and Diarrhea Together. (2013). *Path, 1*, 8.

Wallerstein, N., & Minkler, M. (2008). Community-based Participatory Research for Health from Process to Outcomes. 2nd ed. San Francisco, CA: Jossey-Bass. Print.

Wennberg, D. E., Marr, A., Lang, L., O'Malley, S., & Bennett, G. (2010). A randomized trial of a telephone care-management strategy. *The New England Journal of Medicine, 13*, 7.

Wiggins, M., Austerberry, H., & Ward, H. (2012). *Implementing evidence-based programmes in children's services: Key issues for success* (Vol. 1, p. 51). London: Department for Education.

Chapter 4
Assessing and Promoting More Progress in Health; the Role of Health as a Tracer Sector at the OECD

Elisabeth Sandor

This chapter aims to briefly review the origins and concept of aid effectiveness (1), the rationale for looking at health and operationalization of aid effectiveness in the health sector (2), the main lessons from the work done by the OECD Task Team on Health as a Tracer Sector (HATS) (3) and, finally, it formulates few ideas about possible follow-up to this work stream (4).

Health is a complex sector characterized by large unmet needs, outcomes that depend on many other sectors; powerful lobbies for specific causes; private contributions which often equal or exceed public finance; and competition between levels of service, curative versus preventive and public versus private provision of care. Aid for health is similarly fragmented. In quantity, it has multiplied by five between 1995 and 2009[1] and Development Assistance for Health has quadrupled over 10 years, between 1990 and 2010.

Much of the recent increase is attributable to the significant political and financial emphasis placed upon specific diseases, particularly HIV and AIDS, with few bilateral (such as PEPHAR) and multilateral organizations (Global Fund to fight HIV/AIDS, tuberculosis, and malaria) benefiting from the bulk of the increase. Moreover, the channels through which both funds and commodities are supplied have multiplied rapidly. The growing complexity of the global health architecture is often attributed to a growing number of global partnerships such as the global funds (the most prominent of which are the Global Fund to fight AIDS, TB and malaria, and the GAVI Alliance) or advocacy-based multiple stakeholder partnerships. However, it is important to note that there are over 100 other major international organizations involved in the health sector with varying degrees of financing.

---

[1] ODA commitments increased between 1995 and 2009, from 3.9 to 19.9 billion respectively, in 2009 in USD constant prices.

E. Sandor (✉)
Independent Consultant
e-mail: Elisabeth.sandor@gmail.com

© Springer Science+Business Media New York 2015
E. Beracochea (ed.), *Improving Aid Effectiveness in Global Health*,
DOI 10.1007/978-1-4939-2721-0_4

Global Programs (both bilateral and public–private partnerships) may add to existing fragmentation, but have also been an important source of innovation in the way aid is provided.

Ineffective health aid[2] was a major concern of the High Level Forum on the Health MDGs—a series of meetings organized by WHO and the World Bank in 2004 and 2005. Dialogue with the OECD/Development Assistance Committee began in 2006, leading to a meeting on aid effectiveness in health co-organized with the DAC and its secretariat on 4 December, 2006.

By 2007, a Task Team on Health as a Tracer Sector (TT HATS) was created by willing partners, under the initial co-piloting of the WHO and the World Bank and with the support of the OECD Development Co-operation Directorate, with the view to promote more progress in the implementation of the Paris Declaration in the health sector. From 2007 to 2011, this Task Team has been small in order to be operational and output-oriented, with senior technical participation from selected countries and organizations[3] and a limited number of focused-oriented physical meetings (9[4]). The TT has worked as a coalition of the willing, selecting, and organizing knowledge and analysis generated by each of its member, bridging the discussion on aid effectiveness at sector level (in particular through the International Health Partnership/IHP+), with the global partnership on aid effectiveness hosted at the OECD, called the Working party on aid effectiveness. The TT HATS deliberately used a cross-cutting approach with a view to promote aid effectiveness as a whole. The TT HATS has produced three reports[5] and prepared several inputs for the WP EFF.[6] These have provided public and clear recognition to the remaining bottlenecks for promoting more effective aid and are available for policy makers, beyond the health sector, to improve the management and use of aid to health management.

The final report of the TT HATS further analyzed some of the elements from the previous reports with additional perspectives and recommendations on selected topics including ownership, alignment, and aid architecture.

---

[2] In the context of these previous discussions, ineffective discussions would be illustrated as unpredictable, not aligned and generating too much transaction costs in developing countries.

[3] The current membership of the Task Team includes representatives from WHO and Mali (as co-Chairs), Ghana, Madagascar, GFATM, GAVI Alliance, UNICEF, UNFPA, UNAIDS, IHP+ Results, Action for Global health, African Development Bank, Belgium, Sweden and IFC.

[4] 23/06 2008, 24/11/2008, 2/04/2009, 16/10/2009, 12/02/2010, 22–23/03/2010, 26/10/2010, 20/08/2011 and 12/09/2011.

[5] One for HLF3 in Accra ("Effective Aid—Better Health", September 2008) which served as a background for a high-level Side event on "Predictability of Aid: Challenges and Responses—Experience in the health sector" (2 September 2008, Accra), an interim report ("*Aid to better health—what are we learning about what works and what we still have to do*", November 2009) and a final report "Progress and challenges in aid effectiveness: what can we learn from the health sector?" (24 June 2011).

[6] Including a proposal for a high-level discussion in Busan, a building block on "Who runs health?" and inputs for the Mali "focus country initiative".

Promoting More Effective Aid Is Critical to the Broader Development Agenda

Aid effectiveness is part of the development finance conferences cycle which accompanied the Millennium Development Goals process: the 2002 Monterrey Conference on financing for development was followed by the 2003 Rome declaration on aid harmonization and the 2005 Paris Declaration on Aid Effectiveness.

The 2005 Paris Declaration on aid effectiveness was meant to address the quality aid issue. One could argue that the process was about effectiveness (which means mobilizing all resources to reaching out to specific objective, without caring much about the means) as much as about efficiency (which means maximizing the resources through a cost-effective approach). Indeed, in the current environment marked with increasing constraints on budgets in both donor and recipient countries, the pressure is on ensuring more efficiency, results, and impact with same or even less resources.

In March 2005, around 100 participants endorsed 56 partnership commitments which are expected to support the five pillars of the Declaration (ownership, alignment, harmonization, managing for results, and mutual accountability).

The commitments made by governments from both donor and recipient countries focused on government-to-government relations. Some progress was made towards a more inclusive process in 2008, with the significant contribution from a broad network of NGOs to the Third High-Level Forum in Ghana and the recognition in the Accra Agenda for Action of the critical contribution of non-government actors such as the civil society to country broad ownership and sustainable development.

The Fourth High-Level Forum on aid effectiveness in Korea (29 November–1 December 2011) has deepened the process and ensured even more inclusiveness and broad partnership by focusing on common ground rules that were adopted by the traditional donors, but also by the private sector and new or non-traditional providers of development assistance in order to support more collective action and support more effective country development processes. This change represents a major opportunity while carrying on real challenges.

As highlighted by the second phase of the evaluation of the Paris Declaration,[7] the Paris process has been proven to be very useful and is largely supported by developing countries as a powerful and useful accountability mechanism. The process has promoted progress in the way aid is channelled in countries, particularly in areas such as country ownership and the reduction of transaction costs for countries. But in other areas such as alignment, progress remains insufficient and calls for political willingness to change behaviour. Building on the experience and lessons learned among the initial Paris group, HLF-4 aimed to expand and enhance the development partnership with more and new actors while responding to the remaining concerns from developing countries around more effective aid.

---

[7] As part of the Paris Declaration process, two rounds of independent evaluation have been conducted (2008 and 2011) to review and assess the impact of the Paris Declaration with a strong focus on developing countries.

We are living in a time of opportunities. HLF-4 aimed at achieving critical objectives:

The first one was to re-energize the development community around aid and development goals. As stressed by Brian Atwood, the former Chair of the OECD DAC, "the HLF-4 is the best and last chance to improve the quality of our partnerships for achieving the MDGs".

Secondly, we needed to recognize that aid is the junior partner in development finance. Official Development Assistance has increased between 2009 and 2010 (+6, 5 %), reaching out to 128 billion USD. OECD is well placed to remind the donor community about its commitments and stress the unfinished business. But there was also a need to look at better synergies between ODA and other sources of development finance and to continue to stimulate domestic funding.

Thirdly, it was important to achieve progress towards sustainable development, moving from aid to development effectiveness. We needed to acknowledge the contribution from emerging economies, the private sector, various sources and forms of development finance, including innovative finance for development. Aid can play a more effective leverage effect to stimulate more and better development assistance. We needed to collate and share more regularly and openly information and make better use of existing experience and partnerships.

Fourthly, in the ongoing constrained fiscal and budget environment, we needed to address the increasing demand for results and development impact, clarifying what these concepts mean and promoting more effective collective, long-term, and predictable action in support of country progress.

HLF-4 has been a success in the sense that a new inclusive global partnership has been created. Commitments were officially made to achieve more results through more effective collective long term and predictable action in support of country progress.

Health contributed to the outcomes, although may be too marginally, through sharing the results of its four-year work on health as a tracer sector.

Why Looking at Health as a Tracer Sector?

The OECD DAC decided to create a workstreath on hats after considering five critical issues. It is an issue of effective economics: Health is critical to growth which requires healthy workforce. See the evidence from the 2003 world bank development report on "Investing in health" and the report on macro economies and health. Proportionally higher health and education status than in Sub-Sahara African Low Income Countries has made the difference for countries like Korea to move from the status of developing country and aid recipient to the status of developed and OECD donor country, as stressed by several comparative studies.

It is an issue of credibility for the development cooperation community: Health is central to the MDGs, out of which at least three are directly about health. If we fail to achieve the Health MDGs, the whole MDGs agenda is failing. The final review of the MDGs in 2015 will be critical for development and for the credibility of international partnerships for development. The strong support brought by Canada, the G8, and the UN Secretary General for more progress towards MDGs 4 and 5 demonstrated the willingness of the international community to make one last big push in favour of progress in a very sensitive, visible, and political domain.

It is an issue of donor accountability: the bulk of the increase for sector ODA in the past decade has benefited to health, when other sectors such as agriculture or infrastructure are desperately calling for more funding. In this context, there is an increasing request for accountability and demonstrating what has been done with this money.

It is an issue for countries' independency: aid to health has been representing a very significant part of health spending in the poorest countries: in 1990, 12 % of total health funding in Low Income SSA countries came from external resources; in 2006, this percentage went up to 31 %. At the same time, too few African countries meet the Abuja target of 15 % of their national budget being dedicated to health.

It is an issue of aid architecture: aid to health has increased and it has also become more complex with new actors (Foundations, around 100 global health programmes and partnerships) and new sources of funding (non-for-profit and for-profit private sector funding, Innovative financing mechanisms). At the same time, in-country capacities to manage and make the most out of these various forms of aid have not always increased in same proportions furthermore mandates of international organizations have sometimes become duplicative, for instance in the area of Health system strengthening. The aid landscape needs to be rationalized.

Finally, there is a strong competition for access to donor funding across sectors. Climate change has emerged as a key priority with early estimates by UNFCCC of needed 370 billion USD by 2030 for mitigation and adaptation. Complementarities and better synergies across sectors must be found at global and country levels, including for ensuring more effective health outcomes to which improved water and sanitation, gender equality, accessible and quality infrastructure and services, improved nutrition are all important supportive factors.

The Lessons from Four Year of Review and Practice on Aid Effectiveness and Health (HATS)

The final report of the Task Team on HATS[8] was released on 24 June, 2011. It builds on 4 years of candid and constructive process for reviewing and promoting progress in the implementation of the five principles of aid effectiveness in the health sector. The key messages from the final TT HATS report are summarized below (Box 1).

---

[8] "Progress and challenges in aid effectiveness, what can we learn from the Health sector?" OECD Working Party on Aid Effectiveness Task Team on Health as a tracer sector, 24 June 2011. Accessible at: http://www.oecd.org/dataoecd/61/22/48298309.pdf.

Box 1. Key Messages from the Final Report of the TT HATS

There have been significant achievements in the health sector but more needs to be done

The health sector has made significant progress in aid effectiveness, spearheading innovative approaches such as the IHP+ to improve harmonization, alignment, and monitoring mechanisms. Further progress is needed, particularly to address the gap between commitments at global level and practice in countries and to bring about sustained changes in the behaviour of both countries and donors. Experience from health informs other sectors and wider development. Monitoring progress in aid effectiveness commitments in health and continuing to capture lessons from the health sector remain highly relevant and should continue beyond HLF-4 in Korea.

Effective aid creates conditions for success

There is evidence that aid effectiveness improves sector planning, budgeting and governance capacities, strengthens national systems, and contributes to health results through more efficient and sustainable implementation of national health policies, plans, and strategies. In fragile and post-conflict situations, streamlined and coordinated policy and management processes are providing the basis for improving health and service delivery systems. An ongoing challenge in the health sector is striking the right balance and finding better complementarities between programs that score well on delivering short-term measurable results, though often at the expense of aid effectiveness and longer-term transformational change, and more sustainable whole-of-sector approaches that focus on greater alignment with country needs, institutions, and priorities, but are more challenging to measure.

Health provides unique insights and lessons into the complexities of aid architecture

Aid to the health sector has increased substantially over the last 20 years from $5 billion in 1990 to $21.8 billion in 2007 (IHME 2010). Greater investment and programmatic scale-up has significantly improved some health outcomes. These developments have been accompanied by a growing number of actors and increasingly complex governance and aid management arrangements. While diversity brings many benefits, it poses challenges for country ownership, alignment, and national systems and leads to duplicative and fragmented approaches at global and national levels. Using health as a "tracer" sector has deepened understanding of the risks and benefits of diversity and has leveraged action for a more coordinated and coherent approach to the global aid architecture. This was recognized by the G8 in the May Deauville Declaration in May 2011. Important lessons from health can inform global efforts to tackle issues such as climate change and food security which show signs of following a similar path, including strong political commitment, significant needs, and the launch of new initiatives and funding channels, and similar aid architecture challenges.

More specifically, the review of each of the Paris Declaration principles provides important and useful findings which need to support more effective decision for the financing, channelling, monitoring, and evaluation of aid to health.

Regarding country broad ownership (partner countries, including government and non-government actors, should exercise effective leadership over their development policies and coordinate actions), the report found that there is progress of partner countries in the quality of their national development strategies. For instance, reviews of countries such as Zambia, Tanzania, Cambodia, and Mali show that Programme-Based Approaches such as Sector Budget Support and Sector Wide Approaches (SWAPs) are strengthening country ownership of national health plans, policies, and strategies. Documented experiences of preparing IHP+ country compacts also suggest that country ownership has been strengthened in the case of Benin, Nigeria, Sierra Leone, Mali, and Uganda, through constructive dialogue with and involvement of wider stakeholders (non-health ministries, CSOs, ...). Also, the Joint assessment of the health national strategy (JANS), which is part of IHP+, has added legitimacy to some existing aid management practice at country level (for instance in Ethiopia) by involving several agencies in a unique process.

Regarding Global Programs, they are credited with supporting a broader and more inclusive notion of country ownership through the Country Coordination Mechanisms of the Global Fund and the GAVI Health System Strengthening funding progress. GAVI and the Global Fund are increasingly contributing to national strategies (SWAPs or pool funding).

There is also progress in supporting non-state actors to exercise ownership, as part of the country broaden dialogue which is encouraged in the Accra Agenda for Action. Significant progress has been made in strengthening the debate about civil society engagement and ensuring formal civil society participation in global and country health discussions. This positive trend is illustrated at the global level where CSOs now actively contribute to discussions related to aid effectiveness (TT HATS, IHP+ Consultative group with CSO, IHP+ civil society health policy access fund). Also, IHP+ compact preparation process and JANS have involved non-state actors and the participation of non-State actors in Global Fund national strategies on AIDS process has increased in countries like Kenya or Rwanda.

There is initial evidence that more active participation of non-State actors in the dialogue with the government has improved the quality of policies, resource allocation processes, and even preliminary results: for instance, in rural districts in Tanzania, increased immunization rates and improving child health have been supported by pooled funding, decentralization, and participation of communities to decision including on budget allocation.

But challenges remain in strengthening CSO's participation in health sector policy process and there is evidence that participation of CSOs is uneven and not always meaningful. The mixed experience also depends on the political context.

In the area of alignment (donor countries base their overall support on partner countries' national development strategies, institutions, and procedures, they committed to use and strengthen countries' systems and to put their aid on budget and plan), there is evidence that greater efforts are being made by country partners, donors, and Global Programs to support and strengthen selected country systems.

Partner countries such as Ghana, Burundi, Zambia, Ethiopia, and Madagascar are providing evidence that their national procurement systems either reflect good practice or that reform is underway. Critical factors for success include institutional stability, dialogue between MOH and donors. Some of these countries and others like Nepal or Cambodia have also reported about strengthening public and financial management systems in order to reflect good practices.

Global Programs are making greater efforts towards more aligned support on plan and on budget, as demonstrated by GAVI ISS and HSS Funds in Ethiopia. They are adapting their policies to facilitate participation in SWAPs and pooled funds, as illustrated by the Global Fund in Ghana, Tanzania, and Nepal. Efforts are underway to implement the Health Systems funding platform whereby partners (WHO, the World Bank, GAVI Alliance, and the Global Fund) are working jointly in several countries to streamline funding, align their performance indicators with those of the government, and strengthen national Monitoring and Evaluation. Also, the Global Fund has introduced policies to better use or support national procurement systems.

There is also progress on the side of other bilateral and multilateral donors: For instance, the Australian Aid Agency has joint pooled funding mechanisms in Nepal. There are also several examples of UN agencies strengthening country and inter-agency systems: UNFPA in Cambodia; Four UN organizations join efforts to support cash transfer in Mali; WHO is leading a working group on the alignment of procurement standards for medical goods between international organizations.

However, as highlighted more generally in the last Paris Declaration Monitoring survey and the evaluation phase two of the Paris Declaration, the efforts remain patchy and insufficient in the health sector. Even in the context of well-established SWAPs, for instance in Malawi, Cambodia, Zambia, or Mali, or where PFM systems are reported as good, as this is the case in Rwanda, use of country systems should be reinforced. Too slow progress is linked more with political than with technical reasons.

There are critical challenges for moving forward on alignment. Weak capacities, high staff turn-over, and lack of experience in developing results-oriented work programs in countries can all diminish trust in sector-based plans and systems. Some major donor including the United States and Global Programs still prefer to operate with parallel systems, as evidenced in countries like Mali, Nepal, or Ethiopia. High-levels of off-budgets funds from traditional and new donors can, in turn, undermine the formation and integrity of country systems themselves.

The Paris Declaration and Accra Agenda for Action call for more harmonization (donors' activities are more harmonized, transparent, and collectively effective; more joint missions and efforts to reducing transaction costs for partner countries). There is progress in the implementation of common arrangements.

There is evidence that there has been an expansion of mechanisms for donor coordination and harmonization, such as development partner forums and sector working groups. There has also been development in the use of PBAs, such as pooled funds, Sector Budget Support, and SWAPs. Country's positive examples include Bangladesh where Sector Budget Support represents now 42 % of the budget.

A 2009 World Bank review of SWAPs in Bangladesh, Ghana, Kyrgyz republic, Malawi, Nepal, and Tanzania concluded that SWAPs are helping to coordinate and strengthen sector plans.

In the United States, the 2010 Global Health Initiative emphasizes coordination and collaboration within US agencies and calls for 5 years joint strategic frameworks for cooperation with partner countries. On the UN side, the UN HACT (Harmonized Approach to Cash Transfer) system has been introduced in Mali to harmonize all interventions by UN Agencies.

These trends are positive, although the efforts are sometimes limited to internal or domestic only change. Transaction costs of harmonization are high, especially for donors, as demonstrated in the PD evaluation phase 2.

Project aid and vertical funds continue to present challenges for harmonization, as illustrated in Cambodia which manages 115 active health projects, in Mali where only 14 out of 50 donors have signed the IHP+ compact, or in Mozambique where half of main donors, so 22 % of aid to the sector in 2008, participate in the health common fund.

Also, increasing pressure to demonstrate attribution and address accountability in donor countries are disincentives to donor harmonization.

There are important remaining challenges for more harmonization. First of all, recipient countries are not always supportive of increased donor harmonization and coordination, as highlighted in the Paris Declaration evaluation phase 2. Some countries prefer to diversify external support and don't want to be dependent on a handful of donors. In the case of fragile situations, harmonization is sometimes challenging, as demonstrated in Democratic Republic of Congo by a UW review in 2010.

Progress in improving harmonization and coordination of technical assistance is mixed: at the global level, there is progress, for instance with improved coordination of technical assistance for HIV/AIDS between PEPFAR, UNAIDS, and the Global Fund. But progress remains hampered by the lack of national technical assistance plans and ownership, and remaining donor own incentives and preferences.

Finally, harmonization remains challenging with non-traditional donors whose practice for funding, channeling, and reporting development finance differs from traditional donors.

Is aid allocation and division of labour effective in the health sector? Aid allocation methods vary widely across donor governments and institutions. As a result of this, some countries with important needs benefit from limited or no aid when others, which are better off, attract external funding in significant proportions. There is also evidence of imbalances and inequities in donor support. No serious study has been undertaken yet at the level of the health sector, but there is much literature to highlight that aid for health has increased significantly, much of the increase benefiting to HIV, tuberculosis, and malaria. This can contribute to stress the lack of a whole health sector approach, with some imbalance across regions and countries, and remaining unfunded needs on non-communicable diseases or other sub-sector activities.

Country-led division of labour within country also needs to improve. Overall there has been progress with few European Union countries actually applying the EU Code and concentrating their aid in fewer sectors. Nine countries of the PD evaluation phase 2 identify some progress in reducing duplication and increasing rationalization at sector level. The EU Code of Conduct is cited as having played an important role in Malawi and Mali (where Sweden and Spain for instance are "silent partners"). In Rwanda, strong ownership and leadership have conducted to both division of labour and rationalization of aid across all sectors, including health. But withdraw does not always mean rationalization and positive gains for countries. Moreover, there remain questions about the consequences of donors' withdrawal in the context of increasing budget and fiscal constraints in donor countries.

Through the fifth pillar of the Paris Declaration calls for managing for development results, partner countries commit to improve the management of their resources and the decision making for results, while donors commit to support results which are defined, managed, monitored by countries, and to contribute to—rather than attribute their intervention to—specific outcomes.

The current context, with more constraints on donor aid budgets and more scrutiny around results and impact, provides a more challenging context for progress in this area.

As highlighted in the IHP+ 2011 Results Annual report, "a single performance assessment framework[9] is central to governments' efforts to measure health outcomes, monitor progress and identify areas of under-performance". Seven of the ten countries surveyed by IHP+ in 2010 reported that they had a single performance assessment framework in place. There is also evidence in countries including Mali, Nepal, and Uganda that there is increased results that focus in health sector plans and budgets and greater emphasis on measuring impact and strengthening related performance reviews and M&E systems. In Mozambique, results-based reporting on the health sector takes place in the context of indicators embedded in the PAF that are updated annually. These indicators rely on a national health information system of data collection that has served as the foundation for regular joint reviews of health sector progress.

There is some evidence of increasing donor use of PAFs. IHP+ Results report that more than 60 % of development partners active in the ten countries surveyed in 2010 claimed to use the national PAF as the primary basis to assess the performance of their health aid.

But it is worrying to see that some donors do not draw on PAFs for their results reporting. They still require parallel reporting and/or reporting on additional indicators outside the national PAF (Ethiopia, Mali and Niger). In Uganda, the Joint Assistance Framework and Annual Health Sector Performance Report are increasingly seen as useful tools to scrutinize performance in the health sector, but some donors believe that it remains necessary to commission external monitoring reports because they don't trust the government reporting.

---

[9] A single performance assessment framework, as opposed to several donor reporting and assessment mechanisms, would better support country ownership and capacity building.

In addition, many countries are still reporting on a large number of indicators and are required to submit multiple reports. At the 2010 Global Health Information Forum, the WHO reported that more than 1,000 health indicators are currently in use across a variety of health programs from child and adolescent health to HIV and malaria, while multiple databases on single disease issues operate in isolation.

More fundamentally, the quality of national health M&E systems remains variable and there is a need for more capacity building in this area. Challenges concerning the quality, comprehensiveness, and timeliness of health information remain. And greater efforts are required to strengthen systems for both generation and use of data. Paris Declaration phase 2 Evaluation found that in Mozambique, for example, while PAFs exist at national level and for sectors such as health, which have common funds, there is a need to increase investment in government capacity and systems strengthening for M&E.

Similarly, in Malawi, efforts have been made by the Ministry of Development Planning and Cooperation to build M&E capacity at sector level, but "most M&E systems remain weak" and this is "coupled with lack of quality data and access to such data by stakeholders". In five of the six countries included in the 2009 World Bank review of SWAPs, "the neglect of Monitoring and Evaluation capacity building and use, relative to the strong emphasis on procurement, disbursement and financial management, has resulted in an insufficient results focus".

Donors continue to conduct separate review missions. The increase in the number of countries that have established joint annual health sector review mechanisms does not appear to have significantly reduced the number of separate and uncoordinated donor review and M&E missions. A UNAIDS review of the Three Ones in West and Central Africa (2010) found that reviews and analyses are not always conducted jointly, and several countries reported multiple simultaneous or parallel missions, sometimes with similar objectives.

In most cases, uncoordinated missions are initiated by donor headquarters and relate to implementation of non-delegated budgets or to additional M&E and audit requirements.

Global Programs also appear to be less likely to participate in joint missions. For example, in 2007, only 14 % of Global Fund missions were conducted with other partners.

Finally, the ongoing pressure for results in donor countries and increase in the use of results-based financing by donor agencies is raising some fundamental questions.

There is as yet limited evidence of impact. For example, Global Fund and GAVI funding is dependent on results. GAVI performance-based Immunization Services Support (ISS) funds are only disbursed on demonstrating results achieved. The Global Fund rewards strong-performing grants with a higher percentage of funding than poor-performing grants. But we still need more experience, robust evaluations. We also need to be cautious about potential risks of distorting effects and clear about the incentives of results-based funding mechanisms.

Some experts have stressed the need to be particularly careful about key conditions for effective results-based approaches. For instance, it is very important to focus on the right interventions and results which should be pro-poor, cost-effective,

Box 2. Key Recommendations from the Final TT HATS Report

- Reaffirm commitments to the principles of aid effectiveness and promote them among new actors
- Step up efforts to put commitments into practice, in particular in areas of alignment, managing for development results and harmonization
- Increase support for country leadership and capacity development
- Agree on realistic results to be achieved through aid effectiveness and realistic timeframes for achieving change
- Strengthen the evidence base on the links between more effective aid and improvements in health service delivery and health outcomes
- Improve coordination of the global aid architecture through high-level leadership, greater alignment of accountabilities and incentives, and a stronger mandate for existing mechanisms such as the OECD DAC, rather than the creation of a separate global coordination initiative
- Revisit aid effectiveness frameworks, structures, and processes in fragile states, and to engage a wider range of actors

and equitable. Also, results-based financing is not a simple solution to attribution. The current context pushes donors to demonstrate even more "value for money". Sustainable progress is typically achieved through a package of approaches and it is very challenging to determine which factors are responsible for what progress. Then, results-based financing needs to comply with the aid effectiveness principles and countries need to be in the driver seat to decide which results, how they will be monitored, and what will be the consequences of the assessments. It should not be a new way for donors to "do their shopping" in countries. Moreover, results-based financing should involve payment for results rather than payment by results. Rewarding commitment to achieving results is different from rewarding results achieved. Often, the focus is on the latter. Finally, capacities and systems issues are important to be considered and results-based financing should be part of a comprehensive and consistent health package, not done in isolation and with the support of parallel results measurement industry.

Emerging from the final TT HATS report, seven recommendations have emerged. They are summarized below (Box 2).

What Should Happen Next?

The concept of HATS was time-bound and it has worked very effectively. The TT HATS was linked to the Paris Declaration cycle (2005–2010) and came to an end with the forthcoming Fourth High-Level Forum on Aid Effectiveness in Korea (29 November–1 December 2011).

At the same time, the members of the TT HATS shared the concern that progress remained uneven and insufficient towards the Paris Declaration targets and that much more was to be achieved to scale up towards the review of the Millennium Development Goals, in 2015. The TT HATS has provided a very significant and fruitful experience in terms of regular monitoring and consensus building. Building on this experience, more remains needed to provide more regular, comprehensive knowledge sharing, and decision-oriented analysis on aid and development assistance to health. Recommendations from the TT HATS should be carried on in the future through an appropriate process working at both country and global levels.

Further monitoring and active promotion of more effective aid could take place through a multi-sector or cross sector approach. This consideration stems from both the evidence that the achievement of development, including health, is multisectoral in nature and from the ongoing pressure on aid budget and call for more strategic and synergetic aid interventions. Illustrations and inputs from sectors/ areas, including through a selected and balanced set of sectors and areas contributing to growth and sustainable development, could support country-grounded and results-focused dialogue and action. In addition, discussions at the sector level might appear as some of the best avenues for defining common ground rules with non-traditional partners.

Key Lessons from Monitoring Aid Effectiveness in Health at the OECD (2007–2011)

Who Will Lead the Agenda Next?

For more than 4 years, the OECD has led a senior-level multi-stakeholder working group to regularly review and promote progress towards more effective aid in this sector. This was achieved in support of a broader effort to encourage more progress towards the implementation of the Paris Declaration across sectors. The work on health culminated with the production of a final report of the Task Team on HATS and a debate as part of the Fourth High-Level Forum on Aid Effectiveness in Korea (29 November–1 December 2011) which focused on progress made, including in specific areas such as maternal and child health, but regrettably no specific commitment or reference to health can be found in the Busan partnership agreement.

Few months after this forum and as the work at the OECD DAC on HATS closed down, what are the lessons learned and who will take the lead in driving the agenda for better health now? Most countries are still struggling to further advance donor coordination and alignment and more effectively use available resources for health, mobilisation against ebola has been effective but can we say that health systems are stronger and better supported by donors? Is the aid effectiveness agenda better implemented at country level? What is the impact or what are the early lessons of some of the changes that took place in global health organisations (i.e. global fund new funding model)?

It is worrying that, as of today, there is no permanent global-level policy forum anymore for regularly debating issues related to aid to health, sharing perspectives, and promoting more effective collective action to support country-led efforts. This article is reviewing the main lessons from the work on HATS. In doing so, it is calling for more open and active debate so that countries, and more particularly the populations affected by poor health conditions and policies in developing countries, continue to benefit from global, coordinated, and country-led efforts towards better health for all.

Bridging aid effectiveness and sectors has been paradoxically challenging: Coordination and mutual understanding between aid policy makers and sector experts has often been challenging, although the aid effectiveness agenda was increasingly been translated at the level of sectors and areas (see the use of the Paris Declaration indicators in health with the IHP+ and in education through the Fast Track Initiative-Education For All Initiative). On one side, there was often a lack of appetite from policy makers for focusing on health, one (already well-funded) sector over others. At the same time, health experts were challenged by the concept of the "tracer" which aimed to formulate issues and recommendations in a language to be easily understood by non-experts or other sectors' experts.

Sector-level monitoring of aid effectiveness is key for providing substantive and relevant evidence of and opportunities for results. Both partner country and donor governments are organized by sectors, and so is aid. Sectors remain pivotal for policy design and implementation, budget allocation, and results measurement. Aid effectiveness needs to further trickle down to practitioners and be mainstreamed in all aid activities, at the level of sectors or areas. Only then would it be possible to change behaviour on a wide scale, improve the life of people, and make an impact on development. Measuring progress in health continues to be important because: (1) health remains very politically sensitive; it is a complex sector, with various sectors and interventions contributing to health outcomes; (2) the strong focus on results (see initiatives on each MDGs) calls for more investment in systems and capacities. Yet, most of the discussion on aid is largely focusing on processes with, from time to time, one or two areas of particular interest. The time of health seems to be over. Now, most of the attention is benefiting to climate change, food security, or water, with no appropriate attention to the intrinsic linkages between these and health.

Health as a "tracer" sector offers useful lessons for health and other areas: There is evidence that effective aid is improving sector planning, budgeting and governance capacities, strengthening national systems, and contributing to health results through more efficient and sustainable implementation of national plans. It is difficult to strike the right balance and find better complementarities between programs that score well on delivering shorter-term measurable results, through often at the expense of aid effectiveness and longer-term transformational change and whole-of-sector approaches that are more sustainable, focus on greater alignment with country needs, institutions, and priorities, but are more challenging to measure and report. Also, using health as a "tracer" sector has deepened the understanding of the risks and benefits of diversity and proliferation of new aid providers and it has leveraged action for a more coordinated and coherent approach to the global aid architecture. Important lessons from health can inform global efforts to tackle issues such as climate change and food security, which show signs of following a similar path, including strong political commitment, significant needs, and the launch of new initiatives and funding channels, with similar governance challenges.

The 2011 Busan partnership for development cooperation builds on the lessons from health but without saying it: There has been significant disappointment among health experts and NGOs about the absence of direct reference to health in the Busan partnership for development co-operation. It is true that in the Busan document the word "sector" is used only in reference to the public and the private sector, but commitments made to address the issues of fragmentation, lack of predictability and of coordination of aid and to improve results and mutual accountability all build on the evidence and recommendations from the health sector and can further improve aid to health. The global partnership for effective development cooperation should continue to benefit from the lessons from health. Stakeholders, including developing countries, international organizations, donors, NGOs who wish to do so, can still influence decisions. The ongoing international health partnership (IHP+) which works mainly at country level and has just achieved its fourth round of monitoring progress aid effectiveness in selected countries brings back very interesting lessons which should feed the Busan partnership. But, as of today, it's not clear how much IHP+ can influence the Busan partnership and who will deal with the whole issue of aid and development effectiveness in health. That includes the role of the private sector, aid architecture in a true global and cross-country perspective.

A lot has been achieved through the TT HATS with clear recommendations. These need now to be taken up by policy makers: The TT HATS has developed very valuable dialogue and mutual understanding of issues and concerns among bilateral, multilateral, countries, and civil society organizations. Regular reviews and recommendations have been formulated by the group which came to an end with the Fourth High-Level Forum in Korea end of 2011. They need now to be taken up in appropriate form for a by policy decision makers. The final report of the task team on HATS highlighted that progress achieved so far should not be lost and that significant progress remains to be done to fulfill the PD targets. The implementation of the Busan agenda, the review of the MDGs and finalization of the post-2015 agenda all call for more strategic reviews and decisions on how aid can best encourage progress to improve the well-being of people across the world. Who is ready to take the lead?

Conclusion

There is a unique story to tell about aid to health. But it is not a simple, straightforward, or an all-positive story. The impact of more effective aid in terms of health outcomes also needs to be further documented. We know that the global decline of child mortality can be attributed to more and more coordinated aid, but more evidence of sustainable health outcomes is still needed. Also, a more rationalized aid landscape needs to be put in place together with increased support to capacities so that countries can make the most of the various forms of assistance for health. Long-term perspective, flexibility, and inclusiveness need to be carefully combined with a legitimate search for country-led results and domestic and mutual accountability.

Because health is the initial condition to any development and growth, specific continued attention and support to more and even better aid/development assistance to health is needed towards 2015 and beyond. We hope that the readers of this story, beyond the health practitioners and advocacy community, can take the lessons learned forward and make sure that, in a more constraint financing environment, evidence-based and results-oriented good practice can be scaled up and more widely applied to ensure broader and more equitable progress to meet the needs of the most vulnerable populations.

Chapter 5
The US Government's Efforts to Improve Effectiveness

Carl Mabbs-Zeno

What is the Scope of US Health Assistance? US global health assistance through the Department of State and the US Agency for International Development (USAID) is focused on nine global health challenges.[1] It also recognizes the primacy of building health systems, but uses the more specific listing of challenges to plan funding and report performance. There is overlap among the categories of health assistance, particularly with maternal and child health, and the other categories, but the gaps in apparent coverage are more important. Accidents, mental health, cancers, and aging are among the sizeable health problems that are not targets for assistance programs. Although this selection of priorities can be justified on the basis of the need to focus resources where US assistance can have the most impact in developing countries, it is not expressly defended and represents a longstanding, albeit informal, compact between both major parties in Congress and the Administration.

The United States has long been a global leader in funding international health assistance programs, with budgets rising from $354 million in 1986 to $658 million in 1994 and $1,940 million in 2003. The $2 billion in the 2004 budget for the President's Emergency Plan for AIDS Relief marked the start of several large initiatives that placed health at the top of US development assistance funding. These programs were essentially brought together in the Global Health Initiative (GHI) announced in May 2009. The GHI initially set out global health targets and a 6-year budget, but also soon defined seven principles to guide all US health assistance.

---

[1] HIV/AIDS, malaria, tuberculosis, maternal and child health, nutrition, family planning and reproductive health, neglected tropical diseases, water and sanitation, and pandemic influenza and other emerging threats.

C. Mabbs-Zeno (✉)
Independent Consultant
e-mail: mabbszenoc@yahoo.com

© Springer Science+Business Media New York 2015
E. Beracochea (ed.), *Improving Aid Effectiveness in Global Health*,
DOI 10.1007/978-1-4939-2721-0_5

79

These principles formed the core of the eventual GHI Strategy[2] and USAID's Global Health Strategic Framework.[3]

Most US foreign assistance for global health is appropriated to USAID or the State Department through annual appropriations[4] to fund assistance authorized by the Foreign Assistance Act of 1961,[5] as amended. The 2014 appropriation included $5.67 billion to State and $2.75 billion to USAID specifically for health. An additional $0.84 billion was budgeted by State and USAID for health assistance from the 2014 appropriation.[6] The total of over $9 billion for global health constituted more than a quarter of the foreign assistance budget for State and USAID.[7] Over half of these health funds were budgeted for use for Africa and more than 20 % was for support to international organizations, such as the Global Fund to Fight AIDS, Tuberculosis, and Malaria. Health assistance funded by other agencies is less clearly designated, but efforts to identify such assistance have identified 11 other US Government agencies that effectively address global health, accounting for 14 % of the total US funding for this purpose.[8] Most (64 %) of the funding outside of State and USAID was for research, by the National Institutes of Health, targeting disease treatment or prevention of importance to global health.[9]

Why Is Aid Effectiveness an Important Issue for Health Assistance? Ultimately, the effectiveness of international aid for health is important because there exist preventive and remedial health technologies capable of substantially extending the length and quality of life for billions of people. The aggregate effect of health assistance cannot be confidently estimated, but comparisons of health statistics in assisted and unassisted locations that are otherwise similar, and other research approaches,

---

[2] The *United States Global Health Initiative Strategy* is available at http://www.ghi.gov/resources/strategies/159150.htm.

[3] *USAID's Global Health Strategic Framework*: *Better Health for Development* is available at http://transition.usaid.gov/our_work/global_health/home/Publications/docs/gh_framework2012.pdf.

[4] Division K, Department of State, Foreign Operations, and Related Programs Appropriations, Consolidated Appropriations Act, 2014, H.R. 3547 (2014).

[5] P.L. 87-195; 22 U.S.C. 2151, *et seq.*

[6] Funds mandated for use in health assistance are appropriated to an account currently named Global Health Programs. In 2014, funds in six other accounts were budgeted for health assistance, most notably $379 million from the Economic Support Fund, $151 million from Food for Peace Title II, and $147 million from Development Assistance.

[7] Other large shares of the assistance budget are usually designated for peace and security (about 30 %), economic growth (usually 10–15 %), and humanitarian (emergency) assistance (about 10–15 %).

[8] A report required by Congress to describe all international health assistance was submitted in late 2011 but it did not quantify spending levels for all agencies because health assistance is not a budget category recorded by agencies whose mandates do not specify health assistance.

[9] *The U.S. Government's Global Health Policy Architecture*: *Structure, Programs, and Funding*. The Henry J. Kaiser Family Foundation, April 2009.

clearly establish the dramatic potential of present technology.[10] The control of infectious disease also benefits those who are not recorded as experiencing a disease, in some cases extending to international reductions of health risk. The ongoing efforts to eradicate polio, for example, are offering a global return on investment. In addition, the effect of improved health on the performance of other development sectors is well documented, extending the importance of aid effectiveness for health programs. Malnutrition can permanently impair a child's productive potential. Controllable tropical diseases can greatly reduce school attendance, limiting opportunities for the affected individuals and their contributions to society. The intrinsic importance of health and the extensive improvement possible in health with available resources are the most compelling arguments for aid effectiveness in this sector.

The relative focus on global health within the US foreign assistance budget ensures there will be intense public scrutiny of performance in this sector. Political support for health assistance has relied on evidence that shows its effectiveness. In the competition for US Government funding, it is critical that this evidence is robust and is sensitive to the concerns of American voters. How well the Paris Principles correspond to the American view of aid effectiveness is the challenge for the analysis in this chapter.

How Does US Policy Address Aid Effectiveness for Health? US policy is expressed in a hierarchy built on the National Security Strategy and expanded in the Presidential Policy Directive (PPD)[11] on Global Development.[12] Treaties, international agreements like the Paris Declaration, Presidential speeches, and other Administration statements constitute policy, but the details that control budgets and programs, like health assistance, vary among Federal agencies. Most relevant for assessing health assistance are policies affecting the State Department and USAID. The substantial funding implemented by the Centers for Disease Control and Prevention (CDC) to fight HIV infection is appropriated to the State Department and is, therefore, largely subject to State policies, although it may not be consistent with USAID policies. As one of the three core agencies leading the GHI,[13] CDC helps formulate and follows GHI policy.

The PPD on Global Development references some of the Paris Principles among the six components of its "new operational model", but it is not closely tied to all of them. The major policy statement on development from the Department of State during the present administration was the first Quadrennial Diplomacy and

---

[10] Recent relevant statistics are provided in *Global Health and Child Survival: Progress Report to Congress 2010–2011*, USAID, 2012, available at http://transition.usaid.gov/our_work/global_health/home/Publications/docs/csh_2012/csh_2012_results.pdf.

[11] The fact sheet on the PPD for Global Development is available at http://www.whitehouse.gov/the-press-office/2010/09/22/fact-sheet-us-global-development-policy.

[12] U.S. policy on any topic is conceived as separate from and subject to law.

[13] This permanent leadership structure of the GHI was announced on July 2, 2012.

Development Review (QDDR).[14] It cites the Paris Declaration and the Accra Agenda for Action as sources for its "foreign assistance effectiveness principles."[15] Each of the Paris Principles is clearly represented in the QDDR, in addition to principles on sustainability, transparency, and gender equality. This high level, explicit recognition of the Paris Principles ensures that programs subject to State Department guidance, including those of USAID, will be consistent in general with the Paris Declaration, although they integrate many other concerns in ways that nuance the interpretation of aid effectiveness.

Country Ownership: Since application of the first of the Paris Principles has been the most controversial within the US Government, it was especially significant that the PPD specified "The United States will… underscore the importance of country ownership and responsibility" among its operational principles. However, the inclusion of the familiar phrases of international discussion does not ensure US programs will follow the Paris Principles. The fact sheet from the White House on how to apply the PPD to global health refers twice to this principle, each time accepting a limited role for the principle. It is viewed, in part, as an approach to the Paris Principle of mutual accountability: "[GHI] supports country ownership and donor coordination by treating health assistance as a shared responsibility of the partner country, US government, and other donors." The other reference may appear to limit country ownership to US priorities, but is better understood as a reflection of US interpretation of country ownership, consistent with the Accra Agenda, as the eventual replacement of donor assistance by host country institutions: "GHI strengthens US government engagement with partner countries to support national ownership and priorities that are aligned with GHI objectives."[16] This is essentially to say that the GHI builds the capacity of the host country to fund and implement, i.e., own, the objectives that GHI is now funding.

A broader concept of country ownership was embraced in the QDDR: "The United States will focus on country ownership, with partner countries taking the lead in developing and implementing evidence-based strategies, as appropriate." The significant issue of what entities represent the host country is embedded in the same QDDR policy statement: "In those countries where governments are strongly committed to development and democracy, country ownership means working much more closely with and through those governments; in all countries it means working closely and consulting with organizations and the people most directly affected by programs and activities."[17] The case for governments as partners is further justified: "Our aid is most effective when it is least disruptive to the bond of accountability that links governments to the people they govern, and when we tailor our approaches to fit specific country contexts and needs."

---

[14] Available at http://qddr.state.gov/materials/qddr-report/.

[15] *QDDR*, p. 110.

[16] The fact sheet on the implications of the PPD for global health is at http://www.whitehouse.gov/sites/default/files/Global_Health_Fact_Sheet.pdf.

[17] *QDDR*, p. 14.

The QDDR was followed by a series of policy cables from Secretary Clinton, giving detail for implementing the broad policy prescriptions in the QDDR. The July 2012 cable on diplomacy and development called for US missions to "incorporate expectations of our partner governments into multi-year mission plans and track progress against them." However, the cable immediately follows this guidance with a statement suggesting the need to pursue reforms as well: "Ensure there are coordinated incentives for reform by partner countries and encourage adherence to international standards."[18]

In the USAID Policy Framework,[19] the principle is present but not prominent, being an elaboration of the operational principle to "build in sustainability from the start." The language of the statement reflects the QDDR concern with who represents the country: "Only launch programs and projects where there is demonstrable local demand and ownership, and where a broad segment of the community has a stake in ensuring that the activity or service continues after the USAID program or project ends."[20]

Even as the GHI was being designed, country ownership was regarded as a key aspect of its approach. The eventual GHI principles include "Encouraging country ownership and invest in country-led plans," and like the QDDR, clearly identify a wide range of host country actors in addition to the government. The description of this principle in the GHI Strategy reveals the emphasis on country ownership to mean host country funding of health programs, i.e., the policy carries a connotation of support for host countries replacing donor assistance rather than for host countries to guide donor assistance. "Ultimately, governments—together with non-governmental organizations (NGOs), civil society organizations (CSOs) including affected communities, faith-based organizations (FBOs), the private sector and others in countries—must decide upon their countries' health needs and strategies. They are responsible for making and sustaining progress, and they must be accountable to those served by their health systems. Accordingly, a core principle of GHI is to support country ownership, encouraging governments to engage with stakeholders at the national, provincial, district and community levels as they develop and implement their country health plans and strategies."

The GHI view of country ownership as largely an alternative to donor assistance is followed by the USAID Global Health Strategic Framework. It calls for sustainability efforts to "be integrated with health system strengthening and country ownership… to serve the poor and vulnerable without dependence on foreign assistance." Nonetheless, the GHI Strategy also expresses a US commitment "to aligning GHI investments with partner country plans and strategies, primarily through technical

---

[18] Department of State, Secretary Clinton's Fifth Policy Guidance Cable: Modernizing U.S. Diplomacy to Better Support Development, July 2012, paragraphs 22–23. Available at http://telegrams.state.gov/aldac/view_telegram.cfm?teleid=10369823.

[19] The *USAID Policy Framework* is available at http://transition.usaid.gov/policy/USAID_PolicyFramework.PDF.

[20] *USAID Policy Framework*, p. 12.

assistance, project-level support, and capacity-building of governments and other local institutions." Accepting the leadership from host countries was also highlighted in Secretary Clinton's July policy cable on development and diplomacy: "Where partner governments are undertaking credible reform campaigns, our efforts must respond to and reinforce their priorities."[21]

The approach within HIV programming to country ownership shifted very substantially in July 2008 with legislation to reauthorize the President's Emergency Plan for AIDS Relief (PEPFAR).[22] PEPFAR's Five-Year Strategy, issued in 2009, made "transition from an emergency response to promotion of sustainable country programs" its first goal and "strengthen partner government capacity to lead the response to this epidemic and other health demands" its second of five overall goals.[23] The revised approach includes establishing Partnership Frameworks built on a 5-year joint strategic framework for cooperation between the US Government, the partner government, and other partners to combat HIV/AIDS in the host country through service delivery, policy reform, and coordinated financial commitments. By the end of 2011, over 20 partnership frameworks had been signed.[24] The Guidance for PEPFAR Partnership Frameworks and Partnership Framework Implementation Plans details how to ensure coordination among partners and support of the host country for the Frameworks and includes an annex summarizing the Paris Declaration and Accra Agenda.[25]

Alignment: Alignment under the Paris Principles implies both agreeing with the host country and other donors on what to do in a country, and using local systems to implement assistance. The first point is largely addressed with respect to the host country in the discussion of country ownership. The second point constitutes an area where real reform has recently occurred in US policy.

The PPD refers to building long-term partnerships with assisted nations, but does not give direct guidance on alignment. However, the QDDR is conscious that "Effective assistance requires cooperation between donors and host nations and among donors and other partners," and requires focus on strategic coordination with other donors on objectives, programs, and projects, and to the extent possible, reporting processes. It is also explicit in promoting the role of US assistance by "strengthening country systems and capacity by investing in host country systems and implementing partners to the extent practicable."

The USAID Policy Framework expresses the policy shift toward use of local systems. It states that "In the past, the Agency has channeled few resources directly to and/or through local institutions in our partner countries, and this has reduced our

---

[21] Department of State, Secretary Clinton's Fifth Policy Guidance Cable: Modernizing U.S. Diplomacy to Better Support Development, July 2012, paragraph 21.

[22] Tom Lantos and Henry J. Hyde United States Global Leadership Against HIV/AIDS, Tuberculosis, and Malaria Reauthorization Act of 2008.

[23] http://www.pepfar.gov/strategy/document/133251.htm.

[24] http://www.pepfar.gov/press/121652.htm.

[25] http://www.pepfar.gov/guidance/framework/120739.htm.

incentives to help the capacity of those institutions."[26] Under the overall policy called USAID Forward, a set of implementation and procurement reforms were taken to make more extensive use of partner country systems. The objectives of these reforms are to "Strengthen partner country capacity to improve aid effectiveness and sustainability by increasing use of reliable partner country systems and institutions to provide support to partner countries."[27] The USAID Administrator set a target to implement 30 % of its development assistance through local mechanisms by 2015 from a base of 10 % in 2011. For this target, local mechanisms include use of partner country systems and direct engagement with local nonprofit organizations and the local private sector.[28] To reduce the risks of government-to-government financing, in 2011 USAID developed a new public financial management assessment tool that helps determine which partner countries and which specific Ministries can directly program foreign assistance funds with acceptable accountability.[29]

The GHI Strategy acknowledges the central role of the host country with its expectation that "where possible, country-owned health delivery platforms will be the basis for providing comprehensive health services." This approach has been actively embraced. Health strategies at the country level, including those for GHI, PEPFAR, and BEST Action Plans (which focused on maternal and health, family planning, and nutrition programs), have been prepared for most major recipients of US health assistance. These are reviewed by several Washington offices and commonly emphasize the importance of alignment and building on local systems.

Harmonization: US policy has long held that donor coordination, to share information and avoid duplication, was an essential aspect of development assistance. The main focus of this harmonization has been in the field where donor meetings are held regularly in most posts. In addition, regional and global conferences and multilateral organizations are directed toward harmonization. Global coordination is amply demonstrated in the health sector through, for example, the International Health Partnership and the Joint Platform for Health Systems Strengthening, developed by the World Bank; the GAVI Alliance; the Global Fund to Fight AIDS, Tuberculosis, and Malaria; the World Health Organization; the annual International AIDS Conference; STOP TB, and the Child Survival: Call to Action.

The PPD raises harmonization policy as one of its three pillars: "A new operational model that positions the United States to be a more effective partner and to leverage our leadership." The term "leverage" suggests that this policy will result in additional support from development partners in the areas where the US Government makes its greatest efforts. The new operational model is described in six components, including

---

[26] *USAID Policy Framework*, p. 35.

[27] http://forward.usaid.gov/node/317.

[28] Internal USAID communication.

[29] Remarks by USAID Administrator Dr. Raj Shah at the "DRG 2.0: Promoting Democracy, Human Rights, and Governance in 2011" Conference in Arlington, Virginia, June 20, 2011. Available at http://www.usaid.gov/news-information/speeches/remarks-usaid-administrator-dr-raj-shah-drg-20-promoting-democracy-human.

that "the United States will… forge a deliberate division of labor among key donors, …strengthen key multilateral capabilities, [and] …leverage the private sector, philanthropic and nongovernmental organization and diaspora communities."

The 2010 QDDR is also clear to incorporate harmonization, stating the US Government "will partner with other donors—both public and private—to amplify overall effectiveness, allow donors to build and utilize their respective comparative advantages, while still ensuring overall coordination."[30] The USAID Policy Framework includes it among its seven operational principles in the form: "Leverage 'solution holders' and partner strategically" in order to "magnify results and deploy resources strategically while avoiding duplication of effort." The USAID guidance for Country Development Cooperation Strategies promotes harmonization to implement this Government-wide and Agency policy.

Within the health sector, the GHI Strategy calls for "exploring and learning from different models for harmonizing country and donor efforts." The PEPFAR Strategy similarly calls for "strong and robust engagement with multilateral partners and other external partners." It provides more detail that demonstrates its full acceptance of the Paris Declaration interpretation on this principle: "The challenges posed by the global AIDS crisis must be addressed as part of a shared global responsibility. PEPFAR is engaging in enhanced coordination with multilateral, regional, and bilateral partners, ensuring that USG efforts are not duplicative, and that donors are truly sharing the burden of the epidemic. In an affirmation of high level principles of the Paris Declaration, PEPFAR is working with its multilateral and bilateral partners to harmonize and align responses and support countries in achieving their nationally-defined HIV/AIDS goals."

Results: Focusing on results as a guide to planning assistance resources probably constitutes the strongest convergence between US policy and the Paris Principles. The PPD includes it among the six components of the new operational model: "The United States will… drive our policy and practice with the disciplined application of analysis of impact." The QDDR emphasizes it in one of its six foreign assistance effectiveness principles: "Investments must be focused to achieve measurable results. The United States will promote results-based, focused investments through:

- Adaptable approaches, tailoring strategies to fit country contexts.
- Sustained commitments, taking a long-term planning horizon with multi-year funding guidance to sustain commitments over time.
- Focus on outcomes and impact rather than inputs and outputs, and ensure that the best available evidence informs program design and execution."[31]

The policy cable from Secretary Clinton on diplomacy and development refers to a stronger focus on results within its listing of what the State Department needs to do differently under the heading "Focus relentlessly on results": "We must validate our strategies with regular, clear-eyed evaluations of results. This requires defining, up front, specific, measurable, and time-bound benchmarks and expected outcomes

---

[30] *QDDR*, p. 94.
[31] *QDDR*, p. 110.

that correspond to our development objectives, including those related to policy reform; regularly reviewing results; and making necessary adjustments to strategic and program plans."[32] This additional focus had already been written into planning guidance and into the first Department of State policy on evaluation.[33]

The USAID Policy Framework raises it among its seven areas of reform: "Measure and evaluate impact." It is similarly recognized as one of the seven areas of reform in USAID Forward: "Strengthening monitoring and evaluation." Even before these policy statements were drafted, the concept was institutionalized through the creation of the Bureau for Policy, Planning and Learning, and its Office of Learning, Evaluation and Research. The first formal policy of the new Bureau was on evaluation.[34]

Within the health sector, additional policy guidance may not have been necessary since the heightened focus on results largely originated with the PEPFAR program. A detailed system for planning and reporting with review in Washington of every country program was developed for PEPFAR and a similar, albeit less detailed, approach was established for the President's Malaria Initiative. When the head of PEPFAR became the Director of Foreign Assistance, the system was adapted for use across all USAID- and State-funded assistance. The importance of results to planning is brought out in the PEPFAR and GHI strategies.

Mutual Accountability: This principle is not as commonly brought out in US policy, but is clearly and directly recognized in the QDDR: "We will promote mutual accountability by prioritizing investments where partner nations have demonstrated high standards of transparency, good governance, and accountability—and where they make their own financial contributions to development, by making our own commitments transparent to our partners."[35] It is also cited among the ten central tenets of the USAID Policy Framework: "External partners can open doors to expertise, technology, relationships, trade, and financing, but this support cannot substitute for the efforts and sustained commitment of local communities and leaders."[36]

The health sector within US assistance is recognized for having relatively reliable data on health performance in recipient countries. The quality of these data is widely considered to be a positive factor in attracting Congressional support for health assistance. However, the most commonly used health data do not attempt to attribute specific effects of US programs. The 47 qualitative and qualitative GHI targets given in the GHI Strategy are consistently expressed as the intended outcome of collaboration with other partners.[37]

---

[32] Department of State, Secretary Clinton's Fifth Policy Guidance Cable: Modernizing U.S. Diplomacy to Better Support Development, paragraph 29.

[33] *Program Evaluation Policy*, February 2012, available at http://www.state.gov/s/d/rm/rls/evaluation/2012/184556.htm.

[34] Released in January 2011 and available at http://transition.usaid.gov/evaluation/USAIDEvaluationPolicy.pdf.

[35] *QDDR*, p. 95.

[36] *USAID Policy Framework*, p. 3.

[37] *GHI Strategy*, Annex A.

What Challenges Does US Aid Effectiveness Face? Although the Paris Principles are well known and respected in the design and implementation of US health assistance, numerous competing priorities are balanced against them. Thus, the support given to the Principles in statements at all levels of US policy does not form a comprehensive guide for those who design and implement assistance. A core issue for US programming is how to interpret and weigh the mandates for aid effectiveness in relation to other mandates, such as rapid and conspicuous results, efficient use of funds, or utilizing US-based providers. Major components of this balance must be reached jointly by the Congress and the Administration, greatly complicating the consistent application of broad principles. Although the formal mechanisms of Congressional effect are largely limited to authorizations and appropriations, these are sufficient to direct resources toward priorities that are rarely considered in international discussions of aid effectiveness.

In the lead up to the Fourth High Level Forum on Aid Effectiveness, held in Busan, many Paris Declaration signatory countries, including the United States, prepared evaluations of their progress toward implementing the Paris Declaration principles. The study of US progress relied heavily on interviews with officials across the US Government to determine their awareness of and active engagement with the Paris Principles. The report concluded

> It is unlikely the U.S. Government will ever achieve full compliance with the [Paris Declaration] and [Accra Agenda for Action]. To do so would require a sea change in the way U.S. interests influence both domestic and foreign assistance policy and practices. Full compliance would also require a profound change in the behavior and capacity of the regimes now in place in some partner countries in the developing world. However, the present US Administration clearly is motivated by the normative challenge presented by the USG's commitment to the PD and appears determined to continue to take specific steps to move toward PD-like aid effectiveness.[38]

Despite this broad conclusion, the report acknowledged compliance in many aspects of US policy. Typically, these were the result of US program managers agreeing with the merits of the Principles rather than any directive to follow them. The major disincentives to compliance came from US regulations which place priority on accountability of US programs over building the capacity of host country accounting. Similarly, dependence on other donors was seen as too risky.

Ownership: US assistance is frequently designed in support of country ownership, although the term is used by the United States in a more limited sense than is common in international parlance. Three issues constrain the US usage.

First, US programs are designed to serve purposes defined by the US Congress and the Administration. Practical and ethical imperatives encourage program designs that are consistent with host country wishes, but the starting point is US objectives. As stated in the QDDR: "The cornerstone of our policy is the restoration and application of American leadership."[39] This is well illustrated by the multi-lateral Child

---

[38] *Evaluation of the Implementation of the Paris Declaration: USG Synthesis*, USAID, 2011, p. ix.
[39] *QDDR*, p. 19.

Survival: Call to Action. This effort to direct host country funding toward child survival programs was largely initiated by USAID, but does not involve additional US funding. It describes the role of donors within its notion of host country ownership: "Government, civil society, and private sector leaders in these countries should be supported as they define their own country roadmaps and targets, commit their own financial resources, and pioneer new ways to accelerate progress toward ending preventable child deaths."[40]

Second, US policy and regulations recognize the risk of granting authority over US programs and funding to entities outside US control. The US evaluation found that corruption in host countries is seen as a permanent bar to ownership.[41] This finding is consistent with the interpretation applied in US policy where country ownership refers to a longer-term goal of shifting funding responsibility to the host country rather than ownership of US-funded programs. Clearly, the US policy implies assistance should be consistent with host country wishes in order to reach that long-term outcome.

Third, the United States has emphasized more than most donors that countries are represented in development efforts by many entities in addition to their governments. The QDDR recognizes "that country ownership does not mean government ownership and control in all circumstances, especially in countries whose governments show little commitment to or interest in development or democracy."[42] Although US policy has long held this interpretation, the QDDR states "the Department of State will begin an unprecedented effort to strengthen its cooperation with partners beyond the state. These steps are part of a broader commitment to make engagement beyond the state a defining feature of US foreign policy."[43]

A recent example is provided in the health sector. US assistance to strengthen the private sector in provision of health services has been more extensive than any other donor.[44] Other donors are moving in the same direction, as shown by the formation in 2010 of Harnessing Non-State Actors for Better Health for the Poor (HANSHEP) by USAID and a group of government and private development agencies, along with a few recipient countries to improve the performance of the non-state sector in delivering better healthcare to the poor by working together, learning from each other, and sharing this learning with others.[45]

Alignment: Coordination with other donors is an essential component of US assistance, but alignment in the sense of agreeing among donors and the host country is not given a high priority. It is difficult to agree on purposes in any detail given the

---

[40] Child Survival: Call to Action, Summary Roadmap, June 14, 2012 http://5thbday.usaid.gov/pages/ResponseSub/roadmap.pdf.

[41] Evaluation of the Implementation of the Paris Declaration: USG Synthesis, p. vi.

[42] QDDR, p. 95.

[43] QDDR, p. 59.

[44] Bowers, Gerard, Frank Feeley and Betty Raven Holt. A Review of USAID's Experience with the Private Sector in Health: 1968–2009, QED Group, February 2010.

[45] http://www.hanshep.org/.

differing pressures on the various partners to report their priorities to their constituencies. Just as there are principles competing in US policy with the Paris Principles, host country goals often diverge from US interests, including US interpretation of development priorities. Host countries may not lead the donor community in placing priority on providing broader opportunities for women, ethnic minorities, or the poor. The priorities of the elites, such as higher education and tertiary healthcare, tend to be overrepresented as the interests of the host country.

The aspect of alignment that utilizes host country systems to implement assistance is complicated by the immediate concern in using experienced and familiar providers as well as the political importance of maintaining US contracting. The QDDR discussed this situation: "To succeed in building local capacity and strong systems to advance our broader development goals, we will continue to work with and through the best and most effective US NGOs, non-profit organizations, and private contractors. As we pivot to a greater focus on working with local entities, we are confident that the best US organizations will adapt and continue to be effective partners in supporting these goals as they, too, build stronger partnerships with local governments, NGOs, and businesses."[46]

Nonetheless, host country contracting has expanded and is seen as part of building lasting capacity. Historically, USAID's host country contracting was used predominantly for large infrastructure projects, particularly in the Middle East region where USAID's budgets were large enough to engage in infrastructure building. Increasingly, USAID programs seek to use partner country systems to promote sustainable development, rather than forcing conventional systems and procedures judged more likely to achieve short-term outputs and quick results. USAID is particularly focused on employing this strategy in countries like Pakistan. The USAID Mission to Pakistan has strengthened its working relationship with the Government of Pakistan to identify, design, and implement "on-budget" activities. As a result, the Government of Pakistan has become directly responsible for program development, contracting and implementation.[47]

Harmonization: While the US assistance consistently maintains the priorities from Congress and the Administration, it recognizes the value of coordinating with other donors to avoid redundancy and close gaps in needs. This coordination is often built around the concept of having each donor work in the area it can do best, but may also be responsive to where each donor has the greatest interest. The United States, for example, typically places a higher value on strengthening NGOs than European donor nations and even has a different view of how to do this. Rather than aligning to the view taken by existing host country representatives or donor partners, US assistance tends to accept leadership where civil society is weak.

The Accra Agenda included a general guide to keeping the aid architecture as simple as possible: "As new global challenges emerge, donors will ensure that existing channels for aid delivery are used and, if necessary, strengthened before

---

[46] *QDDR*, p. 99.
[47] *QDDR*, p. 95.

creating separate new channels that risk further fragmentation and complicate co-ordination at country level."[48] Under the Bush Administration, the two largest for-eign assistance initiatives were instituted in newly formed US agencies, the Millennium Challenge Corporation and the Office of the Global AIDS Coordinator. More recently, the joint themes to focus and concentrate assistance resources have been dominant. They were raised as principles in the PDD and made into opera-tional principles in the USAID Policy Framework.

Similarly, US assistance readily addresses the Busan call to "make effective use of existing multilateral channels …[and] work to reduce the proliferation of these channels."[49]

In health, the United States participates in many multi-lateral organizations, but they typically focus on particular health issues, such as HIV, tuberculosis, family planning, or child survival, so there is not much overlap in their objectives or direct competition for resources.

Harmonization in the health sector is best demonstrated by the US–Japan Partnership for Global Health. Every 2 years since June 2002, USAID and the Japanese aid agencies (JICA and the Ministry of Foreign Affairs) have reaffirmed their interest in coordinating health assistance and jointly prepared global action plans, evaluations, staff exchanges, and field visits. These interactions have contrib-uted to exchanges of assistance technology, geographic sharing of responsibility, and enhanced collaboration in international global health meetings at the UN and elsewhere.

Results: In concert with the policy statements for increased attention to results, foreign assistance programs are being more extensively measured and reported. Most notably, a foreign assistance dashboard, called FA.gov,[50] was created in response to the Paris Declaration and President Obama's Open Government Initiative. FA.gov currently contains foreign assistance budget planning data for the Department of State, and budget planning, obligation, and expenditure data for USAID and the Millennium Challenge Corporation. Future versions will incorporate budget, financial, program, and performance data in a standard form from all US Government agencies receiving or implementing foreign assistance, humanitarian, and/or development funds. The site presents foreign assistance investments through a variety of user-friendly graphics, including funding by country, by sector, by agency, and by year. Further, the data are sorted in a variety of additional ways and users are able to generate their own tables.

Within the health sector, the GHI was initially designed to study as well as imple-ment the seven GHI principles, including one to improve metrics, monitoring, and evaluation. For this study, eight GHI Plus countries were designated. The planned GHI Strategic Reserve Fund that was to finance additional attention on these coun-tries was not funded, so the effect of the GHI principles was not given intensive analysis. In effect, the cost of focusing on results constrained that effort.

---

[48] *Accra Agenda for Action*, p. 19c.

[49] *Busan Partnership for Effective Development Co-operation*, paragraph 25(b).

[50] Access at www.ForeignAssistance.gov.

The staff time required to focus on results has been accepted as a constraint on collecting results data. The extensive reporting required of the annual PEPFAR process became a model for USAID in some respects, but the heavy staff burden contributed to a new emphasis on "streamlining." The QDDR set up the Joint State/USAID Streamlining Project, which led to the establishment of the State/USAID Streamlining Program Management Office. This office oversees the joint State/USAID Governance Committee, which manages requests for the collection of foreign-assistance-related information not previously or regularly collected. Thus, new data can be requested only after approval of the request by this committee.

Different views on what results to measure are inherent to health assistance programs. As there is greater interest in adjusting funding according to performance, relatively short-term and transparent, narrow results are favored. GHI promotes an outcome- and impact-based approach rather than an expenditure- or input-based approach to measure progress in achieving and sustaining health improvements, but such measures are difficult to define and document. The effect of prevention efforts tends to lag behind service delivery programs. The impact of strengthening health systems is especially difficult to measure in the short run and to attribute to specific programs.

Mutual Accountability: This principle constitutes an acknowledgement of a fundamental fact of foreign assistance. The acknowledgement has practical effect during planning because the process too often leaps from an analysis of a country's development shortcomings to a program proposal. The role of development partners is substantial since US assistance is nearly always far less than what is needed to resolve development problems. In addition, accepting responsibility only for the portion of development that is directly targeted by US assistance misses the overall purposes of assistance. The GHI Strategy points out that "GHI success will be measured by improved access to and utilization of quality health services and changes in key health outcomes, particularly for marginalized and disadvantaged populations."

The MCC uses data on country performance, not program performance, to determine eligibility for MCC assistance. Its underlying rationale is both that country performance demonstrates that a country is likely to be a good development partner and that the prospect of getting an MCC program can serve as an incentive for a country to perform better on its own. In these ways, MCC is placing most of the responsibility for performance on the host country.

Similarly, the State Department's Office of US Foreign Assistance Resources has provided data on more than 30 indicators of country performance to all Missions planning assistance since fiscal year 2013. The guidance with these data asked program designers to consider the relative performance of each sector in choosing where to direct resources, along with the capabilities and likely efforts of development partners. Again, the concept behind this approach to requesting resources was that country performance on development goals is the shared outcome of various host country entities and international donors.

Chapter 6
Assessing the Effectiveness of Health Projects

Richard Blue, John Eriksson, George Grob, and Kelly Skeith (Heindel)

International Evaluation and USG's Participation

The Paris Declaration on Aid Effectiveness (PD) was endorsed in Paris at the Second High Level Forum on Aid Effectiveness in March 2005 by 90 developing and donor countries, including the United States. In addition, 26 multilateral and intergovernmental organizations participated. Fourteen civil society organizations were present, but were not involved in the negotiations of the PD, nor were they signatories. Since March 2005, a number of additional countries have endorsed the PD and the USG continued to participate in the process, including considerable staff work to monitor and report on USG PD implementation and prepare US officials for subsequent meetings.[1] Intended to address growing donor and partner-country concerns about the quality and effectiveness of development assistance, the PD is a distillation of the development cooperation experience of a half a century. It brings together key principles and conclusions that have emerged from international development conferences and research over the last decade.

---

[1] The original list of signatory countries and other organizations is given at the end of the PD (see: Organization for Economic Cooperation and Development. The Paris Declaration on Aid Effectiveness and the Accra Agenda for Action. http://www.oecd.org/dataoecd/11/41/34428351. pdf. Accessed September 2012).

R. Blue (✉) • K. Skeith (Heindel)
Social Impact, Inc., Arlington, Virginia, USA
e-mail: rblue@socialimpact.com; kelly.heindel@gmail.com

J. Eriksson
World Bank, Washington, DC, USA
e-mail: johneriks@gmail.com

G. Grob
Center for Public Program Evaluation, Washington, DC, USA
e-mail: georgefgrob@cs.com

© Springer Science+Business Media New York 2015
E. Beracochea (ed.), *Improving Aid Effectiveness in Global Health*,
DOI 10.1007/978-1-4939-2721-0_6

Paris Declaration Principles

Ownership—Developing countries set their own strategies for poverty reduction, improve their institutions, and tackle corruption.
Alignment—Donor countries align behind these objectives and use local
systems.
Harmonization—Donor countries coordinate, simplify procedures, and share
information to avoid duplication.
Results—Developing countries and donors shift focus to development results
and results get measured.
Mutual accountability—Donors and partners are accountable for development results.

The PD remains a dominant statement on aid relationships; its initial "Statement
of Resolve" of 12 points is followed by 56 commitments, organized around five key
PD principles: (1) country ownership; (2) country alignment; (3) donor harmonization; (4) managing for results (MfR), and (5) mutual accountability.[2]

The Accra Agenda for Action (AAA) issued by the Third High Level Forum,
held in Ghana in September 2008, reaffirmed the PD and gave particular emphasis
to developing country ownership over development; building more effective and
inclusive partnerships for development; and delivering and accounting for development results.

The Evaluation of Progress Under the Paris Declaration

The PD highlights the importance of independent evaluation as well as monitoring
PD implementation. It states that the evaluation process should provide a more
comprehensive understanding of how increased aid effectiveness contributes to
meeting development objectives. The Organization for Economic Co-operation and
Development (OECD) commissioned an independent two-phase evaluation beginning in 2006. Phase I included 8 partner-country, and 11 donor, case studies that
reviewed the experience of implementing the PD.[3] Conclusions, lessons, and

---

[2] The complete text of the PD can be found at: Organization for Economic Cooperation and
Development. The Paris Declaration on Aid Effectiveness and the Accra Agenda for Action. http://
www.oecd.org/dataoecd/11/41/34428351.pdf. Accessed September 2012.

[3] Four crosscutting, thematic studies were also completed: (1) "Statistical Capacity Building;" (2)
"Untying of Aid and the PD;" (3) "Applicability of the PD in Fragile and Conflict-affected
Situations;" and (4) "The PD, Aid Effectiveness, and Development Effectiveness." See: Dabelstein,
Niels. The Evaluation of the Paris Declaration (PDF). http://www.oecd.org/document/60/0,3343,
en_21571361_34047972_38242748_1_1_1_1,00.html. Published March 2012. Accessed
September 2012.

recommendations were presented in a Synthesis Report, submitted to the September 2008 High Level Forum in Accra. Phase II, recently completed, includes over 20 partner-country case studies and 7 donor case studies, including the US Government (USG) donor case study discussed in this chapter.

Survey on Monitoring the Paris Declaration. Selected Comparisons of the US with Other Donors

The PD identified 12 indicators of aid effectiveness based on the PD principles and commitments. These were measured by an international team in 2006 and 2008 (data for 2005 and 2007). The US played an active role in this exercise, including chairing the 2008 effort. The results for the US are mixed.

- The percent of US aid to the public sector using country systems decreased from 12 to 5 %, but increased from 39 to 43 % for all donors.
- US disbursements on schedule improved from 27 to 32 %, but for all 31 donors, performance increased from 41 to 46 %.
- The share of US aid reportedly program-based grew from 29 to 37 %, while the share for all donors increased from 43 to 47 %.
- The percent of US missions coordinated with other donor missions declined from 20 to 9 %.
- OECD/DAC, Better Aid: 2008 Survey on Monitoring the PD: Making Aid More Effective by 2010.

The donor case studies assess leadership and commitment, capacity to implement the PD, incentives, and disincentives to implementation, and coherence or integration of the donors' foreign assistance objectives and programs across the organization as factors influencing PD implementation. The developing-country case studies assess the effect of PD implementation on development outcomes and impact, as well as progress and constraints in implementing the PD. The results of all case studies have been incorporated into a Synthesis Report and presented to the Fourth High Level Forum on Aid Effectiveness in December 2011 in Korea.

Introduction to USG Participation and USG Study

The purpose of the current study was to review and assess implementation by the USG of the principles of the Paris Declaration on Aid Effectiveness. The evaluation team, through Social Impact Inc., conducted the study over a 14-month period beginning in February 2010. The methodology included an examination of relevant documents from each of seven US government agencies, including the Department of Health and Human Services (HHS) discussed in more detail in this chapter, that manage Official Development Assistance (ODA); key informant interviews at the headquarters levels of each of the agencies; a questionnaire survey of overseas staff of four agencies; and selected interviews of staff in cross-cutting "apex" entities in executive and legislative branches that play important roles regarding development assistance policy and resource allocation.[4] The synthesis report brings together the main findings from these sources, grouped by the factors or conditions identified by the framework for the PD evaluation as enabling donor implementation of the commitments and principles of the PD. These enabling factors are: Leadership, Awareness, and Commitment; Capacity; Incentives and Disincentives; and Coherence.

Limitations to Our Methodology

We use the term "USG" to refer collectively to those policies and actions which influence or affect US foreign assistance programs, processes, and procedures in general. It is important to note that there is no single USG agency with authority over all seven agencies included in this assessment, although the President with the advice of the National Security Council (NSC) does set overall policy. However, the US Congress plays a major role through the appropriations process, frequently mandating agency programs as well as setting specific limitations and conditions on how and for what purposes foreign assistance is to be provided.

It is also important to note that the agencies we evaluated manage a wide variety of foreign assistance funds and mandates. The evaluation found little evidence that the overall management of ODA funds differs significantly from the management of other foreign assistance funds. In cases in which it does differ, we note this, including reasons for the difference.[5] Therefore, we used information collected from interviews with this range of offices and bureaus to more fully describe the context in which the USG implements its ODA and total foreign assistance budget. We also attempted to highlight instances in which the PD principles would not apply.

The data-gathering phase extended over several months, during which USG aid effectiveness policies and pronouncements emerged at an ever-increasing pace, including references to the PD principles in the new Senate foreign assistance draft

---

[4]Case study agencies, DOS, USAID, MCC, TREAS-OTA, HHS, DOL, and USDA, were determined in the SOW provided by the report commissioners. Interviews were conducted with selected staff in the National Security Council (NSC) and the Office of Management and Budget (OMB) in the executive branch and the Government Accountability Office (GAO), the Committee on Foreign Affairs and the Committee on Appropriations of the US House of Representatives, and the Committee on Foreign Relations of the US Senate, in the legislative branch. The names of the seven case study agencies and the study authors are given in the Preface to this report.

[5]DOS comments on its agency case study report also outline the difference they see between all foreign assistance and ODA: "In some cases, the principles of the PD cannot apply in a rigid sense to all foreign assistance programs. We would still argue that flexibility in these nuanced situations is the key. There are offices that have mandates that do not necessarily have economic development/ODA at their core. We believe that the application of PD principles needs to be more flexible in these cases as the programs conducted by these offices often have limited development goals and restricted ability to fully implement the precepts of the PD."

bill and the new foreign assistance global initiatives, including Feed the Future (FtF) and the Global Health Initiative (GHI). This made for a very dynamic period during which information collected at the beginning of the process may well have evolved by the end of the data collection phase, rather like trying to provide a conclusive picture of a hurricane forming in the Atlantic Ocean.

USG Evaluation Results

Main Findings

Leadership, Awareness, and Commitment

After endorsing the PD in March 2005, the USG continued to participate in the process, including considerable staff work to monitor and report on USG PD implementation and prepare US officials for subsequent meetings. The United States Agency for International Development's (USAID) initial PD guidance to the field was issued in March 2006. An Interagency Working Group on Aid Effectiveness (IWG-AE), succeeded by the Aid Effectiveness Sub-Policy Coordinating Committee (AE-PCC), met as an interagency committee under the aegis of the Policy Coordination Committee on Development and Humanitarian Assistance in subsequent years to marshal USG support for PD actions, including a USG Action Plan (2007), the monitoring surveys of PD implementation, and preparing for USG participation in the Third High Level Forum in Accra in September 2008. However, its efforts to raise awareness of and commitment to the PD principles among program management staff were not very effective, according to the case studies. With the exception of the Millennium Challenge Corporation (MCC) and Department of Treasury Office of Technical Assistance (TREAS-OTA) respondents, the case studies revealed that very few program managers in other USG departments—Department of State (DOS), Health and Human Services (HHS), Departments of Agriculture (USDA), and Labor (DOL), and USAID—had an intimate understanding or knowledge of the PD or the Accra Agenda for Action (AAA).

Beginning in 2008, a new USAID Administrator actively began to support the PD and AAA, taking steps to expand awareness and examine constraints. The current USAID administration has accelerated this process by issuing specific guidance for strategic planning, undertaking a serious examination of how to improve aid effectiveness, and identifying constraints that can be relaxed without congressional action as well as those that will require new statutory authorities. The 2011 US Global Development Policy (also referred to as the Presidential Policy Directive on Global Development) focuses on policy and structural reforms necessary to increase the effectiveness of USG assistance. This, and the Quadrennial Diplomacy and Development Review (QDDR) released by DOS and USAID in 2011, represents the results of nearly 2 years of intensive study and discussion by senior staff and policy makers in the NSC, DOS, and USAID. Both documents are informed by PD principles, and the QDDR specifically cites the PD and the AAA as the source for its development assistance principles.[6] The guidance provided by these policies give management structure to three previously announced initiatives: Food Security (FtF), Global Health, and Climate Change.

Based on the evidence collected, these seven US government agency case studies may be organized into three groups:

- *Agencies expressly committed, with policies specifically aligned with PD principles.* In our case studies, MCC and TREAS–OTA come closest to this standard.
- *Agencies that follow practices highly consistent with PD principles.* Among our case studies, HHS comes closest to this standard.
- *Agencies within which some practices conform to PD principles, but for which the constraints imposed by external and internal factors,* such as organizational mandates, USG accountability and contracting procedures and agency practices, or competing organizational *cultures present severe disincentives or constrain movement towards greater compliance with the PD.* DOS, USAID, Department of Labor, Bureau for International Labor Affairs (DOL–ILAB), and USDA make up this grouping of our study cases. As demonstrated in the USAID case study, DOS and USAID leadership is directly confronting many of these constraints, especially through the USAID Forward reforms and to some extent the three major program initiatives—FtF, the GHI, and the Global Climate Change Initiative (GCCI).

However, as noted in all the case studies, the majority of key informants are conversant with aid effectiveness principles, in general, and can describe efforts to improve their own program's effectiveness (though not labeling the construct PD, as such).

Capacity

The capacity required in the reviewed agencies to implement the PD principles effectively tended to be underestimated in almost every case, with the exception of some MCC and USAID respondents. As a corollary, only a few agencies mentioned the need to acquire or develop improved capacity in order to help strengthen host country capacities in areas such as financial management, procurement management, and monitoring and evaluation. Instead, as noted above, agency capacity strengthening tended to focus on meeting USG requirements rather than strengthening host country capacities.[7] HHS and TREAS–OTA are notable exceptions to this

---

[6] The United States Department of State and the United States Agency for International Development. *The Quadrennial Diplomacy and Development Review.* The United States Department of State and the United States Agency for International Development. www.state.gov/qddr, 2010. Accessed September 2012.

[7] Both the PD and the AAA give considerable emphasis to the need for donors to strengthen host country development capacities (six PD commitments and nine AAA commitments). These statements also recognize the need for donors to strengthen their own capacities. Commitment 14 (a) of the AAA states that "Donors will strengthen their own capacities and skills to be more responsive to developing country needs."

finding. Both agency case studies noted that interviewed officials pointed out that strengthening host government capacity is a prime objective of their programs.[8]

Incentives and Disincentives

Efforts to find evidence of PD-like foreign assistance processes yielded positive results, especially for the HHS and MCC case studies, and to some extent, mid-level program managers in DOS. No specific incentives for implementing PD principles were mentioned in any of the case studies. Instead, respondents referred to their professional commitment to improve the effectiveness and impact of the programs they managed. Disincentives derived from the constraints embedded in USG procedures for doing business and for being accountable for how public funds are used. However, the lens through which respondents viewed their compliance varied. Generally, compliance was more influenced by the general laws, policies, and regulations of the US Government, like the Government Performance and Results Act (GPRA) or Federal Acquisition Regulations (FAR), than by an understanding of the PD principles. This was especially the case for procedures related to Managing for Results (MfR) and mutual accountability. The PD principles of mutual accountability and country ownership were largely missing from these discussions. The commitments under the principles, if followed, would impose a very different set of procedural requirements and practices on US government foreign assistance managers. On the other hand, in HHS the PD-like assistance was influenced more by a long-standing culture of public health officers that emphasized partnership-like technical assistance whose goal was sustainability of public health systems improvements.

The agency case studies did not say much about the PD principle of harmonization. Perhaps this is because little need is seen for it, as in the case of the financial and economic advisors fielded by TREAS–OTA—but a more significant reason is that risk-averse cultures in agencies like USAID and DOS militate against joint efforts with other donors to reduce the aid delivery transaction costs imposed on host countries, or to work toward a division of labor among donors.[9] Another factor militating against harmonization is the felt need, expressed by both HHS, DOS, and USAID staff, to attribute their success in MfR to USG efforts and resources, rather than to a harmonized approach with other donors. At the same time, the relatively large field presence of USAID and DOS staff has facilitated informal coordination with other donors.[10]

---

[8] While not a prime objective, capacity building has received increased attention in MCC Compacts and implementing entity agreements. It is implicit in the smaller MCC threshold programs, to the extent that capacity strengthening is required for a country to meet compact eligibility criteria.

[9] For example, the USAID case study suggests that perceived ceding of responsibility by a USAID staff member to another donor would expose the staff member to prosecution and punitive action.

[10] Explicit priority is given to harmonization by the "Presidential Policy Directive on Global Development" (PPD) as well as by the initiatives at USAID, including in the following guidance: The United States Agency for International Development. *Building Local Development Leadership and Country Development Cooperation Strategies*. The United States Agency for International Development. August 2010.

Coherence

US foreign assistance has expanded, both in dollars and in the number of issue areas and objectives, over the last 20 years, in large part due to the emergence of a variety of global issues, negative externalities, and the concomitant expansion of America's global engagement after the end of the Cold War. USG commitment to providing humanitarian assistance has remained strong, but the combined increase in the severity of natural disasters and the persistence of internal conflict in many states has resulted in the engagement of the US military with other USG departments, in association with the international non-governmental organizations (NGO) community, in providing relief. The US government has elevated development to an equal status with defense and diplomacy, but tensions remain among the three objectives, as well as with the economic and trade interests of the several of the US domestic agencies now involved in the development process. Each of the case studies noted examples of where specific amendments to the US Foreign Assistance Authorization and related appropriations bills placed limitations on the foreign assistance programs, most notably in the promotion of agricultural products that compete with US agricultural exports, or in "source/nationality/origin" provisions which may raise the costs of assistance in some countries. Less explicit sources of tension also arise from what we have termed "values-based" program objectives such as support for human rights advocacy groups and the desire to have alliance relationships with important countries for security or diplomatic objectives, especially when some of these alliances are with regimes that have a poor record of protecting human rights or for tolerating political dissent.

Implementation

Respondents across the board, but especially in USAID, were somewhat skeptical of the US Government ever moving toward full compliance with the PD principles—in large part due to the perceived weakness of, and incidence of corruption in, host government institutions, but also because of the very detailed legal responsibilities imposed on USG managers by FAR and other US statutes. Managers are simply unable to take the risk of losing control of funds or of the procurement/contracting process.

Key Conclusions

These conclusions are based on the research conducted mainly in the period of March to September 2010. By late September, the administration's ongoing efforts to develop a new global development policy, to address the issue of policy and operational coherence, and especially to reform and rebuild USAID began to bear fruit. The release of policy and reform-related documents accelerated, and with the

GHI and FtF Initiatives, implementation protocols and practices are being tested. While much of this effort has been driven by a more general recognition that, to serve US interests, US foreign assistance has to become more effective and focused, there is little doubt that the PD, AAA, and the Rome Principles (with regard to food security) have had a major impact on the direction of US aid effectiveness reforms. However, as any student of organizational behavior well knows, the transformation of reform policies into reformed implementation procedures and practices is not automatic. For this reason, many of our conclusions focus on the operational constraints that must be overcome if the new policies are to produce the desired results.

1. US foreign assistance has lacked an overall conceptual and organizational architecture, in spite of efforts to give it conceptual unity under the "Three D" mantra: Defense, Diplomacy, and Development. It involves many federal agencies and is heavily earmarked and influenced by the US Congress and a variety of interest groups. It is therefore difficult to develop generalizations about the degree of PD and AAA compliance.
2. Respondents in US government agencies that did follow assistance management practices consistent with the PD tended to stress country alignment, engagement with host country institutions, capacity building through extended technical assistance, and efforts to gradually shift program implementation responsibility to host country institutions. HHS perhaps shows the greatest responsiveness in this regard. One of the reasons for this degree of alignment is an already-extant global network of public health professionals, as well as a close affiliation between public health development experts and the larger health research and scientific community
3. Within DOS, the Office of the US Global AIDS Coordinator is responsible for coordinating the major USG commitment to fighting HIV/AIDS, and other major global health threats. The oldest and largest commitment has been the President's Emergency Plan for AIDS Relief (PEPFAR) program, which since 2009 has made significant progress in developing operational and strategic guidance for moving PEPFAR towards explicit adherence to PD principles, including country ownership and harmonization with other donors, although it is too early to tell whether this new approach will produce desired improvements in aid effectiveness.
4. There are conditions under which certain PD principles, or aspects of them, may not fully apply. For example, aspects of country ownership and alignment may not apply in situations of fragility, lack of accountable governance, or immediate post-conflict situations. Even aspects of harmonization, managing for results, and mutual accountability may be difficult. However, close coordination among donors at the information-sharing level and some kinds of joint efforts, such as fact-finding missions, will be essential in post-conflict situations. MfR and mutual accountability in these circumstances may need to be multilateral among donors, rather than joint with the country.
5. A key conceptual issue for many respondents and case study analysts is whether "host country" means host government (especially those without credible representative claims), or whether it applies more broadly to all sectors, including civil

society, the private for-profit sector, universities, and more.[11] Moreover, are assistance programs that work directly with civil society or the private business sectors, without host government involvement, permissible under the PD principle of host country ownership, or is some direct involvement of the host government a necessary requirement of country ownership? The 2011 "US Global Development Policy" clearly anticipates working with host governments by stating: "Investing in systemic solutions for service delivery, public administration, and other government functions where sufficient capacity exists; a focus on sustainability and public sector capacity will be central to how the United States approaches humanitarian assistance and our pursuit of Millennium Development Goals (MDGs)," bringing back into balance a US assistance approach that had moved too far toward circumvention of the state and use of intermediaries, as recognized by the managers' report of the 2010 DOS-Foreign Operations legislation.

6. It is unlikely that the US government will ever achieve full compliance with the PD and AAA. To do so would require a sea change in the way US interests influence both domestic and foreign assistance policy and practices. Full compliance would also require a profound change in the behavior and capacity of the regimes now in place in some partner countries in the developing world. However, the present US administration clearly is motivated by the normative challenge presented by the USG's commitment to the PD and appears determined to continue to take specific steps to move toward PD-like aid effectiveness.

Department of Health and Human Services (HHS) Case Study

USG Global Health Programming

Though international work is on the periphery of such a domestic agency as HHS, there are nonetheless six offices with responsibilities to address global health challenges through direct assistance, technical and program support, training and capacity building, and research:

- Office of Global Health Affairs (OGHA) within the Office of the Secretary
- Centers for Disease Control and Prevention (CDC)
- National Institutes of Health (NIH)
- Food and Drug Administration (FDA)
- Health Resources and Services Administration (HRSA)
- Substance Abuse & Mental Health Services Administration (SAMHSA)

Although not officially tracked in the HHS budget, we estimate total HHS funding that could be considered to be for international programs was $2.2 billion in FY 2009, the largest share by far through the Centers for Disease Control and Prevention, with $1.8 billion.

---

[11] One agency stated that this is a settled issue in the PD/AAA that country means more than just government. However, discussions with the US international NGO member organization, InterAction, raised this issue as a major concern.

HHS agencies receive funding for international programs from various sources, including congressional appropriations for budget line items for global health, allocation by agencies from broader appropriations, and transfers from the President's Emergency Plan for AIDS Relief (PEPFAR) and the President's Malaria Initiative (PMI). The latter two account for $1.7 billion, or 78 %, of the total $2.2 billion in HHS international assistance activities. This is particularly important to this study, since the use of these transferred funds are governed, not by HHS administrative procedures, but by those issued by the US Global AIDS Coordinator for PEPFAR and by USAID for Malaria.

Overview of CDC's International Health Programs

Congress appropriates funds to CDC for its global health efforts through five main budget lines: (1) global HIV/AIDS; (2) global immunization; (3) global disease detection; (4) malaria; and, (5) other global health. CDC addresses these priorities mainly via technical assistance to health ministries and field training programs. CDC also receives and leverages other resources to respond to global requests for technical assistance in outbreak response, prevention and control of injuries and chronic diseases; emergency assistance and disaster response; environmental health; reproductive health; and safe water, hygiene, and sanitation. Most of CDC's GHIs were consolidated in 2010 under a new center, the Center for Global Health.

Findings

Based on our analysis and assessment, we assess the HHS implementation of the Paris Declaration Principles as follows:

- Knowledge of the Paris Declaration itself is generally limited; HHS has not been provided with implementation guidance and, in turn, HHS has provided no formal announcement, explanation, or commitment to its component agencies, separate from what the US government as a whole and the lead USG foreign assistance agencies have announced or published.
- Commitment to its principles is strong, nevertheless, especially among those responsible for day-to-day management of HHS global health programs. Almost all work in collaboration with international organizations and under international standards. The Public Health Practice Principles align well with Paris Declaration principles.
- The strongest incentive for HHS staff to embrace Paris Declaration principles is the inherent value of effective and sustainable international aid.
- The most commonly expressed disincentives are the difficulty of implementing it and the time it takes get results.
- Major disincentives and obstacles to *alignment and mutual accountability* include:
  - The lack of capacity of some countries to serve as true partners
  - The possibility of corruption

- Difficulties resulting from disconnects between the United States' and foreign governments' policies and goals
- The major disincentive and obstacle to *harmonization* is the required accountability of government agencies to their program offices, the president, and Congress.

Consistency of the PD Principles with the Principles of the US GHI

On May 5, 2009, President Obama announced his new GHI: a 6-year, $63 billion plan that uses an integrated approach to fight the spread of infectious diseases while addressing other global health challenges. All of HHS's international health programs are subject to the principles articulated in this initiative.

HHS's top leadership has cited the initiative as a driving force behind the agency's global health activities. At a World Trade Organization meeting in Geneva in May 2010, HHS Secretary Kathleen Sebelius praised the initiative, saying: "This is part of what we call our 'whole-of-government' approach. It means that HSS will work closely with USAID, the State Department, and other US government partners to achieve our global health goals."

In each country receiving global health assistance, USG experts work with partner governments and counterparts from other countries to strengthen and support country-led, national health plans. The process of implementation begins with an assessment of existing national health plans, health systems, current financing gaps, and the capacity to use additional resources effectively. Based on this assessment, the GHI works with partner governments and other development partners to identify goals, strategies, and approaches to which it can contribute, including identification of a plan to build an evidence base and capture progress.

The GHI highlights five foundational principles for US Global health programs that directly correlate with the Paris Declaration, as illustrated in Table 6.1.

Table 6.1 Global Health Initiative—foundational principles

Global Health Initiative principles	PD principles
Increase impact through strategic coordination and integration—including joint programming among US government agencies, other donors, and partner country governments, and other institutions to increase efficiency and effectiveness	Results
	Alignment
	Harmonization
Strengthen and leverage key multilateral organizations, global health partnerships, and private sector engagement	Harmonization
Encourage country ownership and invest in country-led plans	Ownership
	Alignment
Build sustainability through strengthening health systems	Ownership
	Alignment
Improve metrics, monitoring, and evaluation	Results
	Mutual accountability

Key Considerations for HHS and Other USG Agencies That Support International Health Development Programs

HHS could benefit from guidance by USG lead agencies in the implementation of the Paris Declaration as to the formal policy regarding the importance and applicability of the Paris Declaration, and the Office of Global Health Affairs could be tasked with assuring that all HHS operating divisions and staff divisions are aware of the USG policy on implementation.

Issuance of such formal guidance would reinforce principles of international partnership that are well engrained in the culture and practices of HHS global health agencies.

The above policy should provide practical guidance regarding realistic expectations and appropriate actions to be taken in dealing with potential problems such as those relating to:

- The proactive development of the partner country's management capacity and adaptations to joint project plans to accommodate the country's ability to participate in planning, budgeting, financial control, monitoring, and project management
- The potential for fraud
- A disconnect between fundamental policies or priorities of the US government and that of the partner country
- Accountability to senior HHS program officials, other executive branch officials, and the Congress, and; improvement of monitoring and evaluation, including impact evaluation, as inherent features of international programs, including the development of the host country's participation in the project evaluation and the general development of its evaluation capacity

Matters for Consideration

The findings and conclusions presented generate ideas and suggestions for improvement and raise additional questions and issues that require further review. These matters for consideration are based on the enabling factors laid out in the SOW and identified in the paper.

Overarching Considerations for US Government Executive and Political Leaders

The operational and procurement reforms already under way in USAID should be monitored for success and their applicability to other agencies.

Capacity

As part of the USAID Forward reform process, USAID is analyzing and developing guidance to address a variety of operational constraints to improving aid effectiveness. This effort should be broadened to require all agencies to prepare an inventory of their substantive capacities and skills in order to assess training, recruitment, placement, orientation, mentoring, and other approaches required to adequately implement the PD principles. This should include assessing the capacity required to provide effective capacity-strengthening assistance to enable host countries to carry out the PD principles, including planning and/or implementing fiduciary systems, donor coordination, and monitoring and evaluation for MfR. Once the key capacity constraints are identified, agencies can begin to develop targeted capacity building programs relevant to each agencies' mandate and responsibilities in 'the whole of government' process.

Incentives and Disincentives

- All USG agencies managing foreign assistance accounts need very specific guidance on acceptable conditions and arrangements for promoting host country ownership, alignment, and greater donor harmonization. Agency officials should be provided with the appropriate means and incentives to ensure appropriate risk taking in developing and utilizing host-country capacity, while being protected from legal or bureaucratic repercussions if problems of accountability or mismanagement do arise.
- The administration, on behalf of USG agencies managing foreign assistance accounts, should ask Congress to eliminate or ameliorate those requirements that inhibit implementation of PD principles.
- Detailed PD guidance should include an analysis of favorable and unfavorable conditions for implementation of the different components of PD principles. USAID currently is preparing guidance for the use of country systems under the alignment principle of the PD. Guidance should also address the role of capacity strengthening in helping to improve conditions for PD implementation. It should be made clear, however, that these detailed considerations are part of a serious USG effort to move toward compliance with the PD principles.

Coherence

- Building on the PD and the Presidential Policy Directive on Global Development, agencies should establish a continuing mechanism to ensure the greatest degree of coherence possible among policies and programs affecting the developing countries.

- The USG executive should dialogue with the US Congress on the potential incoherence among legislative restrictions, trade protection amendments, mandates, and earmarks, and the need for greater policy coherence as a critical part of the overall aid effectiveness reform effort. As noted in the QDDR, some of the degrees of freedom afforded the MCC legislatively should be provided to USAID and other implementing agencies. The US Government should resolve the definitional confusion about what kind of foreign assistance is included in the effort to strengthen its aid effectiveness, consistent with Paris Declaration principles.

Part II
What Is Being Done
to Improve Effectiveness?

Chapter 7
The International Health Partnership

Tim Shorten and Shaun Conway

Progress towards achieving the health MDGs remains inadequate. In Africa, for instance, while the maternal mortality rate (MMR) (the number of women who die per 100,000 live births) fell from 850 in 1990 to 620 in 2008, it is off track to reach the target, which requires a 5.5 % annual decline. In South-East Asia, while the MMR fell from 580 to 240 during the same period, it is also still some way off reaching the MDG target (WHO 2010b).

Many of the key constraints facing health systems are still not being *addressed*.

- Each year, 100 million people are pushed into poverty as a result of out-of-pocket expenditures on health (http://www.who.int/health_financing/documents/pb_e_05_2-cata_sys.pdf).
- There are extreme shortages of health workers in 57 countries, 36 of them in Africa (http://www.who.int/workforcealliance/about/hrh_crisis/en/index.html).
- It is estimated that half of all medical equipment in developing countries is not used, either because of a lack of spare parts or maintenance, or because health workers do not know how to use it (Howie et al. 2008).

T. Shorten (✉)
Independent Consultant
e-mail: tjshorten@gmail.com

S. Conway
e-mail: shaun@9needs.net

© Springer Science+Business Media New York 2015
E. Beracochea (ed.), *Improving Aid Effectiveness in Global Health*,
DOI 10.1007/978-1-4939-2721-0_7

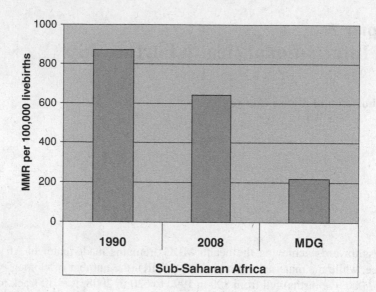

Although the last two decades have seen a substantial increase in development assistance for health from $5 billion in 1990 to $21.8 billion in 2007 (Institute for Health Metrics and Evaluation 2009), global and domestic investment in health is *insufficient*. Estimates of funds needed to reach the health MDGs and ensure access to critical interventions in 49 low-income countries suggest that, 'on average (unweighted), these countries will need to spend a little more than US$ 60 per capita by 2015, considerably more than the US$ 32 they are currently spending' (WHO 2010a). International funding is also *unpredictable*. For example, in Burkina Faso, per capita health aid fluctuated from US$ 4 to US$ 10 and back down to US$ 8 between 2003 and 2006. Lack of predictability is an important problem, both in terms of timely disbursement of aid and the tendency for donors to make short-term financial commitments. Lack of predictability is damaging not only because it reduces the value of aid by 15–20 % (Kharas 2008), but it can also increase fiscal and monetary instability in recipient countries, which can heighten inflation (Osakwe 2008).

Increases in health aid have occurred in parallel with a proliferation of global health actors. This has brought with it concerns about harmonization and alignment of donor programs with country priorities. Dodd et al. (2007) state: '… *there are now well over a 100 major international organizations involved in health, far more than in any other sector, and literally hundreds of channels for delivering health aid*'. Most donors have their own approaches and procedures that place substantial demands on fragile recipient country health systems (McCoy et al. 2009), which risks fragmentation of services and duplication of effort (see diagram below (DFID 2008)).

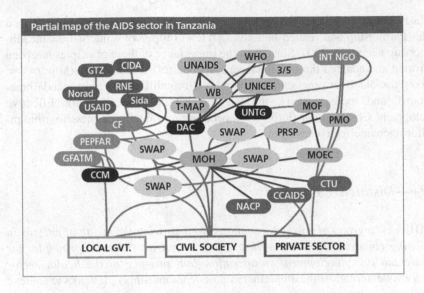

Partial map of the AIDS sector in Tanzania

The International Health Partnership (IHP+) as a Solution

Paris, Accra, Busan

Many national and international initiatives have been launched with the objective of addressing the issues described above. The Paris Declaration on aid effectiveness set out five key principles for improving aid effectiveness.

Five shared principles with actions to make aid more effective

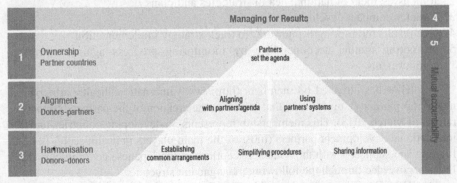

Source: AID EFFECTIVENESS 2005-10: PROGRESS IN IMPLEMENTING THE PARIS DECLARATION (OECD), pp18

The health sector adopted the Paris Declaration with the launch of the International Health Partnership and related initiatives (IHP+) (http://www.internationalhealth-partnership.net/en/) in 2007. Since then the importance of these principles has been reaffirmed and adapted through the Accra Agenda for Action (2008) (http://www.oecd.org/dac/aideffectiveness/theaccrahighlevelforumhlf3andtheaccraagendaforaction.htm), and more recently, through the Busan Partnership for Effective Development Co-operation (http://www.oecd.org/dac/aideffectiveness/fourthhighlevelforumonaideffectiveness.htm).

IHP+—Distinctive Features

The IHP+ is '*a group of partners committed to improving the health of citizens in developing countries. Partners work together to put international principles for effective aid and development co-operation into practice in the health sector* (http://www.internationalhealthpartnership.net/en/about-ihp/)'. It works to achieve the following outcomes:

- Better use of existing funds through improved partner coordination; increased investment in national health strategies
- Country ownership—stronger government leadership in sector coordination
- Reduced burden on developing countries, allowing increased focus on implementing the national health strategy
- And through all of the above, to contribution to better results

It seeks to achieve these through increasing support for one national health strategy, through five distinct workstreams:

1. Support to national planning processes
2. Joint assessment of national health strategies and plans
3. Country compact development
4. One results monitoring framework, to track strategy implementation
5. Promoting mutual accountability by monitoring progress against compact commitments

The IHP+ has attracted 63 members (http://www.internationalhealthpartnership.net/en/ihp-partners/), up from 26 that joined at the creation of the partnership (accurate as of March 2013). This membership represents 36 developing countries and 29 international development partners (most of the main players in health sector policy, funding and support—with the notable exceptions of the Japanese government). The IHP+ is governed through the following managament structure:

The IHP+ Core Team is co-hosted by WHO and the World Bank. It manages the IHP+ work plan, budget and communications, under the oversight of the Steering Committee. It takes forward Steering Committee decisions, organizes Steering Committee, Reference Group and Country Health Teams Meetings, and facilitates Working Group meetings. IHP+ mainly works through staff of partner organizations to implement the agreed "http://www.internationalhealthpartnership.net/fileadmin/

uploads/ihp/Documents/About_IHP_/mgt_arrangemts___docs/IHP__work_ programme_2014_2015.pdf" plan of work.

The IHP+ Steering Committee is responsible for setting overall strategic directions and oversight of IHP+. It approves the IHP+ work plan and budget. It approves IHP+ Working Groups, reviews their recommendations and agrees on actions to be taken. It meets twice a year and has 16 members including six countries, four multi-laterals, four bi-laterals and two CSOs.

The IHP+ Reference Group supports the IHP+ Core Team in implementing the IHP+ work-plan. It serves as a forum for information exchange and collaboration. Members include senior technical staff from the institutions on the Steering Committee and others. Teleconferences are held alternate months.

IHP+ Working Groups are time-limited groups of technical experts, drawn from countries, agencies and CSOs. The group develops collective guidance and/or recommendations on specific topics related to development effectiveness in health. The Country Health Teams Meeting is a meeting of all IHP+ signatories at least once every two years. Partners review progress to improve development effectiveness in health, share lessons from experience and debate new issues. Through its membership and governance structures, the IHP+ provides a unique platform for the promotion and implementation of aid effectiveness principles in the health sector. It is valued for the safe, impartial space that it provides for a broad range of stakeholders to engage in dialogue, learning, and mutual accountability.

The concept of compacts, which is at the heart of the IHP+—both through the IHP+ Global Compact and through country compacts—is important in one of the key defining features of the IHP+: its focus on accountability. To become a member of the IHP+, a government or organization must sign the IHP+ Global Compact, and in doing so agree to a set of principles and commitments, including to be held accountable for implementation of those commitments. This was intended to happen through two mechanisms: (1) annual ministerial level review of progress (last held in February 2009), which has subsequently been replaced by Country Health Sector Team meetings (held approximately every 2 years, most recently in Cambodia in December 2014); (2) an annual independent assessment of individual and collective progress in implementing the Global Compact commitments—which has been undertaken by IHP+ Results since 2009, and results of which are summarized below.

IHP+ and SWAps

Many have asked what is the difference between the IHP+ and health Sector Wide Approaches (SWAps). The IHP+ has responded to this through acknowledging the similarities—the basic principles are the same, and recognizing that in some cases the IHP+ has helped revive an existing SWAp. But the IHP+ has also stressed that the IHP+ is different in a number of important ways:

- It is intended to foster more debate
- It is explicitly built around compact commitments to support the national

- It facilitates the inclusion of new partners
- It works to enable greater harmonization across agencies through the development of tools and procedures
- It includes a stronger emphasis on mutual accountability—including through global leverage via the IHP+ Global Compact

It is clear that the principles are broadly the same, as are the objectives. But the IHP+ offers the possibility of greater collaboration, not least at the international level and, through its governance structures and commitment to mutual accountability, provides additional levers that can give 'teeth' to SWAp like arrangements.

Transparency and Accountability

Background

The IHP+'s commitment to mutual accountability led to the creation of an agreed framework for monitoring IHP+ implementation (described below), which has in turn promoted transparency. At the same time, there has been an increasing recognition about the importance of transparency and accountability as means through which aid or development effectiveness can be improved. This movement may have been driven by growing recognition that the Paris Declaration principles of mutual accountability and managing for results had been given least attention (http://www. oecd.org/dac/aideffectiveness/2008surveyonmonitoringtheparisdeclaration.htm; http://www.oecd.org/development/evaluationofdevelopmentprogrammes/dcdndep/ evaluationoftheimplementationoftheparisdeclaration.htm), by a growing body of evidence showing that the Paris Declaration targets were off-track, and by downward pressures of the economic crisis on aid budgets. It has though contributed to the emergency of a number of initiatives related to transparency and accountability:

- The International Aid Transparency Initiative (IATI) (http://www.aidtransparency.net/)
- The UN Commission on Information and Accountability for Women's and Children's Health (http://www.everywomaneverychild.org/resources/accountability-commission)

The Accra Agenda for Action also emphasized the importance of predictability of aid (The Paris Declaration on Aid Effectiveness and the Accra Agenda for Action, p. 21), in order to enable developing countries to effectively plan and manage their development programmes over the short and medium term. Lack of accountability and transparency are critical shortcomings: many development agencies reveal little about how and why decisions are made and are more accountable to donors and tax payers in high-income countries than to recipients or beneficiaries in low income countries (Haan 2009). Many commentators further suggest that donor government national security, economic, and foreign policy interests drive and explain donor behavior rather than the health needs of people in low-income countries (Labonte and Gagnon 2010).

Predictability can be ensured through a number of means, including through greater transparency (reporting aid on governments budgets), as well as longer-term commitments and disbursing funds in line with agreed schedules. Predictability is particularly important in the health sector as key constraints on achieving better health outcomes, such as health worker salaries, rely on long-term investments and interruptions in financial flows can have catastrophic consequences.

References

Collier, P. (1999). 'Aid dependency': A critique. *Journal of African Economies, 8*(4), 528–545.

DFID. (2008). *Achieving universal access—Evidence for action* (p. 81).

Dodd, R., et al. (2007). *Aid effectiveness and health: Making health systems work* (Wolfensohn Centre for Development, Working Paper 3). Geneva, Switzerland: WHO.

Haan, A. (2009). *Aid: The drama, the fiction, and does it work?* (Working Papers General Series No. 488). Institute of Social Studies.

Howie, S., et al. (2008). Beyond good intentions: Lessons on equipment donation from an African hospital. *Bulletin of the World Heath Organisation, 86*(1), 54.

Institute for Health Metrics and Evaluation. (2009). *Financing global health: Tracking development assistance for health.*

Kharas, H. (2008). *Measuring the cost of aid volatility* (Working Paper No. 3). Wolfensohn Centre for Development. Washington, DC: Brookings Institute.

Labonte, R., & Gagnon, M. (2010). Framing health and foreign policy: Lessons for global health diplomacy. *Global Health, 6*(14), 1–22.

Lancaster, C. (1999). Aid effectiveness in Africa: The unfinished agenda. *Journal of African Economies, 8*(4), 487–503.

McCoy, D., Chand, S., & Sridhar, D. (2009). Global health funding: How much, where it comes from and where it goes. *Health Policy and Planning, 24*(6), 407–417.

Mwega, F. M. (2009). *A case study of aid effectiveness in Kenya: Volatility and fragmentation of foreign aid, with a focus on health.* http://r.search.yahoo.com/

Osakwe, P. (2008). *Aid predictability, ownership and development in Africa.* Washington, DC: OECD. Retrieved March 15, 2011, from www.oecd.org/dataoecd/54/33/40718167.pdf

WHO. (2010a). *Health systems financing, the path to universal coverage* (World Health Report, p. xxi). Retrieved from http://www.who.int/whr/2010/en/index.html

WHO. (2010b). *Trends in maternal mortality: 1990 to 2008, estimates developed by WHO, UNICEF, UNFPA, and The World Bank* (pp. 2 and 39). Retrieved from www.unfpa.org/webdav/site/global/shared/documents/publications/2010/trends_matmortality90-08.pdf

Retrieved December 6, 2012, from http://www.internationalhealthpartnership.net/en/

Retrieved December 6, 2012, from http://www.internationalhealthpartnership.net/en/ihp-partners/

Retrieved December 6, 2012, from http://www.oecd.org/dac/aideffectiveness/fourthhighlevelforumonaideffectiveness.htm

Retrieved December 6, 2012, from http://www.oecd.org/dac/aideffectiveness/theaccrahighlevelforumhlf3andtheaccraagendaforaction.htm

Retrieved December 7, 2012, from http://www.oecd.org/dac/aideffectiveness/2008surveyonmonitoringtheparisdeclaration.htm; Retrieved December 7, 2012, from http://www.oecd.org/development/evaluationofdevelopmentprogrammes/dcdndep/evaluationoftheimplementationoftheparisdeclaration.htm

Retrieved March 25, 2013, from http://www.aidtransparency.net/

Retrieved March 25, 2013, from http://www.everywomaneverychild.org/resources/accountability-commission

Retrieved March 25, 2013, from http://www.internationalhealthpartnership.net/en/about-ihp/

Retrieved March 25, 2013, from http://www.internationalhealthpartnership.net/en/news-events/
    past-events/article/fourth-ihp-country-health-sector-teams-meeting-nairobi-kenya-11-14-
    december-2012-accelerating-progress-sustaining-results-324772/
Retrieved October 12, 2012, from http://www.who.int/health_financing/documents/pb_e_05_
    2-cata_sys.pdf
Retrieved October 12, 2012, from http://www.who.int/workforcealliance/about/hrh_crisis/en/
    index.html

Chapter 8
Paying for Results: The Global Fund and the Role of Civil Society Organizations

Cristina de Nicolás Izquierdo and Ruth Hope

The Global Fund to fight AIDS, Tuberculosis, and Malaria [the Global Fund] was created in 2002 to dramatically increase resources to fight three of the world's most devastating diseases and to direct those resources to areas of greatest need.[1] Ten years after issuing its first grants to country programs, it had become the main multilateral funder in global health, channeling approximately US$ 3 billion annually.[2] Country ownership has been a core principle of the Global Fund since its creation. Initially, the Global Fund established country structures and systems for grant oversight, separating this function from grant implementation—a proven good governance practice. A new innovative structure, the country coordinating mechanism[3] or CCM, that includes representatives from both the public and private sectors, including governments, multilateral or bilateral agencies, civil society[4] (local and international), and private sector, has responsibility for preparing, submitting, and

---

[1] *The Framework Document of the Global Fund to Fight AIDS, Tuberculosis and Malaria* (2001). Key Global Fund documents can be accessed at http://www.theglobalfund.org/en/library/.

[2] Section 1: Overview, *Global Fund Governance Handbook* (2014). http://www.theglobalfund.org/documents/core/guides/Core_GovernanceHandbookSection1Overview_Handbook_en/. Accessed February 27, 2015.

[3] *A note on Global Fund terminology* is available at: http://www.theglobalfund.org/documents/core/guides/Core_GovernanceHandbookVocabulary_List_en. Accessed February 27, 2015.

[4] The GFATM adopted the UN definition of 'civil society' on 8th Policy and Strategy Committee Meeting, Geneva September 2007. Civil society is defined by the UN as associations of citizens (outside their families, friends and businesses) entered into voluntarily to advance their interests, ideas and ideologies. The term does not include the private sector or governing (the public sector).

C. de Nicolás Izquierdo
Independent consultant, formerly with RGH, Yakarta, Indonesia
e-mail: cristinadenicolas@gmail.com

R. Hope (✉)
Center for Reproductive Health, HIV & AIDS, and Gender Equality,
Realizing Global Health, Inc., Fairfax, VA, USA
e-mail: ruth@realizingglobalhealth.com

© Springer Science+Business Media New York 2015
E. Beracochea (ed.), *Improving Aid Effectiveness in Global Health*,
DOI 10.1007/978-1-4939-2721-0_8

overseeing proposals for funding. The CCM applies for funding, governs the distribution of resources, and oversees program implementation by the grant principal recipient and any sub-recipients. In May 2014, the Global Fund updated its Governance Handbook detailing key features of its newly revised Global Funding Model and how to obtain funding.[5]

A Country Coordinating Mechanism in Session

One afternoon a CCM was meeting with two items on the agenda: one, to initiate dialogue about the populations that should be prioritized in the HIV proposal the CCM was planning to submit to the Global Fund; and two, the election of new CCM officers from the various constituency representatives serving on the CCM. After the chairperson had confirmed a quorum was present and opened the meeting, the CCM members approved the agenda and began discussing which key populations the new grant should focus on, with involvement of all the appropriate sectors.

The election of new CCM officers followed facilitated by an ad hoc election committee that the CCM Secretariat had established and guided. Candidates had previously submitted their candidacies and the CCM proceeded with the elections, first of the chairperson, and second of the vice chairperson. All CCM members took their turn to place their ballot papers in the transparent ballot box for each position. While placing his ballot in the ballot box, the representative of the Ministry of Justice looked at his peers with a big smile—obviously excited by the occasion—and said: "This is the second time in my life I voted. The first time was to elect our new Parliament."

The CCM chairperson gave the floor in turn to all the constituency representatives including civil society which was represented by a person living-with-HIV, a man who has sex-with-men, and a sex worker. The one hour discussion concluded that focusing on most-at-risk-populations should be a priority for the country—as reflected in the national strategy—but there was a need to better identify the key priority populations. The civil society representatives advocated for a formal presentation of the country's reported HIV statistics. The presentation showed the most up-to-date epidemiological data and demonstrated the need to prioritize both continuing treatment and giving special attention to prevention interventions for sex workers and their clients.

The representative of the Ministry of Women's Affairs was elected as the new chairperson and the representative from human rights national NGO was elected vice chairperson.

---

[5] *Governance Handbook* (2014). http://www.theglobalfund.org/en/documents/governance/. Accessed February 27, 2015.

The Global Fund: A New Model for Development Assistance

Experiences like that described in the box—increasingly common in many countries now—were totally unknown before 2002 when the Global Fund to fight AIDS, Tuberculosis, and Malaria changed the face of official development assistance (ODA). Traditional multilateral and bilateral mechanisms had failed to contain the three diseases. Mortality was increasing and civil society activists were demanding more funding for treatment of AIDS, as antiretroviral drugs were beyond national ministry of health budgets, and prohibitively expensive for individuals in developing countries to buy.

The Global Fund offers a partnership model for development assistance that has scaled up quickly and effectively to accelerate progress toward the three Millennium Development Goals for health—MDG 4: reduced child mortality; MDG5: reduced maternal mortality; and MDG 6: reduced mortality due to Malaria, Tuberculosis, and AIDS.

Partnership runs throughout the Global Fund governance structures, with the Global Fund Board, committees, and advisory groups each including representatives of the corporate sector, private foundations, nongovernmental organizations, and communities affected by the three diseases who all hold equal decision-making power with government representatives.

In line with Paris Declaration on Aid Effectiveness, the Global Fund grants are:

- Country-owned—country stakeholders have full ownership of their programs and results
- Demand-driven—grants are funded on technical merit, disease burden, and poverty levels
- Performance-based—grant funding is strictly contingent on achieving results. Program implementers identify indicators to measure progress
- Inclusive—governance involves governments, civil society (including affected communities), the private sector, and development partners
- Transparent and accountable with dedication to efficiency—all funding and performance information is placed in the public domain with the ultimate objective of ensuring that the funds allocated to a country are used to serve the populations that most need the services.

The Role of Civil Society on the CCM—Improving Health Program Effectiveness

Civil society participation in CCMs is often regarded as one of the most innovative features of the Global Fund, although it has often presented challenges and difficulties. Civil society is heterogeneous with many alliances and perspectives, thus issues of representation are complex. Those who are most marginalized in any society are rarely represented and may thus be further disadvantaged. For example, too often the rights of key affected populations such as sex workers, men-who-have-sex-with-men, transgendered persons, and injecting drug users are not recognized; their needs are not given priority, in some countries their risk behaviors are criminalized, and they are excluded from crucial information and services. Their representation on CCMs and their ability to influence decision-making can be a huge challenge.

There are countries where representation of key affected populations on the CCM appears *de iure*, but in practice is tokenism.[6] However, globally civil society representatives believe that such challenges are outweighed by the potential benefits of involving key populations, including a public forum to overcome stigma, stronger country ownership, dialogue between government and key populations leading to a better focus for interventions. Communities living with and affected by the three diseases have been at the forefront of advocacy for greater ODA for addressing AIDS, Tuberculosis, and Malaria and in defining effective responses nationally, regionally, and internationally.

The Global Fund itself has progressively advocated for a greater involvement of and the relevance of most-at-risk-populations on the CCM in order to shift the way of thinking about the diseases, and HIV in particular. Their participation directly challenges stigma and discrimination, while at the same time recognizes that people-living-with-HIV and other most at risk populations can be empowered to reduce their risk and take the lead in the grant design and oversight processes, ensuring that national strategies and programs best meet their needs.

That the CCM described in the story above concluded that there was need to prioritize preventative interventions among sex workers and their clients is an example of the active role key populations can play. It also shows how ensuring key populations are always involved in the development of plans and democratic decision-making positively influences the containment of the diseases. Involving key populations also demonstrates democratic practices of inclusiveness, transparency, and participation and is a proof of respect for human rights in global health.

Within the Global Fund governance model, the health sector must work with civil society encouraging dialogue and understanding between people who have not previously had strong working relations. Through working together with civil society, a ministry of health might better develop its services and programs to address the greatest need. Ministries have to work with civil society to both address and draw on the social dimensions of health behavior, to foster wider constituencies for health rights, and to strengthen public accountability and responsiveness within health systems. However, civil society does not speak with one voice and perspectives differ between different interest groups. For diversity not to weaken civil society legitimacy to express differing positions, collaboration has to be close and civil society must engage with government officials to better understand their reality.

---

[6] *Tokenism*—Governments appoint a token woman or token person-living-with-HIV. This token effort is usually intended to create a false appearance of inclusiveness and deflect accusations of discrimination.

Civil society representation brings wide-ranging experience, knowledge, and perspectives to a CCM and, if empowered, its representatives can share their realities with the other constituency representatives. Civil society representatives can contribute the "voice" of marginalized constituencies to governance and strategy development. Governments and their development partners have often previously overlooked this voice—yet engagement of all communities is vital to ensuring full country ownership. Civil society should play an integral role in the design and implementation of country health plans. Civil society involvement can also be crucial to holding development partners accountable for delivering on their commitments and achieving improved health results. The Global Fund, through CCMs, has created effective structures for meaningful engagement of civil society in ownership of improved health results and the means to achieve these results.

In 2007, the Global Fund documented how civil society organizations (CSOs) in Latin America created *El Observatorio Latino* to act as a watchdog over Global Fund projects in the region, to identify technical support needs for CSOs involved in implementing Global Fund grants, and to ensure strong representation of civil society throughout Global Fund processes.[7] In Peru, CSOs played a critical role in delivering treatment to hard-to-reach populations, and in Ukraine, the All Ukrainian Network of People Living with HIV/AIDS played an important role in implementing care, treatment, and support initiatives that were part of a Round 6 grant.[8] NGOs have a good track record as Principal Recipients (PRs) of Global Fund Grants managing grants. Civil society organizations have proven to be effective grant implementers. Year-end figures from 2006 showed that 83 % of civil society PRs were rated A or B1. Civil society received the largest percentage of A and B1-ratings (28 % A-rated and 55 % B1-rated) in comparison to other PRs.[9] In Zambia, the Global Fund had multiple PRs for an HIV grant to spread the workload among governments, NGOs, and faith-based organizations.[10] A peer-reviewed study found Global Fund support to CSOs in the Former Soviet Union resulted in the professionalization of CSOs, which increased confidence from government and increased CSO influence on policies relating to HIV/AIDS and illicit drugs.[11] The International

---

[7] *An Evolving Partnership: The Global Fund and Civil Society in the Fight Against AIDS, Tuberculosis and Malaria* (2007). http://www.theglobalfund.org/documents/civil_society/ CivilSociety_AnEvolvingPartnership_Report_en/ Accessed February 27, 2015.

[8] *Ibid.*

[9] *An evolving partnership: The Global Fund and Civil Society in the Fight Against AIDS, Tuberculosis and Malaria* https://www.google.com/url?q=http://www.theglobalfund.org/documents/civil_society/CivilSociety_AnEvolvingPartnership_Report_en/&sa=U&ei= aLomUeGFCI_J0AGq0IC4DA&ved=0CAcQFjAA&client=internal-uds-cse&usg= AFQjCNHvUd71QvS_eOQ4bC2ab01F4pGkFw. Accessed February 27, 2015.

[10] *Ibid.*

[11] *Has Global Fund support for civil society advocacy in the Former Soviet Union established meaningful engagement or 'a lot of jabber about nothing'?* Harmer et al. Health Policy Plan. (2012). doi: 10.1093/heapol/czs060.

HIV/AIDS Alliance has documented 9 illustrative case studies of effective community systems strengthening in partnership with CSOs in Cambodia, India, Mongolia, Peru, Senegal, Somalia, Thailand, Ukraine, and Zambia.[12] By June 2010, 18 % of Global Fund disbursements for AIDS grants were through civil society PRs; that is more than $150 million on average per year. Most CSO PRs have exceeded performance targets. Indigenous organizations, rather than international NGOs, have managed 57 % of Global Fund disbursements received by civil society PRs.[13]

In many countries, NGOs contribute to improved healthcare by providing services tailored to community needs and adapted to local conditions; they advocate for equity in access to healthcare and some provide services that are more efficient and thus less expensive than government services. Non-governmental organizations may also have technical expertise over a range of areas from healthcare planning to service delivery. Frequently NGOs innovate and disseminate good practices to other NGOs and government providers. Non-governmental organizations often contribute to public understanding of health issues by enhancing both the quality and quantity of information available to people in the community and providing forum for public discussion. The Global Fund disseminates UNAIDS' guidance for supporting community-based responses to AIDS, TB, and Malaria by including community systems strengthening in Global Fund proposals.[14]

Another important aspect that many NGOs bring to healthcare is a human rights approach, viewing access to healthcare as a basic human right. Many NGOs promote and use human rights instruments and actions in health. They monitor health and human rights issues and advocate for patients' rights, women's and children's health rights, reproductive health rights, and reduction of occupational health risks. The Global Fund Strategy 2012–2013 emphasizes human rights through its strategic objective 4, integrating human rights considerations throughout the grant cycle.[15] It seeks to increase investment in programs that address human-rights-related barriers to access and to ensure it does not fund programs that infringe human rights.

Thus, the CCM embodies the Global Fund principles and commitment at country level to civil society engagement in planning, service provision, and governance. Involvement of civil society results in more democratic decision-making for improved and effective programs.

---

[12] *Civil society success on the ground. Community systems strengthening and dual-track financing*: *nine illustrative case studies* (2008). http://www.allianceindia.org/wp-content/uploads/2014/09/2014_AllianceIndia_Civil-Society-Success-on-the-Ground-Community-Systems-Strengthening-and-Dual-Track-Financing-Nine-Illustrative-Case-Studies.pdf. Accessed February 27, 2015.

[13] *Mapping of funding mechanisms and main sources of funding for the community response to HIV and AIDS*, International HIV/AIDS Alliance (2010). http://www.whatspreventingprevention.org/wp-content/uploads/2011/04/CSOandAIDSfunding.pdf. Accessed February 27, 2015.

[14] *Supporting community based responses to AIDS, TB and Malaria*: *A guidance tool for including Community Systems Strengthening in Global Fund proposals*. http://www.theglobalfund.org/documents/civil_society/CivilSociety_UNAIDSCSSGuidance_Tool_en/. Accessed February 27, 2015.

[15] *The Global Fund Strategy 2012–2016: Investing for Impact*. http://www.theglobalfund.org/documents/core/strategies/Core_GlobalFund_Strategy_en/. Accessed February 27, 2015.

Governance: The Democratic Governing Processes to Improve a Nation's Health

Governance has been defined as "the process of decision-making and the process by which decisions are implemented."[16] Good governance of Global Fund grants is an imperative for the CCM to achieve the greatest health gain for the investment through efficient management and effective programming.

> *Good governance* requires transparency, probity, and accountability in decision-making and implementation of decisions

Good governance is a democratic process characterized by participation and inclusiveness—men and women, government and civil society, private sector and development partners; legal frameworks that are enforced impartially; transparency ensuring that decisions follow the rules and law; responsiveness to needs within a reasonable timeframe; consensus—conciliation of the different interests to reach a broad agreement on what is in the best interest of the whole community and how this can be achieved; equity—commitment to providing access to healthcare for minorities and those with the greatest need[17]; effectiveness and efficiency; and accountability—a key requirement. The CCM is accountable for its management of the country's Global Fund grant to the public and to its institutional stakeholders, including the Global Fund. Corruption—the abuse of public authority or trust for private benefit—is closely linked to poor governance. The Global Fund's partnership model of governance mandates good governance of its Grants by inclusion of all stakeholders, not just government, in decision-making and oversight of decision implementation by the CCM at all stages of the grant cycle.

Civil Society Involvement is Central in the Global Fund's Funding Model

The Global Fund's Funding Model (FM)[18] offers stream-lined grant awards for strategic investment for maximum impact to countries with highest disease burden and least ability to pay for the response, with predictable funding for 3 years. Applicants

---

[16]*What is good governance*, United Nations ESCAP. http://www.unescap.org/pdd/prs/ProjectActivities/Ongoing/gg/governance.asp. Accessed February 12, 2013.

[17]Equity is crucial to CCM governance as representative democracy does not necessarily mean that the concerns of the most vulnerable in society are taken into consideration in decision making.

[18]http://www.theglobalfund.org/documents/core/newfundingmodel/Core_NewFundingModel_Brochure_en/. Accessed February 27, 2015 and related presentation:http://www.theglobalfund.org/en/videos/2014-03-06_An_Overview_of_the_New_Funding_Model/. Accessed February 27, 2015.

will submit grant requests within a previously agreed funding envelope in the form of a "Concept Note." The FM will reward high impact, well-performing programs. Whether for health systems strengthening or services addressing the three diseases, to be strategic and attain greatest impact grants must focus on equity: effectively addressing the greatest need within each grant recipient country.

On January 29, 2013, the Communities Living with HIV, TB and affected by Malaria Delegation (Communities Delegation) of the Board of the Global Fund[19] reaffirmed that community involvement has to be central to the FM that streamlines grant awards.[20] Representatives from national, regional, and international networks of communities living with and/or affected by the three diseases identified opportunities and reaffirmed the critical role that communities continue to play in Global Fund processes to ensure that investment focuses on the right interventions for the populations. "The new Funding Model presents a host of new entry points for communities affected by the three diseases to engage and meaningfully participate—both at the national level and globally." "The capacity and expertise of [people living with the diseases] constituencies must be an integral component of making the new Funding Model work and scaling up the successes we have seen in HIV, TB and Malaria." The Executive Director of the Global Fund committed that from 2013, communities living with and affected by the diseases will help monitor and implement the FM, which will better support health and community workers who treat and prevent the three diseases. It will also better advocate human rights in the response to the three diseases.[21]

---

[19] Supported by the Global Network of People Living with HIV (GNP+).

[20] Announcement   http://www.theglobalfund.org/en/mediacenter/announcements/2013-01-29_Community_Involvement_Central_in_Global_Fund_New_Funding_Model/. Accessed February 27, 2015.

[21] *ibid.*

Chapter 9
NGOs Putting the Paris Declaration to Work

James N. Gribble

Key Messages

NGOs and the Paris Declaration

- NGOs have many roles in implementing the Paris Declaration
- While NGOs are generally driven by their institutional missions, their vision can overlap with the Paris Declaration

Country Ownership

- NGOs often work for this goal, focusing on local ownership of issues and solutions
- Technical assistance contributes to local ownership
- Engagement of governments with local stakeholders can be challenging

Alignment

- A focus on a common vision and measures of success are priorities to many NGOs
- NGOs rarely have a place at the table with donors and governments
- Using and strengthening existing systems and strengthening capacity are central to many NGOs

J.N. Gribble, Sc.D. (✉)
Futures Group, Washington, DC, USA
e-mail: JGribble@futuresgroup.com

© Springer Science+Business Media New York 2015
E. Beracochea (ed.), *Improving Aid Effectiveness in Global Health*,
DOI 10.1007/978-1-4939-2721-0_9

Harmonization

- Competing agendas among donors can lead to difficult coordination
- However, there are examples of improved coordination among donors and governments

Managing for Results

- Risk of too much focus on targets and not enough on sustainable development
- Development is not a linear process and results need to be flexible enough to recognize that issues come up
- Results are usually measured at the national level, but increasingly, decisions are made at the subnational level

Mutual Accountability

- Parliamentary oversight is critical to development
- Civil society and stakeholders have a critical role in development, but their capacity needs to be strengthened to improve their effectiveness

Introduction

The Paris Declaration reflects a new way for how development partners think about their work. Yet what happens at high levels—such as the relationships that evolve between governments, donors, and international agencies—can easily stay at that level unless explicit plans are developed to ensure that the agreed-upon principles are actually carried out at an operational level. Governments may agree to and affirm the principles of the Paris Declaration, but the proof of commitment must also be found in the way that development efforts are carried out.

Perspectives from an NGO. Non-governmental organizations (NGOs) play a critical role in carrying out the development agendas of donors and partner governments. They exist to advance missions, taking on roles and responsibilities that the public sector cannot—and often should not—undertake. NGOs come in many varieties, large and small groups, national and international, and they serve a range of functions, including the provision of different types of services, advocacy and watchdog, and capacity building. An NGO like the Population Reference Bureau (PRB), with a mission of "inform, empower, advance", serves a role of synthesizing technical data and analysis and presenting it in user-friendly formats to support informed policymaking in the areas of population and health. This chapter reflects the experience of PRB in responding to the Paris Declaration, examining experiences and insights from the executive level to technical program staff to field staff charged with coordinating and leading program activities on the ground. The view is unique and not intended to be representative of NGOs in general; instead, it reflects how the work of one organization has responded to an emerging paradigm brought on by the Paris Declaration.

Inside an NGO. To understand the perspective presented in this chapter, it may be helpful to understand more about what staff do and how the organization operates—because no two NGOs are alike. Within PRB, the International Programs division includes approximately 20 individuals who carry out a range of activities—from writing, to training, to working with journalists. The staff brings a variety of backgrounds—most have worked and lived overseas, and all bring a commitment to improving the health and well-being of people in developing countries. We work on multiple projects and activities that look at a variety of health and population issues. As I finalize this chapter, I am preparing for two trips to Africa and one to Latin America—far more than my usual travel schedule, but often the schedule is dictated by work needs and opportunities. Many of my colleagues are on the road a lot—it is hard to do work in international development while sitting in at a desk in Washington, DC. And while the workloads may be challenging and the hours long, part of what attracts us to this type of work is that our organization's mission inspires us and challenges us—to inform key groups with information, empower them to act with vision and strategy, and so that they can advance a policy environment of improved health and well-being of communities and nations.

Responding to a Changing Unilateral Environment

Understanding the playing field. As an NGO in the field of population and reproductive health, PRB has been attentive to the international agreements over the past 20 years that have shaped our field's priorities. The 1994 International Conference on Population and Development (ICPD) Programme of Action shifted the way population issues had been viewed—moving away from population control toward a vision of helping women and men achieve the number and timing of children they want to have. More recently, the Millennium Development Goals (MDGs) have provided a framework that has guided priorities, investments, and outcomes in health and development; though population and reproductive health are not explicitly included among the original goals, increasing attention has focused on the role these two areas can play in achieving the MDG targets. As an NGO actor in the population and reproductive health field, PRB has supported the vision and objectives established by both the ICPD and the MDGs.

A game changer? In contrast, the Paris Declaration has received far less attention in the population field, and this may be due to a few reasons. The Paris Declaration focuses on processes rather than specific outcomes. As a new paradigm for how development assistance is carried out, clear guidance for implementing the Declaration needs to come from the donors and governments who have signed the agreement. Because the goals focus on *how* to carry out work rather than *what* to do to address specific development issues, the technical work conducted by NGOs like PRB can easily be unaffected by the Paris Declaration—at least on the surface. Our measures of success relate to seeing differences in policy and programmatic indicators, with much less emphasis on the types of goals included in the Paris Declaration. Yet as we look at the principles underpinning the Paris Declaration, it is clear that its language and concepts are permeating into the ways we carry out our work.

Perspectives inside an NGO. Even though the Paris Declaration was signed into effect in 2005, there has been relatively little emphasis on getting NGOs in the population field to understand it and focus attention on it. In fact, reading the Paris Declaration can easily leave NGO staff wondering what their role in its implementation is: Do we still providing technical assistance? Do we still strengthen systems and improve capacity? Do we still synthesize information and share lessons learned across countries? The experiences of my NGO colleagues reflect varying degrees of understanding what the Paris Declaration is and what it is intended to achieve; their experiences are based largely on their working with national governments. In other cases, my colleagues had little knowledge of the Paris Declaration, but certainly saw how it is being implemented through the work we do and the attitudes and language that donors are increasingly using.

The following sections reflect on the five principles of the Paris Declaration, and examine how they are shaping the work PRB carries out; in some cases, one can see a direct influence; in others, it seems to have little impact because the principles focus on high-level relationships.

Country Ownership

Reaching agreement. Country ownership is one of the principles that has received broad coverage and is well understood and accepted. The ideas of consultation and participation of civil society and the private sector are central to today's efforts to create a more enabling environment for population and reproductive health policies and programs. Stakeholder engagement is critical to advancing development efforts at all levels—national, subnational, and local. And NGOs, civil society, and the private sector are taking on increasingly larger roles because there is awareness that all sectors can make a significant contribution to advancing the population and health development agenda.

Principles take root. The principle of country ownership is one that NGOs clearly appreciate and understand. Efforts to garner public input for World Bank poverty reduction strategies serve as an example of how participation has become a priority among high-level donors. More recently, USAID's Global Health Initiative explicitly calls for ensuring that development efforts reflect the priorities that governments identify for their own countries. In general, since the approval of the Paris Declaration, we have increasingly noticed calls for better engagement of national governments in requests for proposals. While not explicitly calling for the implementation of the Paris Declaration, there is a general acceptance on the part of donors that country ownership is at the crux of development.

An example from Africa. Colleagues working at the regional level in sub-Saharan Africa have long noted that regional efforts have attempted to support existing national policies and would help harmonize strategies and monitoring indicators. In fact, a recent effort among donors and governments of West African countries to prioritize family planning in the region has explicitly used language of the Paris Declaration. At the same time, in our work at the country level, we notice that government officials and local development partners have also appropriated the language of country ownership as part of their roles in carrying out development programs.

Stronger systems. Our goal as an NGO in providing technical assistance is to strengthen systems and capacity so that in-country collaborators can understand the issues, map their own strategies to improve situations, and ultimately take ownership of the challenges and solutions to their own development issues. For example, PRB's work to strengthen the capacity of local media, while not necessarily identified as a national development priority, fits well into creating an enabling policy environment for population and reproductive health by drawing attention to existing evidence, challenging decision makers to take responsibility for the issues, and raising awareness among the general public to understand and speak up for effective policies and programs. This type of work ultimately contributes to better health governance, and thus to better overall governance.

A lack of consistency. At the same time, while in-country partners champion country ownership, they do not necessarily embrace all aspects of it, which further poses challenges to NGOs as they try to carry out their work. National governments are generally willing to engage stakeholders in discussion about policy and program needs—thus upholding that aspect of country ownership, but can also put up barriers to achieving a real solution to the problems: delaying the policy approval process; only putting selective parts of policies into practices; and limiting dissemination of policy documents so that people living outside of the national capital do not understand either what the policy addresses or their rights and recourse as citizens for when a policy is not implemented.

Alignment

Strong capacity. Alignment, through referring to the relationship between donors and partners, reflects an attitude of sharing priorities and creating a common vision for achieving longer-term development goals. NGOs like PRB working on development issues recognize the vital role that development strategies play in setting both the tone and priorities for development programs. Alignment plays a critical role for how we approach our work, for without strong systems and developed human capacity, development efforts will not take root and flourish. At the same time, an important aspect of alignment is coming to agreement on a manageable number of indicators that do not overburden institutional capacity and that provide measures of progress toward annual goals and longer-term objectives.

Not at the table. NGOs rarely end up at the bargaining table when it comes to alignment; those efforts usually take place between governments and donors. Yet, NGOs are challenged with implementing activities that reflect aligned priorities. One of the approaches organizations in family planning and reproductive health take is to align our messages with development strategies and to position our priorities in the language used in the strategy documents. For example, efforts to draw attention to the health and economic benefits of family planning consistently turn to national development strategies and make the case for paying attention to population growth as an important component of reaching the established goals. Similarly, on a global basis, reproductive health organizations draw on evidence to show the benefits of family planning programs to achieving the MDGs, which most countries have taken on as a priority.

Linking goals to funding. It is refreshing to work with a partner that is driven, effective, and productive—and has embraced the principle of harmonization. Our experience with groups in both the public and private sectors that work on target-based annual work plans suggests that fostering this type of alignment is healthy and productive, as the organizations see their annual budget linked to achieving target goals. Our work with Kenya's National Council for Population and Development, which operates on such an alignment strategy, results in the agency's knowing what it needs to get done and by when—which means that they have an appropriate set of incentives that are linked to completing their work plan.

Strengthening not duplicating. One of the challenges of alignment is the need to strengthen national systems rather than duplicate them. Whether supply chains to get commodities to the field or data collection systems to provide information for monitoring and evaluation, donors' commitment to the principle of alignment should result in the longer-term investment in national systems, which make development initiatives sustainable in the long run.

Building local capacity. Within the principle of alignment is the commitment to strengthen capacity, which is also one of PRB's priorities. Having worked for years with individuals and institutions to strengthen capacity for effective policy communication around population and reproductive health, we once again see donors talking about capacity building as a priority, but not necessarily putting sufficient resources into it. One of the biggest development challenges the world faces is staff turnover and brain drain. As a result, there is an ongoing need to build individual and institutional capacity to ensure that locally owned development approaches and efforts succeed. At the same time, one of the challenges of capacity development building is that it is more complex than "training"; people need to hear information and apply it in order to take ownership of it. Many training workshops are so rushed that participants may be exposed to skills or content, but do not get enough practice with it to apply it on their own. Most capacity development building seems to occur at the national level, but as countries move forward with decentralization, decision making authority is pushed out to subnational levels. With such changes also comes the need to strengthen the capacity of individuals and institutions at those levels if we expect to see development efforts achieve sustainability. Working in the field, we increasingly hear about decentralization, but rarely hear about or see resources allocated to putting in place both the systems and capacity needed to support these emerging levels of decision making.

Harmonization

Limited coordination. If donors could better coordinate among themselves and with partner governments, development efforts might be better structured and more effective, with less overlap. As it stands, there may be coordination, but it is often difficult to see. It continues to be a challenge as donors replicate each other's efforts, ineffectively divide up priority regions within a country, and fail to rely on their own institutional strengths. In addition, the lack of coordination within donor groups poses challenges, as priorities and activities from the headquarters office may not be in synch with those that regional offices identify. As a result, there can be duplication of efforts and approval of activities that work at odds with each other, which lead to an ineffective use of resources.

Challenges to harmonization. Efforts to harmonize present challenges at multiple levels. Attempts to reach consensus at a global or regional level can be long and arduous and may not be carried out effectively at the national level. One of my colleagues mentioned her involvement on a regional basis to develop a healthcare protocol and curriculum to be carried out by countries in the region. As it turned out, only those countries that received seed grants to implement the new curriculum made any progress. The lack of a monitoring system to assess how well the curriculum and protocol were implemented also meant that there was insufficient leverage to make the agreed-upon changes. Such an attempt to harmonize represent a wellfounded attempt that proved to be less than successful because of insufficient buyin, and inadequate support and systems to see that the changes actually took place.

Effective multilateral collaboration. One aspect of harmonization that has become more visible is increased collaboration among bilateral donors and foundations. Recognizing the need to be mutually supportive and to better leverage scarce resources, there are very positive examples of donor coordination at a global level. The Reproductive Health Supplies Coalition, a global partnership of public, private, and nongovernmental organizations, receives support from multiple donors who collaborate with member organizations to make significant advances on policy and finance issues related to contraceptive commodities and supplies. Similarly the Ouagadougou Partnership—a group of donors working together francophone West African governments to develop strategies for prioritizing family planning and reproductive health efforts in region—also stands out as a recent example of donor harmonization. Although each donor and country has its own separate agenda, the group is trying to take advantage of each donor's comparative advantage to provide funding for the region, working to avert the risk of fragmentation, and need to balance country demands in evolving political climates of decentralization.

Insufficient attention to cross-cutting issues. What NGOs tend to resonate with is the need to harmonize around environmental impact, gender equality, and other cross-cutting issues. Gender is a crucial development agenda, yet it is often relegated to a very secondary position. And understanding the environmental impact of development recognizes that the world is changing and that we all need to be cognizant of how to minimize the adverse consequences of development on the world. As a population and reproductive health NGO, PRB has been actively engaged in these two cross-cutting development issues since before the Paris Declaration. Yet in spite of global commitments to these issues reflected in numerous treaties and agreements, neither donors nor partner governments sufficiently prioritize these two critical aspects of the development agenda.

Managing for Results

Better decision making. While managing for results is not new to NGOs, the way that it is articulated in the Paris Declaration takes the concept in new directions. At the heart of the principle is the use of information to improve decision making. More specifically, the principle considers the links between development strategies and annual and multiyear budget processes. At the same time, through the Declaration, donors commit to harmonizing monitoring and evaluation requirements.

Emphasis on targets instead of sustainability. Managing for results—linking activity outputs to intermediate outcomes and objectives all the way up to how they contribute to a development effort's strategic objective—has long been a part of NGO's involvement in development assistance. From the NGO perspective, results frameworks create a roadmap that informs how a project is supposed to help contribute to a development objective. Identifying indicators that are measurable and that reflect the project's objectives, developing targets and benchmarks, and conducting baseline measures all fall within the spirit of the Paris Declaration. Yet one of the challenges that development organizations are facing is that, with greater attention to results and indicator targets, they run the risk of focusing too much on reaching targets and not enough on sustainability and capacity to carry out the work after a specific project is finished.

Using evidence. As a development organization, PRB is committed to helping decision makers use current data to make informed policy choices. Whether through publications, building the capacity of individuals and local partners to communicate evidence-based advocacy messages effectively, or working with journalists to understand population and health issues so that they can report on priority issues and promote transparency, the use of unbiased evidence is at the heart of PRB's mission. However, what is not articulated well in the Declaration is that decision makers have regular access to the data they need to make decisions (which will certainly be broader than the results indicators on which they report), understand what the data mean, or have the capacity to translate the evidence-based need into action. This is a critical aspect of capacity building that is frequently overlooked.

Development is not linear. While managing for results is important, there is often a sense that development work is a linear process, with one step following the next. Increasing attention to reporting on indicators and expectation that innovative approaches can be developed and successfully implemented creates a challenge for NGOs and implementing partners. Further impeding managing by results is dealing with political environment that are not enabling, staff turnover within the public and private sectors, and the need for ongoing capacity and institutional strengthening. These factors all add to the NGO's challenge of managing increasingly more complex and demanding results. These challenges must be dealt with for managing by results to take place.

Need for data at subnational levels. At the country level, staff who implement activities note the growing role of evidence-based policies at the national level; however, as subnational areas increasingly assume decision making and resource allocation responsibilities, it is often budgets rather than evidence—and immediate rather than longer-term priorities—that dictate decisions. In one country, a centralized monitoring and evaluation framework facilitates a more common vision for how the country manages its development efforts. Yet donor segmentation can easily fragment the M&E process, as the reporting requirement from donors for NGOs may not be in alignment with those that exist in a national M&E framework.

Tracking fewer indicators. As the Paris Declaration continues to take further root, it is likely that managing for results will continue to be a cornerstone of the Declaration as donors, partner governments, and NGOs strive to make the most of the development resources—demonstrating that they can do more with less. If, in fact, donors and partner governments can reach a consensus on a limited set of indicators and focus attention on creating strong data collection and fewer project-related indicators, the spirit of the Paris Declaration will be achieved.

Mutual Accountability

Stakeholders' roles. For aid effectiveness to improve, it is critical to have the involvement of parliamentarians and a broad set of stakeholders. Although many policies are put forward by the executive branches of government, the legislative branch needs to have a voice in the oversight of policy implementation, ensuring that the goals are achieved equitably. Similarly, stakeholders—civil society—have an important role in advocating for policy change, monitoring policy implementation, and serving as watchdogs to ensure actions are transparent, effective, and lead to the intended objective.

Reaching parliamentarians. From the NGO perspective, it is critical to reach these two audiences with accurate, understandable information. Turnover among members of parliament poses a challenge to advocacy groups as they work to inform new members about the importance of prioritizing population and reproductive health as part of the development agenda. Given the demands on parliamentarians' time, we work to find informative, creative ways that give them the information they need and to identify champions who can advance the issues on the inside, such as members of strategic caucuses and regional leaders who know how national political systems function.

NGOs and CSO contribute. While local civil society organizations and NGOs are also critical to engage in the process of improving aid effectiveness, their role is less clearly defined and their capacity to engage is varied. Given that an important aspect of the Paris Declaration is monitoring budgets, it is critical that there be a segment of civil society that has the capacity to carry out these types of complex, political functions. In addition, civil society needs the capacity to advocate to donors and decision makers; they need to know how to use data, develop messages, and develop communication strategies. Though these challenges remain ongoing, PRB has eagerly engaged in this aspect of the Paris Declaration—promoting mutual accountability through working to inform parliamentarians and strengthening the capacity of civil society. Together these groups can hold the public sector accountable for addressing population and reproductive health issues.

Conclusion

In the spirit of Paris. Increasingly, NGOs are becoming familiar with the Paris Declaration, recognizing it by name and appreciating how it is contributing to improving aid effectiveness. NGOs like PRB, which are involved in providing technical assistance on population and health issues, may not have been familiar with the Declaration in 2005 when it was signed, but are seeing how it is impacting our work through the directions that our donors are taking in their work.

NGO values in line with Declaration. The principles articulated in the Declaration have been, to a large degree, the principles that have guided our philosophy as an NGO. We support country ownership, working with governments and other stakeholders to ensure that the work we do together responds to their priorities. We have worked to support alignment between donors and government partners, helping to position the critical issues of population and health so that they are both incorporated into and respond to priorities included in national development strategies. Alignment also reflects the need to strengthen systems and capacity so that national development goals become a reality. Harmonization, while perhaps residing at a higher level than most NGOs work, incorporates gender and environment as key issues and promotes efficiency through working to avoid duplication of efforts. NGOs are well familiar with managing for results; our mandate is to get information in understandable, easy-to-use formats to decision makers, so that they can make sound policy decisions; without evidence, policies and programs will not address root causes and advance development objectives. And through mutual accountability, we support the engagement of a broad set of stakeholders in the development process—each with a role that advances toward more effective use of aid.

Toward a common vision. Donors are working more closely with governments to advance aid effectiveness and improve collaboration. In recent years, we have seen clearer demonstrations of donors working together to make a difference. They are working to leverage funds and share a common agenda, and their efforts are making a difference. But since much of the communication between donors and NGOs has to do with more specific projects, or donor-led initiatives, the explicit language of the Paris Declaration has been less visible than expected. Even among the staff of PRB, with whom I consulted in preparing this chapter, some people were very familiar with the Paris Declaration, while others had never heard of it. And while we as an NGO do not necessarily incorporate the language of the Paris Declaration into our work, we do see in it new ways of carrying out development work—greater collaboration, use of evidence, and commitment to improved capacity—that correspond with our institutional values.

Discussion Questions

- What does the Paris Declaration mean in light of international development goals, such as the Millennium Development Goals?
- How is the role of an international NGO different from a national NGO in implementing the Paris Declaration?
- There are many types of NGOs—service delivery, education, advocacy, monitoring, and evaluation, to mention a few. How do these different types of NGOs contribute to the Paris Declaration?
- How does the principle of country ownership correspond to and challenge donor priorities for technical assistance? What happens when a donor's priorities are not in line with the governments?
- How does an NGO reconcile donors' multiple perspectives toward the Paris Declaration—from explicit support to tacit agreement, to a strong donor-driven agenda that does not take local consideration into account?
- How does an NGO measure success related to the Paris Declaration when its own measures of success are based on specific indicators and targets?

Bibliography

Hayman, R., Taylor, E. M., Crawford, F., Jeffery, P., Smith, J., & Harper, I. (2011). *The impact of aid on maternal and reproductive health: A systematic review to evaluate the effect of aid on the outcomes of Millennium Development Goal 5*. London: EPPI-Centre, Social Science Research Unit, Institute of Education, University of London.

Monye, E., Ansah, E., & Orakwue, E. (2010). Easy to declare, difficult to implement: The disconnect between the aspirations of the Paris Declaration and donor practice in Nigeria. *Development Policy Review, 28*(6), 749–770.

The Paris Declaration on Aid Effectiveness and the Accra Agenda for Action, OECD. (2008).

Webb, R. (2011). *Aid effectiveness for health: Toward the fourth high-level forum*, Busan. Action for Global Health. Retrieved March 15, 2012, from http://www.actionforglobalhealth.eu/index.php?id=233

Chapter 10
Scaling-Up of High Impact Interventions

Rashad Massoud and Nana Mensah Abrampah

In a discussion with a leader of a global health system, the leader said, "our system is great at everything—just not everywhere. I can name somebody who is a world-class leader in any clinical area in our system. However, I cannot say the same for every part of our system." This reality describes many healthcare systems in the world where excellent practices may take place in one place, but not throughout the system. Achieving excellence throughout the system requires the deliberate spread of such practices.

What do we mean by spread or scale-up? Though some people differentiate between the two, for the purposes of this chapter we will use spread and scale-up interchangeably. Spread is defined as the science of taking a local improvement (e.g., an intervention, a redesign of a process or system) that has demonstrated better results than the current method and actively disseminating it across a system (Massoud et al. 2010), i.e., making an intervention that has proven to be more successful happen at a much larger scale than the initial location where the improvement originally took place. In this chapter, everything we will discuss will relate to an improved practice, a high-impact evidence-based intervention, a better result or a new process of care delivery that has produced a better result. We will discuss this in the context of taking the practice from the scale at which it was originally developed and actively moving it into a much larger geographic area covering a large number of facilities and patients. This is essentially what we mean by spread or scale-up.

There is a notion that if it is known that an intervention or different practice is better, why does it not happen all the time? In reality, there are evidence-based practices and results that are not taken up anywhere nearly as much as we would like

R. Massoud (✉) • N.M. Abrampah
Quality and Performance Institute, University Research Co., LLC., Bethesda, MD, USA
e-mail: rmassoud@urc-chs.com; nana.m.abrampah@gmail.com

© Springer Science+Business Media New York 2015
E. Beracochea (ed.), *Improving Aid Effectiveness in Global Health*,
DOI 10.1007/978-1-4939-2721-0_10

them to be used. For example, 1.4 million people worldwide are suffering from infections acquired in hospitals (Vincent 2003). Evidence-based research suggests that hand hygiene is the single most important factor in the prevention of healthcare-acquired infections and can drastically reduce these infections (Doebbeling et al. 1992). However, compliance with the hand washing guidelines still remains low even in resource-rich settings with compliance levels most frequently well below 40 % and at times even as low as zero percent (Evidence for Hand Hygiene Guidelines 2013). A recent study conducted by Pittest et al. found that in 2,834 observed opportunities for hand washing, non-compliance was higher in intensive care than in internal medicine units during procedures that carry a high risk for contamination and when intensity of patient care was high (Pittet et al. 1999). This is consistent with another example from the Agency for Health Research &Quality (AHRQ). AHRQ researchers looked at physician compliance with evidence-based interventions in the United States. The researchers analyzed that counseling patients against smoking, mammography screening, and warfarin for Atrial Fibrillation was only being done for less than a quarter of the patients. Angiotensin co-enzyme inhibitors for congestive heart failure were only being prescribed for a third of the patients. In reality, evidence-based practices and interventions that have proven to be capable of saving lives are not necessarily implemented in the way that they should be. A major issue in quality of healthcare is that not all the patients receive all the care they need, every time they need it.

Another interesting aspect of this research done by AHRQ looked at the pathway from original research to implementation. The conclusion from this study was that it takes 17 years to turn 14 % of original research to benefit patients. Although medical research serves to benefit the patient and improve health systems, the long time lag from research to implementation often yields a waste of scarce resources and a sacrifice of potential patient benefit (Ward et al. 2009). In the area of improvement, great strides are made to improve the quality of healthcare. These results are often tangible and easier for the patients to see. However, we continue to see islands of excellence, i.e., great results in parts of the system, but not throughout the whole system. Though one will think that it is natural for best practices to spread spontaneously, we do not see that happening as a rule. The uptake of improved interventions to a broader scale continues to be a challenge.

How can we actively work on making sure interventions that have proven to be worthy of scale-up are spread to the largest degree possible? Some of the literature that we have on this comes from the work of Everett Rogers. Rogers described in his book *Diffusion of Innovation* (Rogers 2003) that an innovation is an idea, practice, or object perceived as new by an individual or other unit of adoption. The attributes of an innovation determine how likely or unlikely the innovation is to be taken up by the social system. With this in mind, Rogers described the following attributes of an innovation:

- Relative advantage: if an innovation is not better than the existing model, it will be difficult for a social system to engage with it. We have to be able to show that the innovation is better than what currently exists today.

- Compatibility with existing systems, habits, and belief structures. The more compatible an innovation is with the social context, the more likely it is that it will be taken up in the social context that we are trying to spread it in.
- Complexity: the more complicated the new idea is, the less likely that it will be adopted. As we take new innovations to scale, we need to simplify as much as possible so that their uptake is enhanced.
- Trialability: when taking new ideas to scale, it is essential to allow testing the idea or innovation by the potential adopters. The ability to try something for one's self and see how it works and adjust it is key to the success of the adoption of any new innovation. People are not resistant to change, but they are resistant to being changed.
- Observability: the ability to see that the new way is better than the old one.

Another key issue that Rogers brings up are the different categories of adopters (see Fig. 10.1). Different people lie on different ends of the spectrum of adoption. Rogers' categories of adopters curve (see Fig. 10.1) is a normal distribution curve that has the number of people on the y-axis and time on the x-axis. The further away from 0, the more time it takes for individuals to adopt a new innovation. The figure shows the distribution of people with respect to the adoption of an innovation. Rogers categorizes most people as an early majority or a late majority. He describes early adopters as people who are open to ideas and are also highly interlinked with the system in which they exist. Early adopters are in many ways opinion leaders and are key to the adoption process. They typically are young, educated, and financially savvy. Early adopters tend to be more discreet in adoption choices than innovators. They realize that being an early adopter of innovations will help them maintain a central communication position with their peers (Rogers 2003). A small minority at the top end is classified as innovators. These are the people who come up with the

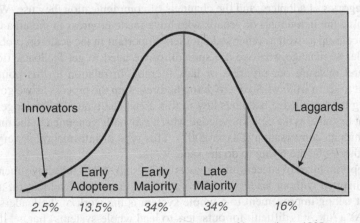

E. Rogers, Diffusion of innovations, 1995

Fig. 10.1 Bridging the Access, Retention, and Wellness gaps

new ideas. Innovators are less connected with the social system in which they operate. Innovators are great for developing ideas, but they do not necessarily lead the way for the majority. Early adopters are much more interlinked with their system, which is also important for the adoption process. The majority of the social system can be divided into an early and a late majority, depending on the timing of the uptake of an innovation. The early majority are influenced by the early adopters. The remainder are known as the late majority, who normally follow after seeing many others adopt the innovation. There will always be people who will not come on board. This group is called the laggards. It is very important for those trying to spread an innovation to identify who are the opinion leaders (early adopters) in the system as they have influence over others. Where a person fits in the categories of adoption will be different for different innovations as well as over time. An individual may lie on the upper left half of the bell-curve for one innovation and may lie towards the tail end of the curve for another. The same person can also change from one category to another with regard to the same innovation over time.

The passive spread of an idea from an individual to another can be accelerated through change agents. A change agent is defined as someone who acts as a catalyst for change. The deliberate spread of improvements we are engaged in builds on Rogers' diffusion theory, but requires additional factors for optimal results. In the case of system-wide spread, directed change in a system requires a framework for spread. The Institute of Healthcare Improvement developed the Framework for Spread (Massoud et al. 2006) which looks at innovations surrounding high-impact interventions on one end, and on the other, the social system in which we want to spread to. The social system consists of multiple people and communities, with actors who are the leaders and messengers, and rules that govern the social system. We must be very cognizant of the way in which communications happen within that social system. In order to get better ideas across to the social system, we must understand the individuals or groups we are going to address, which of them fall in what categories of adopters, and the channels of communication they use. We must also involve the individuals or groups who have made progress in the area that we want to scale-up as well as other stakeholders important in the scale-up process.

In order to manage what we are spreading, we need to get feedback from the system and measure our progress or lack thereof. In relation to this point, it is important to learn from what we are doing and redesign the process as we go along. Managing the knowledge becomes key in this area. The type of knowledge that is important to gather is the tacit knowledge which is usually generated in the moment, through human conversation (Dixon 2002). This type of information is very valuable to others who are trying to do the same work.

An important part of successful spread is leadership. All of the above-mentioned will not happen without leadership. We can develop an improvement on a small scale, but taking improvement to a whole system is the work of the leaders in the system. As a rule, it is difficult for outsiders to lead whole-systems change. It has to be led by the authority that operates the system. Leaders need to set the priorities, align resources to implement the priorities, and garner support from the social system to achieve these priorities. Leadership is also essential for empowering frontline workers and management at all levels within the system. Leaders support teams by making resources available and celebrating and recognizing the hard work and accomplishments of their staff.

In developing a spread strategy, we have to ask ourselves three main questions:

1. What do we want to spread? This can be a superior result, an innovation, a best practice, or a new process of care.
2. To whom do we want to spread? By when? Who are the members of the social system, how many facilities, patients, and setting a timeline is key. The timeline forces us to develop plans that are much more aggressive. Ideally, we would like to spread as much as possible.
3. How are we going to spread? There are multiple ways to spread. Different spread approaches can be more appropriate for different interventions and for different contexts.

There is no one right way to spread. It depends on what we are trying to spread and the context within which we are spreading it. There are several known approaches to spreading high impact interventions. The most successful tend to be those that take the appropriate elements from different approaches in order to contextualize to their setting. There are several ways to spread and a few are outlined below:

- Natural diffusion: also knows as Everett Rogers "Diffusion of Innovation." This is the uptake of new innovation by individuals within the social system.
- Extension agents: heavily used in the agricultural industry in the United States. This spread involves people moving from site to site sharing experiences and best practices. In healthcare, we use coaches as extension agents.
- Emergency mobilization: often used by international organizations in cata-strophic events. Emergency mobilization is done very quickly and at scale to reach a large number of people in the shortest time possible.
- Collaborative Improvement: is a time-limited improvement approach that brings together multiple teams to work on common aims and indicators for improve-ment to change processes of care in order to improve outcomes (Franco and Marquez 2011). Collaborative improvement accelerates the adoption and spread of evidence-based approaches across multiple sites. Collaborative improvement is good for complicated systemic changes.
- Virtual collaborative: this type of collaborative is conducted through the internet. This type of spread works well for simple, well-defined interventions. Those that require systematic changes and more collaboration need in-person interaction.
- Campaign spread: an all-at-once strategy. This is a very effective means of spread. One must be aware what interventions can be spread with this strategy. Simpler interventions are much easier to spread through campaigns (McCannon et al. 2006).
- Wave sequence spread: a type of spread that uses agents from the original sites to spread better care delivery to other sites within the system. We start with a slice of the system, i.e., the number of facilities that are interlinked and cater for

a certain population. This normally represents a system of care that consists of at least one facility that represents the different levels of care (tertiary, secondary, primary, and community levels) (World Health Organization [WHO] 2004). We identify champions (those who excel and achieve great results) within a health facility at the district from the pilot (start-up phase) and use them to spread the new innovation to other parts of their system. Like collaborative improvement, this approach is useful for complicated interventions. This wave-sequence approach should be used if we cannot reach the whole system all at once.

- Hybrid models: this combines more than one element in the above-mentioned strategies. For example, extension agents (otherwise known as coaching visits) may be used in combination with collaborative improvement.

Our experience has led us to believe that some principles tend to hold true for spread:

- Begin with the full scale in mind: consider the full scale you want to reach at the beginning of the design process. If we design with the full scale in mind, the program will be much more conducive to spread at a large scale.
- If you can, reach all at once.
- If you cannot reach all at once, consider a phased approach.
- How factors change in going to scale:

  - Arithmetic scale-up: we must take into account scale up arithmetically. For example, treating 1,000 patients will likely require 10 times as much medication as treating 100 patients (WHO 2004).
  - Favorable scale-up: sometimes economies of scale can be helpful when going to scale. For example, a single machine that is currently performing 10 tests in a day may also be able to perform 100 tests in a day (WHO 2004).

    Information systems: with small pilot projects it is often easy to collect data but with large scale-up projects, data collection and analysis becomes cumbersome. Information systems that catered for pilot phase will not necessarily cater for scale-up phase.

    Communication needs: knowledge must be gathered and shared across the whole system and beyond. This is important both for helping spread what works, energize the members of the social system as well as provide learning from the experience.

    Oversight: when going to scale, the need for oversight becomes different from the pilot phase. Building the oversight for scale-up has to come from within the system.

Key Lessons Learned

1. Results are key drivers: we have to spread proven and worthy results. It is better to show good results early on. This will engage people and they will be more likely to take the innovation we want to spread more seriously.

2. Improvement is about change. Therefore, we must enable people to make changes in their work:

   (a) Equip people with the ability to make changes. A change model such as Plan-Do-Study-Act (PDSA) cycle to test different changes is very useful. (Langley et al. 1996)
   (b) Provide assistance to teams in the form of coaching site visits to help them through the process.
   (c) Systems thinking: understanding all the work that we do in terms of processes and systems in terms of care delivery, and that the level of performance that we achieve is a characteristic of those processes and systems and is critical to the ability to improve and spread improvements.
   (d) Spread has to be led by the managers within those systems. When developing a demonstration on a small scale, it is possible to operate as an external program. However, when going to large-scale, it has to be led and conducted by the leaders within those health systems themselves. This includes leadership at all levels. For example, instructions on what to do and how to do this. This also includes providing technical assistance, training, and capability building.
   (e) Role Modeling: if external assistance is being provided, it is important to be aware of the effect that the change agents can have on the members of the social system through their everyday behaviors.
   (f) Provide normative and regulatory support in the form of written standard operating procedures and policies to support the new systems and their spread.

3. People working under constraints can be creative. There are many examples of creativity, which came out of the unavailability of resources (www.ttwwud.org).
4. Scale-up efforts require meticulous attention to detail. Logistics and organization are key to success in scale-up.
5. The champions who developed the prototype are critical for leading the scale-up in the wave sequence approach.
6. Leadership has to come from within the system.

Measurement of successful scale-up should focus on the degree of attainment of the improved result and increase in the adoption of the improvement at a larger scale, i.e., the number of facilities that have started making improvement, percentage of sites adopting the new intervention, etc. Measurement is particularly important, as you are able to see how many facilities adopt the improvement over time. An indicator of monitoring is the number of facilities who have started with this new innovation over the total number of facilities within the geographic region you intend to scale-up to.

In our experience, using effective spread methods such as wave sequence has enabled us to go to scale in a much more cost-effective way. This was done by using local resources such as spread agents, who are within the system from the initial demonstration phase. Increasingly, donors are requesting improvements at scale rather than demonstrations (http://www.healthsystems2020.org; http://www.usaid-assist.org; http://www.mchip.net). We ask ourselves, how do we get this funding from donors? Donors are interested in proposals that take innovations to scale in an effective and efficient way. Funding for scale-up comes in different ways. Frequently those who demonstrated and showed the better results will be asked to scale-up. More often than not, donors are interested in scaling up cost-effective innovations and not by repeating the same experience over and over.

There have been many successful efforts to scale-up interventions that have worked. These scale-up efforts have used different approaches. The approaches seem to have some common principles behind them. Key to the successful scale-up of interventions has been the degree to which the innovation and the spread method have been appropriately used for the context in which they were spread. There remains a great deal to be learned about how to take successful interventions to scale. Much of this learning will be derived from learning about scale-up experiences that take place.

References

Dixon, N. (2002). The neglected receiver of knowledge sharing. *Ivey Business Journal, 66*, 35–40.

Doebbeling, B. N., et al. (1992). Comparative efficacy of alter-native hand-washing agents in reducing nosocomial infections in intensive care units. *New England Journal of Medicine, 327*, 88–93.

Evidence for Hand Hygiene Guidelines. (2013). Geneva, Switzerland: WHO.

Franco, L. M., & Marquez, L. (2011). Effectiveness of collaborative improvement: Evidence from 27 applications in 12 less-developed and middle-income countries. *BMJ Quality and Safety, 20*(8), 658–665. Published Online First: 11 February 2011 doi:10.1136/bmjqs.2010.044388.

Health Systems Strengthening. (2012). Abt Associates. Retrieved from http://www.healthsystems2020.org

Langley, G., Nolan, K. M., Norman, C. L., Provost, L. P., & Nolan, T. W. (1996). *The improvement guide: A practical approach to enhancing organizational performance*. San Francisco, CA: Jossey-Bass.

Massoud, M. R., Donohue, K. L., & McCannon, C. J. (2010). *Options for large-scale spread of simple, high-impact interventions* (Technical Report). USAID Health Care Improvement Project. Bethesda, MD: University Research Co. LLC (URC).

Massoud, M. R., Nielsen, G. A., Nolan, K., Nolan, T., Schall, M. W., Sevin, C. (2006). *A framework for spread: From local improvements to system-wide change*. IHI Innovation Series white paper. Cambridge, MA: Institute for Healthcare Improvement. Retrieved from www.IHI.org

Maternal and Child Health Integrated Program. (2013). Retrieved from http://www.mchip.net

McCannon, C. J., Schall, M. W., Calkins, D. R., & Nazem, A. G. (2006). Saving 10,000 lives in US hospitals. *British Medical Journal, 332*(7553), 1328–1330.

Pittet, D., Mourouga, P., Perneger, T. V., & The Members of the Infection Control Program. (1999). Compliance with handwashing in a teaching Hospital. *Annals of Internal Medicine, 130*(2), 126–130.

Rogers, E. M. (2003). *Diffusion of innovations*. New York: Free Press.

Turning the World Upside Down—Turning the World Upside Down. (2013). Retrieved from www.ttwwud.org

USAID Applying Science to Strengthen and Improve Systems Project. (2013). USAID ASSIST. University Research Co. Retrieved from http://www.usaidassist.org

Vincent, J. L. (2003). Nosocomial infections in adult intensive-care units. *Lancet, 361*, 2068–2077.

Ward, V., House, A., & Hamer, S. (2009). Developing a framework for transferring knowledge into action: A thematic analysis of the literature. *Journal of Health Services Research & Policy, 14*, 156–164.

World Health Organization. (2004). *An approach to rapid scale-up: Using HIV/AIDS treatment as an example*. Geneva, Switzerland: Author.

Chapter 11
Aid Effectiveness in Working with Private Sector Health Organizations: The Smiling Sun Franchise

Juan Carlos Negrette

Introduction

Bangladesh has been able to greatly reduce maternal mortality in less than one decade, from 322 down to 194 per 100,000 (NIPORT 2011), and increase life expectancy to 69 years; an achievement that took European countries not decades but centuries (http://www.gapminder.org/). Along similar lines, with an economy that has expanded more than 6 % annually in the last years, foreign aid is now hovering around 1.5–1.9 % of GDP (http://www.dfat.gov.au/geo/bangladesh/bangladesh_country_brief.html), just a fraction of country's garment exports (http://www.epb.gov.bd/bdprofiledetails.php?page=56). In spite of its amazing progress, Bangladesh has not been able to leave behind its image of impoverished and overpopulated, basket case kind of country. The reason for the stubborn perception lies in the fact that Bangladesh still has almost half of its population living under $1.25 a day (UNDP 2011), and with close to 160 million inhabitants in just over 144,000 km^2, Bangladesh is one of the most densely populated spots in this planet. So, in the same space and time, Bangladesh conjures great hopes based on impressive results, while still facing huge challenges. This discussion no longer happens in other countries that not long ago were where Bangladesh is today, like Colombia—considered a high middle income country—or the Philippines—low middle income, but that once received much more foreign aid than they do today.

Because of the rapid pace and nature of change, the way aid is implemented in Bangladesh is subject to sometimes intense debate. Where, who, and how should projects work are relentlessly resurfacing topics in a discussion that undoubtedly takes place in other countries as well and that seeks to find the best way, the best

J.C. Negrette (✉)
Global Health - Health Sciences at the University of Utah, Salt Lake City, Utah
e-mail: jcnegrette@hotmail.com

© Springer Science+Business Media New York 2015
E. Beracochea (ed.), *Improving Aid Effectiveness in Global Health*,
DOI 10.1007/978-1-4939-2721-0_11

outcome for the country and persons in need. In that context, implementing an effective project that seeks to expand access for the poor, while attaining financial sustainability, will always attract attention… and debate. This is even more the case, when a project is designed to work not directly with the Government, but with private organizations instead, an approach that was quite common—and in many instances successful—in Latin America in the 70s and 80s.

This chapter will present a reflection on the main success factors of effective aid to the private sector based on the author's perception in leading a project to develop the private sector in Bangladesh as an effective strategy to expand access to quality healthcare.

Private Sector Definition

The term private sector refers here to all non-state providers, who operate on a for-profit or non-profit base, and in a formal or informal way. This term includes service providers, pharmacies, hospitals, pharmaceutical companies, producers and suppliers, retailers, and traditional healers (https://www.wbginvestmentclimate.org/toolkits/public-policy-toolkit/upload/Glossary-4-28-11a.pdf).

Smiling Sun Franchise Program

The Smiling Sun Franchise Program (SSFP) was a USAID-funded project that complements the existing network of healthcare facilities set up by the government of Bangladesh. SSFP utilizes an innovative approach to social franchising that seeks to provide good quality and affordable health services to a vast portion of the country's population, including the poorest of the poor, in a sustainable manner.SSFP works with a network of 26 local NGOs that have received funding from USAID for more than two decades. They serve women, children, and men through a network of 323 static clinics and more than 8,400 satellite clinics in all districts of Bangladesh (http://www.smilingsunhealth.com/About_us.aspx).

A Day in the Life of Smiling Sun

It is a sunny April morning in Chittagong, the second largest city in Bangladesh. Tahmina crosses the busy and noisy street, holding Abeer's head tightly. She enters into the Smiling Sun clinic in West Bakalia. She brings her son to see the doctor, as he has had mild fever and has been coughing lately. The clinic staff knows Tahmina well. She delivered Abeer there. She cannot forget that day. She was in severe pain and she told her husband she needed to see a doctor. Ashok, her husband, initially refused as his mother thought this was just "normal." Finally after insisting obstinately, Ashok gave in and took Tahmina to the Smiling Sun clinic. When she arrived she was immediately examined by the paramedic and was rushed to the OR. She presented a ruptured uterus, but fortunately, doctors could save her as well as her baby.

Today is a different experience. After a proper examination, the doctor in Smiling Sun prescribed Abeer the right treatment according to standard treatment guidelines. She gets the medicines in the clinic's pharmacy, pays 30 Taka (less than $0.5) for the consultation and the medicines and leaves. Abeer will get well a few days later.

The Case for Private Sector Engagement in Health

Smiling Sun provides over 30 million health consultations per year in a catchment area estimated in 20 million persons. In 4 years it has provided over 60,000 safe deliveries and has offered over seven million couple years protection as a measure of family planning services. While still heavily dependent on donor support, its level of cost recovery, or its ability to generate revenue compared to the actual cost of providing services, has gone up from 25 to 40 %. It is interesting to keep in mind that while revenue has increased almost three times in this period, and proportion of poor people served have also increased. Today over 30 % of SSFP clients are poor, up from 26 % 4 years ago.

Perhaps, when assessing the actual private sector contribution in monetary and social terms, monitoring is reduced to track ratios around cost-effectiveness, which is not necessarily negative as it addresses important societal concerns, but in many instances, it leaves on the side other aspects essential to improve quality of life, such as perceived and actual quality of the services offered. It implies that if improvement of quality of care is measurable, and that those quality services—at reasonable levels of service consistency—can be accessed by more individuals at more cost-effective levels, the society as a whole is better off with this type of services than without them. It does not imply that governments cannot do the same; it implies that for the specific case we are analyzing, the program and its outcomes offered a win–win situation for the people of Bangladesh.

The Social Case: Access to Quality Care for All

People like Tahmina appreciate SSFP because it offers good quality services (in a recent survey sponsored by GIZ, over 60 % of the respondents mentioned that they went to SSFP because of the perceived quality of its services). Tahmina is ready to pay for the services she receives, perhaps even pay a bit more than what she would have had to pay in other clinics or what she can be charged in the public sector facilities. This perception of quality is shared by the majority of clients, regardless of their location or socio-economic group. In SSFP, close to 65 % of clients pay full price or a fraction of it, and approximately 35 % receive services for free. SSFP is able to do that because of donor support (although proportionally decreasing) and because paying clients help to cover expenses generated by those who do not pay. So Tahmina, when paying full fare, is not just ensuring she will receive the service she is requesting, but she is also helping the poorest members of her community as well.

Smiling Sun has clinics that generate a surplus (although up to 2010 no single NGO was generating positive net income), which is distributed in such a way that has helped to reduce the overall NGO dependence on donor support.

As clients increased their contributions, it also raises their expectations. A paying client like Tahmina tends to be a more empowered one. SSFP started a program in 2008 to track clients opinions through suggestion boxes placed in every clinic. Some opinions were full of compliments to the clinic staff, but others were candidly demanding something that was lacking, either in the quality of the attention, schedule, doctor's presence, or any other element clients everywhere consider important. The clients exercise their right to expect a certain level of service because they pay and that ensures access to quality care for all. Patients in public facilities rarely demand improvements.

Therefore, in improving access, perceived quality and helping client empowerment were factors that contributed to improve the quality of life of the members served by SSFP in a given community.

The Managerial Case

Managerial innovations, ranging from the invention of double entry accounting to bureaucratic organization, have been essential to manage constantly increasing wealth, while contributing to generate more services, products, and wealth. Improving managerial conditions in healthcare organizations working in the developing world also has the purpose to help them reach always higher levels of performance measured through better metrics, more opportune feedback, or allowing increasingly educated human resources to participate in decision making for quality improvement.

In the case of SSFP since the project's onset, clinic staff and managers received training in new ways to conduct planning and became more attuned with prevalent business practices, than with the regular way of planning for financial resources in the development cooperation world. But new management practices did not stop there; SSFP changed the focus on the patient by putting the patient first in all situations to boost quality throughout the network, through clinic-based quality circles.

Smiling Sun Franchise Model

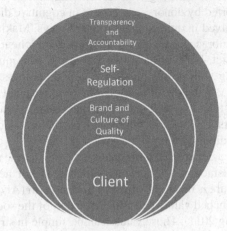

- The client first, really?

  When organizations are heavily donor-dependent, their leaders and their staff understand that the "client" is the one who provides the money. Structures have been consistently put in place to serve the interests of donors, which brings a clear benefit for the parties involved; and clearly donors look to benefit the final user, which for the most part happens as desired. However, this approach is not in alignment with the way "client" is defined in the commercial world and does not consistently deliver quality health services. While the perspective of solving client's needs as the first rule might sound romantic or, to some cynical, the truth is that organizations who provide value and have consistently met real -or not so much-clients' desires have been successful. (Just think of Apple)

  For Smiling Sun, it was a totally new ways of working, when through a series of training exercises and structured meetings, the concept of the user as the (main) client was introduced. The concept might seem a platitude and, in the abstract, who could be or do things against the patient? However, this is reflected in many ways, for example, it was quite common to see the disruption of patient's privacy, when donor agencies' representatives visited and clinic and staff, eager to demonstrate how well they were doing, entered in rooms where patients were not necessarily examined, but having a private conversation with their providers.

  The realization the client comes first started happening when clinic staff are reminded that users like Tahmina are paying their salaries, in some instances, fully. One must continuously bring the image of the barefoot women, wearing a modest, if not so clean sari, and explaining that the one or two Taka they bring to pay for a consultation are related to salary compensation, is one that must be told and repeated. This clearly does not happen overnight, but the focus on the real client eventually sinks in.

- Creating a culture for providing quality of care

  Understanding who the client is, is essential to the concept of quality of care. While doing things right is ethically and morally correct, potentially conflicting agendas (i.e., when reducing costs, or entering new development areas because they are supported by donors) can end up in cognitive dissonances for the staff, which are resolved in quite straight forward ways. Making sure that clinic staff at all levels embraces the idea of the user as the client will not eliminate the potential conflict, but will have two additional consequences that would help them in dealing with it; one, they have now a compass that in case of lack of direction, they can make decisions that favor clients and in favor of the concept of quality and, two, they will make sure that conflicts reach higher decision levels so managers are aware—if they were not before—about unintended consequences some directives might have caused.

Developing a culture that turns quality of care—as the means to ensure patient safety and satisfaction—is not easy, albeit it is not necessarily complicated. Prevailing culture is incredibly difficult to transform (Alvesson and Sveningsson 2008), as entrenched values and beliefs are part of the social tissue of an organization (Denning 2011). Those values can be simple in structure, but can be contrary to what an organization needs to do to survive and thrive when environmental conditions change (i.e., dwindling donor support) (Diamond 2005); so to develop a culture of quality, patience is of the essence, as well as persistence, proper consistent monitoring, and ensuring that a system that rewards positive behavior is in place, as well as one that acts as a disincentive for behavior that strengthens status quo, or does not favor to create a culture around quality of care.

SSFP acted at three different levels. It created a central body on which the overall climate for quality was founded; it was called the *Central Quality Council* (CQC). At this level, the new strategy to attain higher levels of quality of care, the new rules and regulations as well as a new set of expectations was set. Every network NGO was represented in the CQC by a professional and the person responsible for the Smiling Sun program in that particular NGO. The CQC was also a forum in which quality achievements or shortcomings were candidly discussed.

Another quality improvement intervention was implemented at the clinic level through the clinic-based *Quality Circles*. While these were a fad in the 1980s and seemed to disappear, the concept offered an important participatory component that allowed all members in the clinic to address quality issues where they actually happened, without having to wait for directions from higher levels. Clinic (and NGO) staff received training in problem solving and management tools like the Plan-Do-Study-Act PDSA cycle to address critical quality issues in a process of continuous improvement. When using PDSA, the team establishes short-term achievable goals in relation to a specific quality problem that allow ample team participation and quick feedback. If objectives are attained, the team looks for the next related achievable goal and follows this process continuously until structural improvements are achieved (http://www.ihi.org/knowledge/Pages/Tools/PlanDoStudyActWorksheet.aspx).

Equally important was to ensure that quality was measured externally by *independent auditors*; so auditing was done through two main activities, one through medical doctors contracted specifically to visit SSFP clinics randomly to conduct a comprehensive evaluation of all relevant quality aspects using a standard tool. Equally important was to implement a *"mystery client"* activity that ensured the client perspective in the overall clinical evaluation. Simultaneously, clients were encouraged to provide input about their experiences through suggestion boxes placed in every clinic. Tahmina shared once a comment about the service she had received to express her satisfaction.

While these actions did not correct all quality of care shortcomings the network faced, it served to improve conditions across the network as measured by a set of indicators published in the SSFP website (www.smilingsunhealth.com), by much better self-reporting practices, and by improved clients' perception about quality offered.

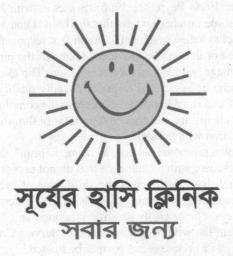

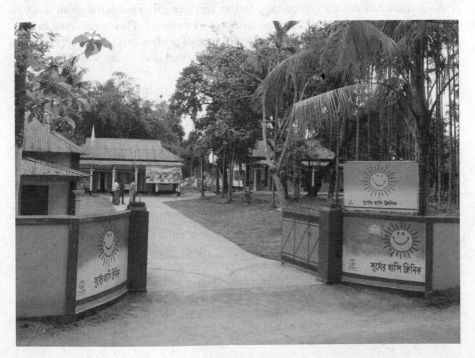

- Branding and its relevance

Since its start, SSFP made conscious efforts to look different in a way areas users could appreciate; quality improvements were made tangible to users. It developed guidelines to paint the clinics with distinctive colors, make sure consultation rooms and waiting areas were clean and tidy, and that even make sure the interaction with providers would be perceived as positive and pleasant. All these were areas where Smiling Sun decided to leave an imprint, a seal users could use for future reference, when talking to others, or when deciding for healthcare services again.

Branding is a concept associated with commercial transactions, but also with trust (Fukuyama 1996; Peyreffite 1996). Societies with higher levels of trust have more — in some instances international — brands than those in which trust is weak. Brands act as an endorsement, a claim that responsibility is taken for the product delivered or the service provided. That was the rationale adopted when developing an image and identity for Smiling Sun. The idea was, and is, that the Smiling Sun name be associated to good, friendly quality, regular people can afford. This was, and is, an important element in the communication between the network and its clients and the concomitant relationship that results from it and the direct interaction with the staff.

Smiling Sun was promoted publicly as "Surger Hashi", the equivalent Bengali expression, to resonate with an audience that do not necessarily speak — or even understand — English well. Towards the third year of the project, there were some copycats emerging in the market, perhaps the greatest compliment a brand can get. In surveys, clients easily identified the logo and name of the organization they were familiar with (Capacity Building Service Group 2008).

- Self-regulation: can a private sector partner be trusted?

As a means to ensure consistency in the services provided throughout a vast network of clinics, a level of standardization is required. This is reflected in the service structure (kind of services offered, type of professionals and support personnel in every clinic), in the way clinics look, and also in the way clinics are managed and regulated.

By applying these common principles, different organizations (and we could define these as "social entrepreneurs") can have access to know-how, discounted products, funds, and certain types of clients such as family planning clients that they, on their own, could hardly get or developing services to attract them would be so onerous that it would not be attractive to pursue them. So the corollary is that it is reasonable to expect self-regulation to occur in a context of standardization in which benefits stemming from following the rules and costs for not doing so are clearly known, and that rules of engagement have been clearly defined at the beginning of the relationship. In the case of Smiling Sun, different dimensions between service provider institutions and the program were guided by grant agreements that have in them explicit conditions that required both parties to provide, on the one hand resources for the adequate provision of health services, and on the other, adherence to clear quality principles, proper brand utilization, and levels of performance — among others — to ensure the continuous flow of resources, as capacity was build and conditions for enduring financial sustainability were constructed.

Within the context of the contract between providers and the network, it is expected for self-regulation to work… to a point. It is also important that partnering organizations, like the NGOs working in SSFP, know that there are external elements, such as audits and "mystery client" interventions that will help to verify whether agreements are followed, and that patients are treated the way they should in an environment in which trust is sincerely praised.

* Transparency and accountability

An important innovation of SSFP was to empower clinic managers and staff to develop their own business plans and become responsible and accountable for achieving what they had actually aimed for. The process to conduct the plan and to verify results was the same for every NGO and for every clinic. A database was created and all organizations involved in the network received the same training and were invited to provide information according to the number of clinics every organization had, to ensure fair treatment. While the process was dutifully followed by SSFP staff, their work was mostly to ensure that network NGO's received adequate support during planning, understanding that things might not come out as planned, but that it was important to be close to the expected results. Clinic staff was expected, and trusted, to conduct a thorough and realistic planning exercise.

An important element of SSFP's strategy to improve accountability and transparency was to convert clinic management into an important, full time job; therefore, providers who wanted to still be managers had to choose between providing consultations or managing the clinic. That helped managers to focus their attention in all tasks from procuring supplies on time and charging adequate prices, to ensuring staff maintain the facilities clean and tidy.

Managerial and service delivery activities—including quality of care—were continuously evaluated and results widely shared (SSFP decided to implement a contest in which the "best NGO director" would be selected, following a commonly understood criteria) to favor transparency and accountability, essential factors in developing a culture of trust inside the organization which should result in lower transactional costs (Fukuyama 1996) and patient satisfaction.

Conclusion

While there is still—and there will be for long time—debate about how to engage the private sector, the question is more about how to do it, instead of whether doing it or not. Working with private healthcare organizations (both for-profit and nonprofit) offers the possibility to expand access to quality health services in cost-efficient ways. Private providers can also offer their clients a value proposition that is centered on quality at prices that can be afforded, as this is an important factor in choosing providers when options are present. At the end, perceived and actual quality is an important factor for sustainability of the SSFP providers.

Quality is a factor that requires monitoring and for that reason, it's important to develop structures that favor this activity either by a contracting agent, or by third party, or both. Developing those structures and conditions, and monitor their proper operation, could be an essential task for governments to ensure that health services delivered through public facilities meet established quality standards. Health networks in the private sector can develop regulatory frameworks that complement those implemented and required by government entities, ensuring compliance through proper monitoring and regulatory mechanisms and with more frequency than the one exerted, in many instances, by government entities.

Modern managerial elements and techniques, performance evaluation, third-party quality evaluations, and patients' perception are interventions that increase transparency, favor developing a culture of accountability, and help to reduce the usual agent problem in the provider-recipient scheme, particularly enhanced when information asymmetry is more a chasm than a mere gap.

The experience of SSFP in Bangladesh might be unique from the culture and specific socio-economic environment and structure. That said, there are precursors to this social franchising approach in countries like Colombia and the Philippines with similar results in terms of quality management, service delivery output and, keeping proportions around countries' economic development and financial performance. Tahmina's experience should not be much different in terms of type and quality of services received than that one of any woman of similar socio-economic exaction in the Philippines or Colombia or any woman for that matter.

Below is a summary of the steps to consider when expanding the role of the private sector and some questions for the readers to continue the debate.

When Implementing Projects Engaging Networks of Private Providers

- Make quality of care the most important subject. Rally all staff around few quality elements: Hand washing, clean bathrooms, or something that can help make quality easily tangible.
- Develop a framework that measures quality inputs, outputs, and health outcomes.
- Make sure that quality can be measured by providers, as well as by others in the network or by third parties.
- Always stress in how important clients are. Remind providers and clinic staff that their salaries are either totally or partially covered by the people who come to the clinic to procure their services.
- Monitor competition and ensure your value equation (quality and affordability) is always maintained.
- Providers are not managers. Facilities can be managed by a medical professional, but in that case, her/his function should be only to manage the facility and not to provide consultation services.

Suggested Debate Questions

- Should foreign aid programs focus on supporting public sector programs? Why should they support private sector programs (and institutions) offering services to elements of the society that in many instances should be served by the government.

- Is self-regulation reliable? As a corollary, are quality assurance programs led by private institutions trustworthy? Is client satisfaction measured by private programs relevant and reliable?
- Is charging for health services immoral? Should health services for the poor provided only for free? Should be provided only by the government, or at least, indirectly paid by the government? What if the "should be of things" and reality do not coincide? Is there space for private intervention? Is outpatient payment a condition that should be avoided for all the subjects all the time? How can societies cover all expenses related?
- Is it "healthy" that providers have to be accountable to their patients and their employers? Do you think financial sustainability objectives for an organization can create cognitive dissonances among providers when serving their patients? How should those dissonances, if present, be solved?
- If "essential factors in developing a culture of trust inside the organization which should result in lower transactional costs and patient satisfaction" can be constructed within public sector institutions, do you still see a role for private sector health service delivery?

References

Alvesson, M., & Sveningsson, S. (2008). *Changing organizational culture: Cultural change work in progress*. New York: Routledge.

Australian Government, Department of Foreign Affairs. Retrieved February 2, 2012, from http://www.dfat.gov.au/geo/bangladesh/bangladesh_country_brief.html. Foreign aid to Bangladesh is estimated to range between $1.5 to $1.9 billion for a GDP estimated around $106 billion.

Bangladesh Exports Promotion Bureau, Ministry of Commerce. Retrieved February 2, 2011, from http://www.epb.gov.bd/bdprofiledetails.php?page=56

Capacity Building Service Group (2008). Market survey report. In this survey the Smiling Sun logo and name were recognized by over 90 % of the respondents.

Denning, S. (2011, July 23). How do you change an organizational culture. *Forbes Magazine*.

Diamond, J. (2005). *Collapse: How societies choose to fail or succeed*. New York: Penguin Books.

For more information, please visit the site of the Institute of Healthcare Improvement where you can see examples about how does the tool work. http://www.ihi.org/knowledge/Pages/Tools/PlanDoStudyActWorksheet.aspx

Fukuyama, F. (1996). *Trust: Human nature and the reconstitution of social order*. New York: Free Press Paperbacks (Simon & Schuster).

Gapminder: Unveiling the beauty of statistics for a fact based world. Retrieved February 2, 2012, from http://www.gapminder.org/

NIPORT (2011). Measure Evaluation/UNC-CH, ICDDRB. *Bangladesh maternal mortality survey 2010* (Preliminary Results Report, p. 19).

Peyreffite, A. (1996). *La Sociedad de la Confianza: Ensayo Sobre los Origenes y la Naturaleza del Desarrollo*. Santiago de Chile: Editorial Andres Bello.

Smiling Sun Franchise Program. Project Webpage. Retrieved August 30, 2012, from http://www.smilingsunhealth.com/About_us.aspx

UNDP (2011). *Human development report*. Retrieved July 28, 2012, from http://hdrstats.undp.org/en/countries/profiles/BGD.html

World Bank Group. Health Policy Toolkit Glossary. Retrieved July 28, 2012, from https://www.wbginvestmentclimate.org/toolkits/public-policy-toolkit/upload/Glossary-4-28-11a.pdf

Chapter 12
Effectiveness in Primary Healthcare in Peru

Laura C. Altobelli

Healthcare in the community of Las Moras in Huánuco, Peru, consisted of a poorly equipped one-room health post staffed by an auxiliary nurse and visited by few patients. Then in 1994 the primary healthcare facility in Las Moras and about 250 others throughout the country were incorporated into a new government-community partnership for the delivery, management, financing, and monitoring of primary healthcare services, called the Shared Administration Program. The program formed committees of locally elected community members, called "*Comunidades Locales de Administración de Salud*" (CLAS), into private non-profit associations to collaboratively manage government funds for primary healthcare services. This gave communities not just a voice in priority-setting and oversight, but also direct control over public funds for expenditures on infrastructure, equipment, and human resources. Since the inception of CLAS, Future Generations, a private non-profit organization, has worked with the government, civil society, and local communities to design the CLAS system and build the capacity of communities to thrive within the CLAS framework.

As a result of participating in the CLAS partnership, the Las Moras health post built additional consultation rooms and a birth center, purchased necessary equipment and supplies in a timely manner, and increased the staff to 36 members, including doctors. It now supports a system of community health promoters, who are trained and supervised by health personnel to do monthly visits to families with pregnant women and children under 2 years old for checkups, referrals, and health education. This system of outreach and support has quadrupled the level of coverage for maternal and child healthcare.

The Paris Declaration envisions a new development paradigm based on broad national ownership of development strategies, capacity building of national actors

L.C. Altobelli, Dr.P.H. M.P.H. (✉)
Future Generations, Future Generations Graduate School,
Calle Las Petunias, 15023 Lima 12, PERU
e-mail: laltobellim@gmail.com

© Springer Science+Business Media New York 2015
E. Beracochea (ed.), *Improving Aid Effectiveness in Global Health*,
DOI 10.1007/978-1-4939-2721-0_12

and institutions, a strong voice for civil society in governance, and achieving the Millenium Development Goals. This paper presents how one country's experience with decentralized primary healthcare (PHC) can provide an example as to how health systems reform can strengthen the organizational and management structures at the local level that contribute to more efficient and effective utilization of public and donor support.

The country is Peru on the Pacific coast of South America including a large section of the Amazon jungle, home to the astonishing 5,000 year-old Caral civilization and numerous other flourishing civilizations culminating in the Inca Empire that ruled the western part of the South American continent at the time of the Spanish invasion in 1534.

This paper will show (1) how PHC in Peru was organized before and after a new system was implemented with local governance by the community, called CLAS (Local Health Administration Committees), (2) what were some of the key factors in these new financial and human resources management processes with local governance that contribute to Aid Effectiveness, and (3) how an enhanced model of decentralized PHC with CLAS further increases Aid Effectiveness.

Prior to 1994, the PHC system had a top-down structure, as shown in Fig. 12.1. Public administration law was cumbersome and bureaucratic for processes such as contracting and purchasing, which resulted in slow management responses and

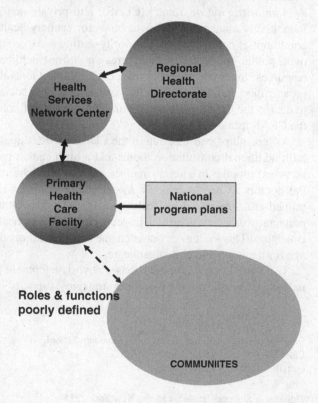

Fig. 12.1 Primary healthcare under public administration in Peru

contributed to corrupt practices. Primary care services were focused on curative care and passively attended the demand for services: their roles and functions in relation to the community were poorly defined. The community had no defined role in health. Production of services and healthcare coverage was poor, and key health indicators were very substandard.

The Shared Administration Program began in 1994 with the normative establishment of CLAS—Community Associations for Local Health Administration, which are private non-profit civil associations that function under private law. This was established as a pilot program and involved legalized community participation in the administration and management of PHC services, with the idea the "those who receive services are the best ones to manage it." Six community members from the catchment area of a health facility were elected by the community as members of the CLAS General Assembly. The chief physician or nurse of the primary care facility was the CLAS Manager. The CLAS General Assembly chose three from among themselves to form the Board of Directors with a President, Secretary, and Treasurer. See Fig. 12.2. A commercial bank account was opened by the CLAS, into which the government treasury, and other entities, deposit funds on a monthly basis. The CLAS Treasurer and Manager sign checks to pay for health personnel contracted by the CLAS and for purchasing equipment, supplies, and infrastructure.

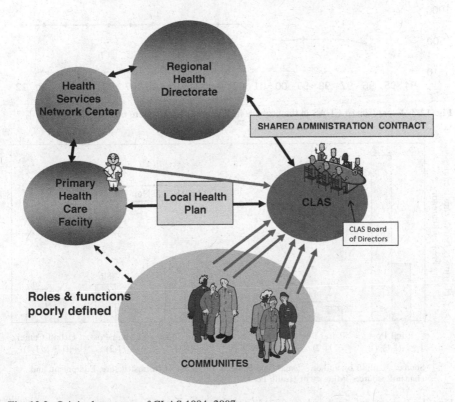

Fig. 12.2 Original structure of CLAS 1994–2007

The CLAS committee was responsible for annually developing and overseeing the implementation of a Local Health Plan for providing preventive and curative services in the catchment area of the CLAS. This plan was financed by the public sector Regional Health Directorate through a Shared Administration Contract signed with the CLAS, through a public to private transfer of funds. This was a bottom-up health reform process that allows direct citizen participation in the management of PHC services. The program was initiated on a small scale in 16 health facilities in 1994 which, by 2002, had scaled up to currently cover one third of Ministry of Health PHC services, or over 2,100 PHC facilities out of a total of 6,700, as shown in Fig. 12.3. The current distribution of CLAS among all PHC facilities is shown in Fig. 12.4.

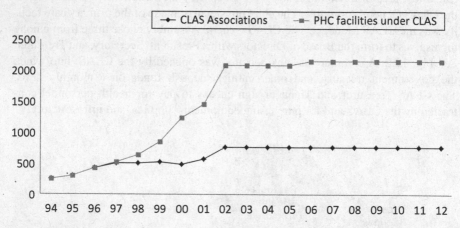

Fig. 12.3 Expansion of CLAS in the primary healthcare (PHC) system of Peru 1994–2012

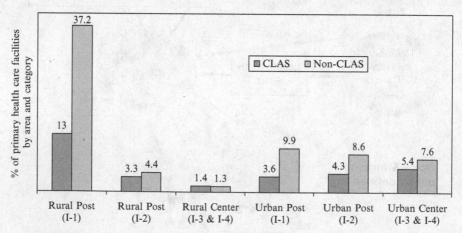

Source: Analysis by author. Data: 2006 National Inventory of Instrastructure, Equipment, and Human Resources. Ministry of Health Peru.

Fig. 12.4 Proportional distribución of 6,871 PHC facilities by category and type of management: 2006

The design of the CLAS program improves accountability and transparency with modifications in public financial management that promote efficiency and reduce corruption. How is this achieved?

Various public and private sources provide resources for CLAS to provide primary health services. The primary source of funding for CLAS is the central public treasury which transfers funds for salaries, goods, and services, and from the public health insurance program through reimbursements. Municipal budgets can transfer funds to CLAS through normal budgeting and through a participatory budgeting process. International donors can deposit funds directly in CLAS bank accounts, as well as any other private entity.

CLAS is authorized to spend resources, based on local priorities and decision-making by community members with transparency and accountability. CLAS selects, contracts, and supervises health personnel. CLAS prioritizes, plans, and purchases equipment and supplies. CLAS contracts building projects and supervises them. A major advantage of CLAS is that it can decide to use discretionary funds to finance community-based health promotion activities and incentives, even though public budgets were and are not always available to finance health promotion. Public as well as private resources are transferred to CLAS, somewhat akin to the principles of a private insurance company: CLAS obligates itself to provide services to a group of people through signing a contract with the DIRESA to complete the Local Health Plan.

To compare financial management mechanisms that improve efficiency in CLAS with non-CLAS PHC facilities that are managed and financed under public sector administration: in non-CLAS, there is no mechanism for local financial management; fees-for-service are deposited into the regional MOH account for them to manage; public insurance reimbursements are deposited in regional MOH accounts; and no purchasing can be effected here. On the other hand, CLAS controls a private bank account into which they receive transfers of public and private funds; fees-for-service are deposited into this account; public insurance reimbursements are deposited into this account; and personnel salaries and purchases are paid by CLAS out of this account.

Human resource management mechanisms in non-CLAS versus CLAS are highly differentiated and are a major reason for the greater efficiency of CLAS. In non-CLAS, health staff who are government payroll employees are not accountable for their work except in serious faults; short-term contract employees are common in non-CLAS, but they receive no benefits; employees are evaluated solely on the basis of number of reported consultations per day, creating a focus on curative care and giving incentive for over-reporting of consultations. Government payroll employees work in both CLAS and non-CLAS facilities: in CLAS these are legally accountable to CLAS members, but they have little local accountability when working in a non-CLAS. The CLAS system allows use of direct private-sector contracts with full benefits: paid vacation, bi-annual bonuses, private pension plan, and health insurance. And these personnel are directly accountable to CLAS.

What are the results of these differences in health sector management? Early on in the program there was already evidence that CLAS was better able to selectively provide exonerations to the poor, as compared to non-CLAS, improving equity of

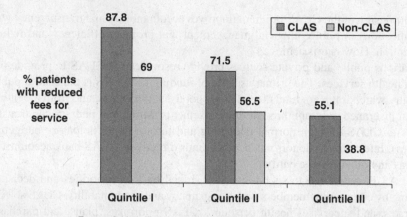

Fuente: LAltobelli (1998) Health reform, community participation and social inclusion: the Shared Administration Program. Lima, Peru: UNICEF. (Data from National Survey for Living Standards, 1998)

Fig. 12.5 Proportion of patients with full or partial reduction in fees for service in three lowest income quintiles, comparing CLAS versus non-CLAS

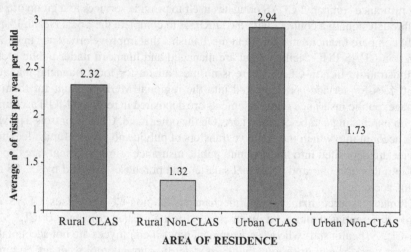

Source: Altobelli L and A Sovero (2004) Cost-Efficiency of CLAS. Lima, Peru: Future Generations. (Data: SIS Health Insurance Program, Plan A, 2002)

Fig. 12.6 Average no. of consultations per child <age 5, by area and type of management in 600 PHC facilities of Cusco, Huánuco, and La Libertad Regions 2002

access, as shown in Fig. 12.5. CLAS was able to provide nearly double the coverage of key child health services for better cost-efficiency as compared to non-CLAS, despite having fewer medical staff, as shown in Figs. 12.6 and 12.7. Other comparative studies on CLAS vs. non-CLAS uses national survey data to have greater utilization due to better quality of service (see Fig. 12.8) and greater impact on child growth (see Fig. 12.9) despite the lower socioeconomic situation of populations in CLAS catchment areas versus that of non-CLAS.

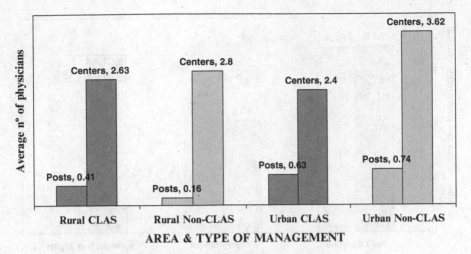

Source: Analysis by author. Data: 2006 National Inventory of Infrastructure, Equipment, and Human Resources. Lima, Peru: Ministry of Health.

Fig. 12.7 Average number of physicians in PHC facilities, by area and type of management 2006

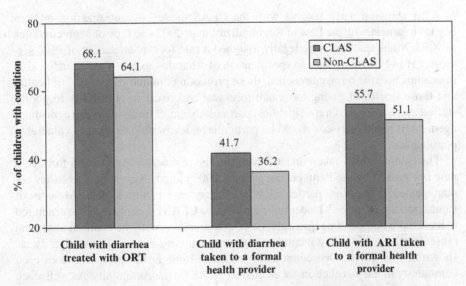

Source: Altobelli, L (2006) Análisis comparativo de impacto en salud y utilización de servicios de salud en CLAS y No-CLAS. Lima: Future Generations. (Data: ENDES IV)

Fig. 12.8 Proportion of rural mothers who sought care for sick child <age 5, by type of management in nearest PHC facility 1996–2000

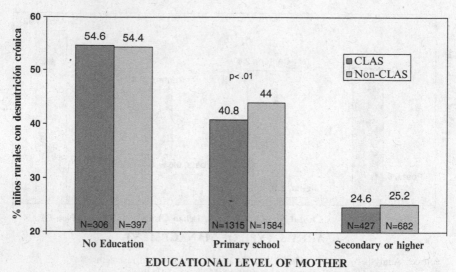

Source: Altobelli, L (2006) Comparative analysis of impact and utilization of health
services in CLAS and non-CLAS. Lima, Peru: Future Generations. (Data: DHS Peru 2000)

Fig. 12.9 Proportion of rural children <age 5 with chronic malnutrition, by maternal education
and type of management of nearest PHC facility 1996–2000

After showing early success with the CLAS model, decentralization in Peru
began in earnest with the Law of Regionalization in 2002 and Law of Municipalities
in 2003. Municipalities were legally assigned a role for "management of PHC services." However, there was no specification of what this meant. Two already existing camps became more entrenched: those promoting "municipalization" of health,
and those fearful of giving too much technical and fiscal responsibility to poorly
staffed and unprepared municipalities, particularly small rural ones where mismanagement of health services would be particularly devastating to already vulnerable
populations.

This situation was taken under control by the restructuring of CLAS through a
new law passed by the Peruvian congress in 2007 called, "Law that establishes co-
management and citizen participation in primary care facilities of the Ministry of
Health and the Regions." Under this new law, the CLAS committee was restructured
to have more democratic representation of communities, with the addition of several
representatives of local government entities including the local municipality, as
shown in Fig. 12.10. One community leader and one health promoter from each
community in the jurisdiction are elected to CLAS by the community. As well, each
social organization that is associated with health or nutrition elects their representative to CLAS. Among government representatives in the new composition of CLAS,
there is one elected representative from among health facility employees, one representative designated by the network or micronetwork management center, one
representative designated by the regional government, and one designed by the

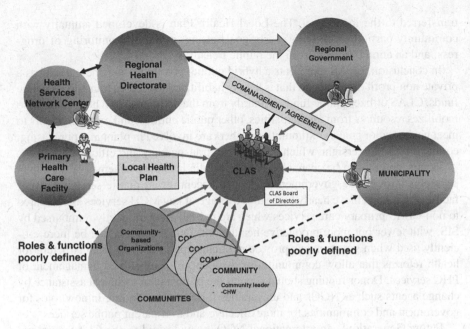

Fig. 12.10 Structure of CLAS under Law No. 29124 of 2007

district municipality (who cannot be the municipal mayor him/herself). This restructuring allows broader representation and more transparency in the decision-making for effective use of discretionary health resources.

Under the new law on CLAS and new decentralization laws, funds can flow from public and private sources to PHC services and eventually to communities for both health and development projects. Starting with a new organizational strategy to link PHC services with communities, financing can flow from any source directly to CLAS bank accounts from which PHC services are administered. Through a community empowerment strategy whereby health personnel help communities to develop Community Work Plans, CLAS can help to finance health activities in communities. Community Work Plans facilitate funding streams from Municipalities, which before had trouble prioritizing their expenditures. In this way, community development needs, identified by the communities themselves, are more appropriately met, thereby improving the quality of expenditure of public and donor financing.

CLAS management is based on results for better effectiveness of both public treasury and donor financing. For PHC services in Peru that are not administered by CLAS, there is no local budget management. CLAS-run facilities, on the other hand, have two results-based management tools: the Co-Management Agreement between the CLAS, the district municipality, and the regional MOH. This agreement is based on the district development plan and has specific goals agreed on that are in line with the Millennium Development Goals. The other is the Local Health Plan that is created by each CLAS on the basis of which public funding is transferred to the local level. The Local Health Plan is developed annually with community participation, with yearly goal setting, monthly monitoring of progress, and an annual budget from the public treasury.

In conclusion, CLAS represents a hybrid public–private management model as a private non-profit organization that is legally habilitated to receive transfers of public funds. CLAS utilizes public funds primarily from the national health budget, but also mobilizes resources from municipalities, other public entities, and external donors to meet health sector goals. Community members are involved in planning, purchasing, contracting, and oversight, which contribute to transparency and efficiency.

Donor funding can be channeled through public insurance schemes or per capita payments through the government system to decentralized public service delivery facilities. CLAS achieve nearly twice the coverage of key MCH services as compared to non-CLAS primary care services which are partially and indirectly reimbursed by SIS, with fewer but more productive health staff. Donor funding can be more efficiently used when governments provide political support and the legal structure for health reforms that allow community-involvement in results-based management of PHC services. Donor funding should support the provision of technical assistance by change agents such as NGOs and universities for capacity building in new roles for government and communities for more effective and transparent public services.

Future Generations, an international NGO, provides aid to the CLAS system's participatory budgeting and local collaborative management by linking both of these functions more effectively with the communities served by CLAS and thereby helping the health system to strengthen its relationship with local municipalities. The goal is to develop an effective and efficient community-oriented health model based on incorporating participatory and results-oriented budget processes into municipal oversight of primary healthcare service delivery.

Future Generations also trains teams of municipal officials, health sector personnel, and community representatives to work with local communities to develop a strategic vision based on local data and community priorities and a work plan to implement the vision. For priorities that require resources from outside the community, projects are presented in the annual participatory budgeting process. Municipal officials have found this an ideal method for ensuring that they satisfy community needs and demands as required by law and learn community organizing skills that bring them closer to their constituents.

The CLAS model of PHC management has been recognized in Peru through a number of national awards and recognitions. Internationally, the OECD identified CLAS in their analysis of Peru as one of the best examples of transparency and citizen participation in oversight of public services. The World Health Organization included CLAS as one of 13 case studies of programs that address social determinants of health in a book published by WHO in 2011.

Acknowledgments The author acknowledges the following persons who have collaborated in the development of CLAS in Peru: Jaime Freundt-Thurne, M.D., Carl E. Taylor, M.D., Dr.P.H., Juan José Vera, Ing., Ricardo Díaz-Romero, M.D., Carlos Acosta-Saal, M.D., Jackeline De La Cruz, M.D., Alexander Tarev, M.D., M.P.H., Luis Espejo-Alayo, M.D., M.S., Jose Cabrejos-Pita M.D., M.P.H., Alejandro Vargas-Vásquez, M.A., M.S., and others not listed here.

Chapter 13
Academia's Role in Improving Aid Effectiveness in Global Health

Padmini Murthy, Amy Ansehl, and Aishwarya Narasimhadevara

Introduction

The role of academia in the past two decades has undergone a great transformation in not only being an instrument of education, and bringing new evidence of effective practice to the field of global health, but also in the development of a work force to promote aid development in various settings globally and implementing projects that improve the health of various populations.

In recent years, there has been a tremendous increase in donor investment to fund projects particularly to fight specific diseases such as AIDS, malaria, and TB in low-income countries around the world. The various donors that include foundations, private sector, and governments are interested in making sure that the allocated funds are being used effectively in promoting sustainable development which is synonymous with aid effectiveness. This proactive stance taken by the donors has been a major contributor to the development of a new field which is known as "evidence-based advocacy" and is being recognized as a powerful indicator to measure aid effectiveness. Donors make decisions about project funding which is

---

Between now and 2015, we must make sure that promises made become promises kept. The consequences of doing otherwise are profound: death, illness and despair, needless suffering, lost opportunities for millions upon millions of people.
UN Secretary-General Ban Ki-Moon

P. Murthy, M.D., M.P.H., F.A.M.W.A., F.R.S.H. (✉)
Global Health, New York Medical College,
School of Health Sciences and Practice, Valahalla, NY, USA
e-mail: minimurthy@aol.com

A. Ansehl, D.N.P., F.N.P-.B.C.
Environmental Health Science, New York Medical College, School of Health Sciences and Practice, Valhalla, NY, USA

A. Narasimhadevara, M.A.
Brussels School of International Studies, University of Kent, Bruxelles, Belgium

© Springer Science+Business Media New York 2015
E. Beracochea (ed.), *Improving Aid Effectiveness in Global Health*,
DOI 10.1007/978-1-4939-2721-0_13

based on the data they receive and review as this indicates the success or failure of proposed projects. The skills and expertise needed for data collection and analysis is usually found in academic institutions (Pierce 2006).

Ruth Katz, former dean of George Washington University School of Public Health, sums up the role of academia aptly in her quote "faculty helps produce the research, the evidence that is the basis for global efforts" (Pierce 2006).

Faculty and researchers at various universities in North America and Europe serve as visiting scholars or consultants on various projects in many low- and mid-income countries.

Similarly, faculty from developing countries visiting the academic institutions in North America and Europe will help to maximize the role of academia in being an important cornerstone for aid effectiveness.

Role of Academia

At present, in lieu of the ongoing conflicts in countries and between nations, the role of academia is crucial in bringing together various players from different diverse ethnic groups and fields in building bridges through peaceful negotiations. To illustrate the power of academia in being crucial for promoting peace and sustainable development, graduates from universities and colleges bring to their communities the knowledge and skills learned at these institutions to develop stable societies. These graduates and alumni often go on to work in leadership positions and can help to bring about effective leadership and good governance, which can be instrumental in attracting donor investment.

Geology for Global Development is a not-for-profit which can be best described as a "think tank" and has been successful in bringing adversarial or warring countries (India and Pakistan) together in working on issues of concern for them through effective academic settings. An example is the recently held conference in June 2014 in Leh, the Ladakh region in the Himalayas, which was jointly organized by the Geological Society of London in collaboration with the Institute of Energy Research and Training at the University of Jammu, India. This initiative in the Himalayan region focused on the education and engagement of students and faculty on the following issues: access to clean water, climate change, and energy conservation. Initiatives such as these are crucial in promoting neutral working environments for mutual cooperation and promoting donor investment (Geology for Global Development 2014).

Examples: Think and Act Locally with Global Outcomes

The authors have been involved with grass roots work highlighting the principle of local action for a global outcome. A partnership effort was established by Dr. Padmini Murthy (one of the authors) with The Callista Mutharika Foundation, which was started by the former first lady of Malawi to promote safe motherhood practices in Malawi. In June 2011, Murthy had the opportunity of meeting HE Callista Mutharika, wife of the President of Malawi, at a high level meeting in the United Nations and learnt about the high rates of maternal mortality in Malawi. This meeting was instrumental in Murthy spearheading the NYMC Safe motherhood project, in which she worked with her colleague Amy Ansehl (co-author) in organizing a student effort to raise funds and supplies for Malawi. In the span of 1 year, the team collected 150 boxes of medical supplies and assembled 250 Mama Kits and USD 13,200 to build a maternity waiting home for high-risk pregnant women in Malawi. Since the team worked with the foundation and the wife of the Permanent representative of the Malawi mission to the United Nations, there were no overhead expenses and the collected funds were completely earmarked for the project.

This project is an example of a success story which illustrates the role academia played in promoting aid effectiveness and efficiency in the arena of global health.

Paris Declaration and Beyond

At the Second High Level Forum on Aid Effectiveness (2005), it was recognized that aid could—and should—be producing better impacts. The Paris Declaration was endorsed in order to base development efforts on first-hand experience of what works and does not work with aid. It is formulated around five central pillars: Ownership, Alignment, Harmonization, Managing for Results, and Mutual Accountability. (Organization for Economic and Social Development [OESD] n.d.)

The power imbalance in the development cooperation is an important issue that needs to be dealt with and academia is an effective catalyst in reducing this imbalance. The commitments in the Paris Declaration advocate for partners in development to cooperate in a mutual partnership, and this translates into the need for recipients to take more responsibility in development strategy (High Level Forum, 2005). The aid effectiveness agenda has been at the forefront at the High Level Forum in 2008, which was the follow-up to the Paris Declaration and which was held in Ghana and Busan (High Level Forum 2008, 2012).

During the events that led to the development of the Paris Declaration and the consequent High Level talks, several local civil society organizations including members from academia were proactive advocate for the inclusion of civil society players to be active partners in the development partnership, since they felt their participation was disregarded in the Paris Declaration. In a retrospective review, the debate on aid effectiveness has been an important item for discussion on the agenda of the international community and this culminated at the high level forum with the outcome being the Paris Deceleration in 2005 (Whitfield and Fraser 2009). However, the year of aid effectiveness started in 2003 at the Rome Declaration where the stakeholders made a commitment to harmonize and align aid. As a follow-up to this, at the High Level Forum 2 the commitments of the Rome Declaration were reaffirmed, and the following five partnership commitments were agreed upon:

1. Ownership—Partner countries exercise effective leadership over their development policies and strategies, and co-ordinate development actions

2. Alignment—Donors base their overall support on partner countries' national development strategies institutions and procedures
3. Harmonization—Donors' actions are more harmonized, transparent, and collectively effective
4. Managing for results—Managing resources and improving decision-making for results
5. Mutual accountability—Donors and partners are accountable for development results (High Level Forum 2 2005)

Academic institutions have been playing an important role in working to reaffirm the five partnership commitments which have been listed above. For example, the CUGH, i.e., the Consortium of Universities for Global Health, has been at the forefront in establishing guidelines and framework to facilitate aid effectiveness for its partners and other stakeholders working in the field. The mission of CUGH as described by the organization is

Dedicated to creating balance in resources and in the exchange of students and faculty between institutions in rich and poor countries, recognizing the importance of equal partnership between the academic institutions in developing nations and their resource-rich counterparts in the planning, implementation, management, and impact evaluation of joint projects. (Consortium of Global Universities [CUGH] 2014)

This statement has been translated into action by its academic partners in North America, who have been instrumental in launching projects in developing countries to improve the health status of communities. Some examples of partnerships which have been effective will be discussed in the section titled partnering with a purpose.

Partnering with a Purpose

Examining the role of academia in promoting aid effectiveness is illustrated in the partnering with non-governmental organizations, foundations, and the United Nations agencies. Aid effectiveness has become a significant buzz word in development rhetoric and academia has emerged as an important player in the arena. In this connection, the concept of "Partnership Approach" has emerged, as a strategy of how to manage development assistance (Andersen and Therkildsen 2007).

As observed, donors base their development assistance on different interests, Hyden (2008) considers the partnership approach, more as a mutual partnership, with focus on both donors and recipient countries commitment to "ownership" and "alignment partnership approach" presupposes a high level of trust between partners, in the sense that there is a social contract rather than a business contract, where partners have more at stake. The recipient countries' strategy has to trust that donors are willing to align to their development strategy. The role of academia as mentioned previously in the chapter is crucial in this process of checks and balances and creation of a favorable environment for the process.

Pfizer has been partnering with universities to train healthcare workers in Rwanda, which is an example of the effective team work between academia and the private sector in promoting aid effectiveness (Pierce 2006).

Another example of partnering with a purpose which has been successful is the HIV Equity Initiative launched in 1998 by Partners in Health (PIH) in Haiti and this has the unique distinction of being the first program in the world to provide free services and HIV/AIDS treatment to the socially disenfranchised populations and members of academia have been active partners in this initiative and many of the other projects undertaken by PIH (Partners in Health [PIH] 2009).

The Academic Response

Academia in recent times has begun to shape global health training programs to educate and empower health professionals through cross-disciplinary didactic and experiential and by providing a hands on learning experience which includes service delivery. As a result, the academic programs in global health have been established in the global north and south and have included a pretty much well-rounded curriculum, which focuses on both qualitative and quantitative research methodology, data collection and analysis, social science (Garrett 2007). These programs also include the principles of behavioral science, technology, and practice of public health incorporating the social determinants of health. Some examples of innovative courses included in the curriculum in schools which train the next generation of global health workers include gold standards for global health practice, training community health workers, and the development and political economy to name a few.

In an effort to bring academics, diplomats, and other stake holders in June 2007, the Graduate Institute of International Studies, Geneva (HEI), welcomed 18 participants, with professional backgrounds in both diplomacy and health and representing ten countries, to the first Summer Program on Global Health Diplomacy.

This program was designed to be interactive and the participants were able to engage with a faculty of health professionals and diplomats to share views and professional experiences from their work. The goals of the course were to focus on health diplomacy as it relates to health issues that cross national boundaries and are global in nature and discuss the challenges facing health diplomacy and how they have been addressed by different groups and at different levels of governance. In recent years, *Health Diplomacy* is seen to play an important role in aid effectiveness as it is instrumental in addressing the interdependence/interface between foreign policy and health, which attempts to create policy coherence between the various stakeholders (Kickbusch et al. 2007).

Academia has an important role to play in shaping the governmental and nongovernmental emphasis on health in international relations at present, especially in lieu of the various conflicts at present; examples include the ongoing armed conflicts and societal instability in Afghanistan, Iraq, and the middle east and recognizing this the

World Health Organization has been working with academic institutions globally to address maternal and child health. This partnership has resulted in the establishment of the maternal and child health division within the Colorado School of Public Health's Center for Global Health and was designated by the World Health Organization (WHO) as a WHO Collaborating Center for Promoting Family and Child Health. This center has been collaborating with WHO and the Pan American Health Organization (PAHO) with a focus on the following areas:

- Assist countries in reducing health inequality and excessive morbidity and mortality among mothers, infants, children, and adolescents
- Accelerate vaccine research and implementation
- Train vulnerable communities and countries in disaster preparedness in ways that will meet the needs of children
- Train doctors, nurses, midwives, and other birth attendants in the Helping Babies Breathe program, to reduce neonatal asphyxia (Center for Global Health n.d.).

The above-mentioned objectives are crucial in making donors aware of the outcome of their investment and also are instrumental in compiling data-driven outcomes, which are needed for monitoring and evaluation and for replication of projects which meet the criteria of being designated as best practices.

The landscape of global health, diplomacy, donors aid recipients, sustainable development, and foreign relations has changed in the past decade and thus the global community needs a new lens on what is effective in global health and how to view the dynamic and fluid landscape of global health. This lens is academia.

Aid workers and academics can collaborate well in enhancing aid effectiveness and sustainable development. Many academic institutions have included the field of developmental studies in their curricula. It is not uncommon to have academics take on the dual responsibility, i.e., teaching at an institution and also of working in the field as aid workers and mentoring students and local stakeholders in data-driven service delivery. The Asia Foundation embarked on a multi-year collaboration in 2012 with the London School of Economics named "Justice and Security Research Program" (JSRP) to look into the "theories of change", which focuses on the ultimate impact on the health status of the global populations. This initiative by the foundation has been instrumental in providing a platform for academics and aid practitioners to engage with each other, both on an intellectual and a practical manner. "On the one hand they allow practitioners to directly tie research to their actual programs on the ground. On the other, they allow academics to look at the relative causality of aid programs in relation to wider social change" (Arnold 2013). This collaborative project has resulted in identifying areas where academia and aid workers can work in teams effectively to strengthen the quality of development assistance provided and maximize aid effectiveness. In addition, the findings provided as a result of such research have started to influence programmatic management, within Asia Foundation country offices, and can be used effectively to attract donor finding (Arnold 2013).

Recognizing the dynamic and powerful resources academia offers, the United Nations in 2009 launched the United Nations Academic Impact and launched a global partnership with universities to promote aid effectiveness and sustainable development. Institutions globally are partnering with UN agencies and donors to ensure aid effectives and sustainable development. One of the mechanisms used is that they committed to advance the following ten principles listed below:

1. A commitment to the principles inherent in the United Nations Charter as values that education seeks to promote and help fulfill
2. A commitment to human rights, among them freedom of inquiry, opinion, and speech
3. A commitment to educational opportunity for all people regardless of gender, race, religion, or ethnicity
4. A commitment to the opportunity for every interested individual to acquire the skills and knowledge necessary for the pursuit of higher education
5. A commitment to building capacity in higher education systems across the world
6. A commitment to encouraging global citizenship through education
7. A commitment to advancing peace and conflict resolution through education
8. A commitment to addressing issues of poverty through education
9. A commitment to promoting sustainability through education
10. A commitment to promoting inter-cultural dialogue and understanding, and the "unlearning" of intolerance, through education (United Nations Academic Impact [UNAI] 2014).

The authors would like to recommend that these ten principles of the UNAI listed above be adopted and incorporated into the service delivery mechanisms by all academic institutions which work in global health as the gold standard of academic practice.

Conclusion

The landscape of global health, diplomacy, donors aid recipients, sustainable development, and foreign relations has changed rapidly since the past decade and thus the global community needs a new lens on what is effective in global health and how to view this dynamic and fluid landscape and this lens is academia. The role played by academia is becoming more prominent in the post 2015 agenda and the United Nations. Recognizing the positive impact academia has in promoting aid effectiveness, the various United Nations agencies have been appointing renowned academics as advisors and consultants to promote this agenda and to take it from theory to practice.

Aid workers and academics can collaborate well in enhancing aid effectiveness and sustainable development. Many academic institutions have included the field of developmental studies in their curricula. It is not uncommon to have academics take on the dual responsibility, i.e., teaching at an institution and also of working in the field as aid workers and mentoring students and local stake holders in data-driven service delivery. The theories of change have focused on the socio economic determinants prevalent in society and have been important in providing a platform for academics and aid practitioners to engage with each other, both on an intellectual and a practical manner. "On the one hand they allow practitioners to directly tie research to their actual programs on the ground. On the other, they allow academics to look at the relative causality of aid programs in relation to wider social change"(Arnold 2013). Arnold's collaborative project has resulted in identifying areas where academia and aid workers can work in teams effectively to strengthen the quality of development assistance provided and maximize aid effectiveness. In addition, the findings have started to influence programmatic management, within the Asia Foundation country offices, and can be used effectively to attract donor finding (Arnold 2013).

Some of the perceived disadvantages of academic partnering in aid effectiveness may include increased costs, narrow research which some donors feel is too complicated and time-consuming. In addition, academic research methods and evaluation may be viewed as being complicated and cannot be shared before translating it into a format which can be easily understood by all the stakeholders. This may contribute to an additional expense and time before a clear picture of the success or failure of the project is known. Some donors may hesitate to seek academic input for the projects they are funding due to the so-called inflexible and impractical outlook of the academic institutions and their faculty.

However, the advantages of partnering with academia in the opinion of the authors outweigh the disadvantages due to its impact in demonstrating evidence-based interventions and preparing the future global health professionals.

In conclusion, academic institutions can be effective partners working at many levels with various stake holders such as the private sector, foundations, private sector in maximizing aid effectiveness and in ascertaining that the funds allocated contribute to the long-term sustainable development of communities. This can be summed up well by this quote "If we can work toward instilling some of the rigor, objectivity and ethics of academia into the more practical, decisive, dynamic world of international development, both will be better off" (Svenson 2001).

Questions for Discussion

1. Discuss why Academia is being recognized as a key stakeholder in improving service delivery and aid effectiveness of global health?
2. Do you agree that students in the discipline of global health needed to be involved in service delivery projects as a part of their curriculum to make them effective leaders in promoting global health advancement and diplomacy?
3. Do you agree with the authors' recommendation of adopting the ten principles of the United Nations Academic Impact for institutions working to promote aid effectiveness in improving global health? How would you apply these principles in your work?
4. Can you share an example of best practice at grass roots to increase targeted aid/aid effectiveness which you have heard of or have been involved in?

References

Andersen, O., & Therkildsen, O. (2007). *Harmonisation and alignment: The doubled edged swords of budget support and decentralised aid administration* (Working Paper No. 2007/4). Retrieved from http://www.diis.dk/sw32922.asp

Arnold (2013). Getting Academics and aid workers to work together. Retrieved from http://asia-foundation.org/in-asia/2013/12/11/getting-academics-and-aid-workers-to-work-together/

Center for Global Health. (n.d.). Retrieved from http://www.ucdenver.edu/academics/colleges/PublicHealth/research/centers/globalhealth/about/Pages/WHO-Collaborating-Center.aspx

Consortium of Global Universities. (2014). Retrieved from http://www.cugh.org/about-cugh

Garrett, L. (2007). The challenge of global health. *Foreign Affairs, 86*, 1–17.

Geology for Global Development. (2014). Retrieved from http://www.gfgd.org/projects/himalayas2014

High Level Forum. (2005). Paris declaration on aid effectiveness. Retrieved from http://www.oecd.org/dataoecd/11/41/34428351.pdf

High Level forum (2008). Third level forum on aid effectiveness. Retrieved from http://www.oecd.org/dac/effectiveness/theaccrahighlevelforumhlf3andtheaccraagendaforaction.htm

High level forum (2012). 4th High level forum on aid effectiveness in Busan, South Korea. Retrieved from http://cso-effectiveness.org/busan-partnership-for-effective,190

Hyden, G. (2008). After the Paris Declaration: Taking on the issue of power. *Development Policy Review, 26*(3), 259–274.

Kickbusch, I., Silberschmidt, G., & Buss, P. (2007). Global health diplomacy: The need for new perspectives, strategic approaches and skills in global health. *The Bulletin of the World Health Organization, 85*, 243–244.

Organization for Economic and Social Development (n.d.). Retreived from http://www.oecd.org/

Partners in Health. (2009). Retrieved from http://www.pih.org/priority-programs/hiv-aids/about

Pierce, O. (2006). The Role of Academia in the Global Aid Industry. Retrieved from http://www.terradaily.com/reports/The_Role_Of_Academia_In_The_Global_Aid_Industry_999.html

Svenson, N. (2001). The academic council on the United Nations System Informational Memorandum No. 2.

United Nations Academic Impact. (2014). Retrieved from https://academicimpact.un.org/; http://hei.unige.ch/summer/healthindex.html

Whitfield, L., & Fraser, A. (2009). Negotiating aid. In *The politics of aid African strategies for dealing with donors*. London: Oxford University.

Part III
Challenges

Chapter 14
When Charity Destroys Dignity and Sustainability

Glenn J. Schwartz

Introduction

I have been involved in cross-cultural missionary work since 1961 when I first went from the USA to Africa. That is now more than 53 years ago. Very early in my missionary career I became aware of the importance of local sustainability—allowing local people to learn the joy and privilege of supporting their own churches and community development work. In the limited training I had for cross-cultural ministry in those days, no one expressly taught me about sustainability issues. What I learned over the years was through gentle nudges from the Lord as I stumbled onto an article or illustration here and there. For the past 30 years, I have been engaged in writing, speaking, and consulting about self-reliance issues in the Christian movement.[1]

One of the earliest stories I heard about came from Vietnam or French Indo-China as it was then called. When the French Indo-China war ended, missionaries returned to see what happened to the church they left behind when they were forced to leave. Upon their arrival back into the country, they discovered much devastation and wondered what they might do to help the suffering church. They noticed that many pastors' houses had been damaged during the war. Their first thought was that they, as missionaries, could help to rebuild those houses. But the church members

---

[1] About the Author—Glenn Schwartz Served as a missionary in Zambia and Zimbabwe during the 1960s. He then served for 6 years in the 1970s as Assistant to the Dean of the School of World Mission (now School of Intercultural Studies) at Fuller Theological Seminary. From 1983 to 2012 he served as Executive Director of World Mission Associates conducting seminars and consultations on sustainability of Christian institutions in the Christian movement. He has done this in many countries around the world. Since 2012 he continues in ministry and holds the position of Executive Director Emeritus of World Mission Associates based in Lancaster, Pennsylvania.

G.J. Schwartz (✉)
Former Executive Director of World Mission Associates, Lancaster, PA, USA
e-mail: glennschwartz@msn.com

© Springer Science+Business Media New York 2015
E. Beracochea (ed.), *Improving Aid Effectiveness in Global Health*,
DOI 10.1007/978-1-4939-2721-0_14

rejected the missionaries' offer, saying, "It is our privilege to repair our own pastors' houses." That incident had a significant impact on me.

A **second** event happened when I was a young missionary working in rural villages in Zambia. By this time, I had a premonition about the importance of local people doing for themselves what they could with their own resources. I learned recently of a succinct way of saying this: "Do what you can … with what you have … where you are." In this particular case, we were sitting under a locally constructed shelter discussing a new church plant in the area. Some of the local leaders asked how much the mission would be willing to give toward the construction of a new church building. I pointed to a nicely built building next to where we were sitting that was made with burnt brick and mortar, complete with a corrugated iron roof. It was a locally owned grocery store. I asked how much came from the mission for that building. They seemed to scoff at the idea that anyone from the outside—like the mission—would need to pay for "their" grocery store. My next question was, "Then why is it not possible to build a church building of the same quality as the store?"

I soon came to live by an important principle: People can have a church building equal to the quality of the homes in which they live. If they have grass-covered houses made of poles and mud plaster, they can have a church equal to that. If they live in houses made with burnt brick walls, concrete floors, and a metal roof, then they can most likely afford a church like that. If they live in western style houses with heating and air conditioning, they can have churches equivalent to that. As you may suspect, dependency happens when outsiders, who are used to a higher level of "brick and mortar," decide what a church should look like—and then offer to put in enough money to make it happen! That is where the dependency syndrome gets a foothold.

But this raises an important question: Why are so many people not able to build their own church buildings, clinics, or hospitals? For quite some years, I have been concentrating on this question, traveling far and wide encouraging church and mission leaders to consider the importance of helping local people discover the joy and privilege of doing things for themselves. I am referring to doing things that they can do with their own resources and creativity.

I also learned that it is quite common for local people to ask for assistance even when they could do things for themselves. While serving as a missionary in Zambia, I was once asked by several church leaders for overseas funding for a project that they were discussing. My question was, "Why do you ask for funding from overseas whenever you begin working on a project?" The response I was given is classic and one that has stayed with me for the past 30 years: "We always ask first, and we are usually given!" So why not ask!

Presuppositions Are Part of the Problem

I have learned over the years that the presuppositions with which we enter cross-cultural ministry often determine whether unhealthy dependency will develop. If we assume that people are too poor to do things for themselves, we will probably be right. On the other hand, if we begin with the assumption that there are local resources within arm's reach which could be mobilized, then we will also be right. Presuppositions determine the outcome and are like small self-fulfilling prophecies. The ideas we begin with will most likely determine the results.

I must quickly add that while unhealthy dependency has developed because of faulty assumptions, this does not mean that the situation is without hope. I believe it is easier to avoid unhealthy dependency from the beginning than to overcome it after it has taken root. I also firmly believe that unhealthy dependency can be overcome where it exists. There are many examples of churches, hospitals, Bible Institutes, and other institutions which have overcome unhealthy dependency and where people learned the joy of standing on their own two feet. Progress in this area is usually a result of someone, somewhere, changing the assumptions with which they carry out their ministry. If I did not believe that such change was possible, then I believe our world would be doomed to live with a growing dependency mentality. We must not assume that nothing can be done about it.

A simple illustration shows what I mean by this. Several years ago I spoke on issues of dependency at a large mission conference in North America. When the conference ended, I was standing by the door waiting for my ride to the airport. A man saw me and said he wanted to share his experience. He said he was a medical doctor and that he and his wife were missionaries in Ghana where they ran a mission hospital. He said the hospital was dependent on him as an American medical doctor, and it was also dependent on money from America to keep it going. Someone recommended that he acquire the eight-hour video series that World Mission Associates (our small organization) had prepared on dependency. After he and his wife watched the videos, they asked themselves what they should be doing differently based on what they learned from the videos. He then said, "That was 10 years ago, and today that hospital is fully staffed by Ghanaian workers and totally funded with local resources." I tell this story to show that one of the ways churches, hospitals, and other institutions become sustainable is through a change in the presuppositions on the part of those who began the work or inherited it from someone else. I will go so far as to say that without this change of assumptions—by both insiders and outsiders—there may be little hope that local sustainability becomes possible.

About 10 years ago, I learned about a medical mission organization that was launched with a worldwide goal of ministry in 4 countries. I shared the platform with them one evening and spoke on the matter of discovering and mobilizing local resources. At the end of the evening, the founders of the new organization began to reassess the number of countries in which they would work. When they took into consideration the availability of local resources that could be mobilized, they adjusted their goal from 4 to 80 countries. Today, 10 years after that event, that mission society is serving in 74 countries—almost reaching their goal of 80. This is a result of adjusting assumptions based on what can happen when local resources are brought into the picture.

Lessons Learned from a Consultation on Medical Institutions in East Africa[2]

At a medical conference held in Nairobi, Kenya, in the year 2000, about 70 medical officers, hospital administrators, and others related to cross-cultural healthcare spent 5 days telling about their successes and failures regarding the sustainability of Christian medical institutions. At the conclusion of the conference, it was agreed that the syndrome of dependency may be widespread, but it is not inevitable or incurable. The following are a few illustrations from the lessons learned.

First, some of the best examples of local sustainability were with hospitals in countries where government subsidy was not available. Two of the case studies from countries outside of East Africa were presented, and both, despite substantial government subsidy, were struggling for their existence. Other hospitals (in places like Kenya) were able to exist almost completely on local resources. This was *in spite of* the fact that government subsidy was not available in Kenya. Conclusion: *Local sustainability is not tied to the availability of government funding.*

Second, there is no substitute for solid local "ownership." Several illustrations are in order. One hospital in Kenya succeeded in recruiting Kenyan-trained medical doctors from an East African university. Hospital staff developed a relationship with doctors in training and followed them through their educational experience until they were ready to serve. The transition from the medical school to the hospital did not allow for an overseas "brain drain" because young doctors went to serve in a Kenyan hospital where they already had a relationship. In this particular hospital, there were four Kenyan medical doctors all supported by the hospital from local resources. The hospital received 95 % of its funding from local resources.

One other factor about that hospital is significant. The financial viability of this Kenyan hospital was helped by the presence on staff of four debt counselors who went into the surrounding villages to counsel those who were asked to pay for the healthcare they were receiving from the hospital.

Tumutumu Hospital (a Presbyterian institution) in Kenya fell into economic difficulties and was threatened with closure. Those providing funding from overseas developed "donor fatigue" and issued an order to close the hospital. Local people rose up and asked, "How can someone from overseas tell us that our hospital should be closed? Let us take it over to see what we can do." This is a vivid example of the transfer of "psychological ownership"—a central issue in promoting local sustainability. But there is more to the story.

The transformation of Tumutumu Hospital is nothing short of astonishing. Local people from the Tumutumu area went back to the place where the Gospel was first brought to Kenya by Presbyterian missionaries at the beginning of the twentieth

---

[2] The next section of this chapter is excerpted and edited from the book When Charity Destroys Dignity: Overcoming Unhealthy Dependency in the Christian Movement—Chap. 23, page 310ff. This 400-page book is available on the website of World Mission Associates at www.wmausa.org.

century. That was in a suburb of Nairobi called Kikuyu, about 150 km from Tumutumu Hospital. A small group of concerned individuals organized a march from Kikuyu to Tumutumu. Among the marchers were medical personnel as well as pastors and other believers. As they marched toward Tumutumu, they held roadside clinics and evangelistic meetings in the evenings. When villagers along the way asked why they were marching they were told. "We are trying to save our hospital. Help us!" Through this effort, the organizers of the march raised awareness and invited others to join them.

So successful was their effort that in a short period of time the hospital went from 95 % foreign funding to 95 % local funding. Facilities were refurbished, and new equipment was installed. It soon became a showpiece for those in other hospitals in Kenya. Staff from other hospitals came to learn about the transformation of Tumutumu Hospital.[3]

A **third** illustration of the transformation of a hospital took place at Clinica Biblica, a mission-run hospital in Costa Rica. This was a mission hospital started by missionaries, but eventually it was overtaken by what one might call "mission fatigue." Similar to Tumutumu, it was the donors overseas that recommended closing the hospital. Upon hearing about this threatened closure in the 1970s, local people in Costa Rica asked if they could take over the hospital in an effort to keep it going.

So successful was the transformation of Clinica Biblica that it, too, became a model medical institution in the region. Several years ago, Clinica Biblica launched an expansion program costing about 23 million dollars. There were several major side benefits of this transition to local ownership.

First, it stopped draining funds from the mission agency—funds intended to be used for the spread of the gospel, not for subsidizing a church or mission-run institution.

Second, services to those in need were significantly increased in both quality and availability.

Third, the new "owners" established a fee scale in which middle and upper class people needing treatment helped to subsidize those who were unable to pay. This is sometimes referred to as "cross-over income" and is similar to North American hospitals that treat the poor either free or at a reduced rate. As much as 40 % of Clinica Biblica's services were redirected to those who were otherwise unable to afford medical care.

A **fourth** Illustration is provided through the experience of Dr. Dan Fountain who served as a medical missionary in Congo for more than 35 years.[4] Vanga Hospital was a small rural mission hospital in the northwestern part of the Democratic Republic of the Congo. It was established in 1912 and struggled to

---

[3] A more complete story about this can be found on the WMA website at www.wmausa.org under the title *The Transformation of Tumutumu Hospital.*

[4] Dr. Fountain wrote this story in a book called *Health for All: The Vanga Story.* It is available through William Carey Publishers, Pasadena, California.

survive as many mission hospitals do. In 1961, 1 year after the country gained independence from Belgium, Dr. Fountain and his wife arrived at Vanga. Initially he was the only physician serving the hospital and the 250,000 people in its surrounding area of 2,500 square miles. Beginning in 1961, church leaders, and a small growing group of Congolese nurses and staff, were able to build a comprehensive African, Christian, and sustainable health service. By 1985, they were able to achieve the World Health Organization's goal of "Health for All by the Year 2000." That was 15 years ahead of schedule. This happened in a country which was in many ways struggling to survive in post-independence Africa. Today, the hospital is a 450-bed multispecialty hospital training family medicine residents and university-level nurse practitioners, and it continues to function well. The decentralized rural health zone serves a population of more than a quarter of a million people with the full range of primary healthcare services and community health initiatives, including agricultural interventions. The creation of rural health clinics was central to the transformation, in large part because treatment was nearer to the villagers needing healthcare, and it was considerably less costly.

The health service developed at Vanga Hospital became the model for the Ministry of Health in the Democratic Republic of Congo and is now used in more than 100 similar programs across the country. Most of those are church-based programs, providing health services for nearly 70 % of the total population of the country. Dr. Fountain acknowledged receiving some funds from the international community, but feels the hospital survives today largely because they were able to mobilize local resources for general operation. In his own words, "From the beginning, the health program at Vanga has operated on a fee-for-service basis in order to maintain a sustainable program. In spite of the economic collapse of the country, this self-financed approach has proven effective."

Regarding the transformation of Vanga Hospital, a key part of the story should be given consideration. For 12 years, there was an expatriate medical doctor (Dr. Osterholm) at Vanga. He wisely taught an African male assistant to do various kinds of surgery and other treatment. When the political situation became more and more unstable in the early 1960s, it became necessary for Dr. Oestrholm to be evacuated from the country. The story of his leaving will be of interest to anyone seeking to understand dependency issues and the need for transfer from foreign to local ownership. The following is the story as told by Dr. Fountain in *Health for All: The Vanga Story*.

When it became clear that Dr. Osterholm needed to be evacuated for safety reasons, he met with Mr. Musiti, the African hospital worker that he had been training to give curative medical care. Dr. Osterholm sat down with Mr. Musiti to discuss the coming change. He told Mr. Musiti that in the desk drawer in the hospital office, there was enough money to pay the staff for one more month. He then said that when the money was used up, Mr. Musiti should simply close the hospital and go home. Thankfully, that piece of advice did not become necessary.

For a start, Mr. Musiti found himself faced with a serious decision. A villager needed a caesarian section operation, and there was no doctor present to do the surgery. Mr. Musiti turned to the local church elders for advice, not knowing what he should do about the medical crisis they were facing. The elders wisely told him that for the sake of the mother and the child, he should perform the c-section. After all, there was no one else who could help. Later on, in the absence of a medical doctor, Mr. Musiti performed a c-section on his own wife. This was clearly a turning point for the medical services at Vanga.

Needless to say, the hospital did not close when the money in the desk drawer ran out. In fact, 18 months later when Dr. Fountain arrived, he discovered that the hospital was still there and still providing services. Mr. Musiti was the link with the past and present to ensure that Vanga had a future. Dr. Fountain stepped into a situation where a transition from a mission-run institution to one locally owned and operated was in process. Dr. Fountain accepted the fact that he, as medical officer, was not in charge as would have been characteristic of the old missionary paradigm. He realized that this was an opportunity to keep the hospital administration in the hands of Mr. Musiti and other Congolese people. The hospital had turned a corner, and Dr. Fountain was convinced that it should not return to expatriate leadership. From that point on, Dr. Fountain and Mr. Musiti were co-coordinators of Vanga Hospital. Each had their own responsibility, and a spirit of true partnership characterized their style of management. One can only imagine how differently the story would read if they had not moved forward when the opportunity presented itself. There is much more to the story which can be found in Dr. Fountain's own words in *Health for All: The Vanga Story*.

Observations on Local Ownership of Christian Hospitals

It is important to remember that not all transitions toward self-reliance are successful. Also, it is important to note that while positive things happen at a particular time, it does not mean that everything will be a rosy picture forever into the future. However, there are a few lessons that can be learned from these illustrations.

In each of the examples above, it is possible to find things that were not ideal. For example, some will say that after the transfer to local ownership, spiritual ministry in the hospital deteriorated. In reality, we should recognize that there is no guarantee that spiritual ministry will be effective simply because outsiders run a hospital with significant outside subsidy. Spiritual renewal is often at the heart of effectively avoiding or overcoming dependency.[5]

The most effective local ownership is where parachurch institutions (including Christian hospitals) are under independent board leadership. One of the first questions to be asked is whether the final authority for the hospital rests with church leaders or with qualified business and medical people. Remember, the church should be designed to run on tithes and offerings. But institutions such as hospitals, guesthouses, and other "businesses" should be designed to run on a profit and loss basis.

---

[5] For the importance of spiritual renewal and overcoming dependency see *When Charity Destroys Dignity* page 127ff.

On a related issue, it is not uncommon for church leaders to want a hospital, clinic, or other development project because of economic side benefits for the church. Indeed, benefits to the church might well be temporary or even counter-productive in the long run. Following a 10-year period of outside funding for development projects, one bishop in East Africa discovered that his church members were giving less than before the outside assistance began. That is characteristic of the dependency syndrome and should not be surprising.

Short-term medical missions (STMMs) can have a positive impact on local healthcare, but too often that impact is minimal or, sometimes, counterproductive. One study done in Central America showed that the amount spent on STMMs in one year—in one country alone—was 14 million US dollars. In spite of this amount being spent, there was no noticeable change in the overall quality of healthcare in the country!

One way the short-term experience can be beneficial in medical missions is through the visit of specialists who are able to bring expertise and respite to overworked medical staff in busy mission hospitals. That kind of help brings true assistance. If those on short-term teams are not specialists or are not medically trained, they may actually end up taking time and energy from medical staff that are already overworked and yet feel obligated to create something meaningful for the visitors to do.

On the positive side, it is possible for short-term medical teams to make a positive contribution in specific areas. Several teams going to Uganda included those who were specialists in Emergency Medical Training (EMT). They were so effective in giving that kind of training that a nation-wide program was started in which Ugandans were trained to provide emergency medical services. Soon after the training began, lives were being saved because local people were trained in emergency care.

Short-term medical teams should be aware that the service they give can sometimes be in competition with local practitioners who may be trying to make a living through a privately owned clinic. Since some short-term medical teams provide medicine and services free of charge, this may have an adverse effect on a private clinic nearby. Remember, the private clinic is a 52-week a year enterprise based on profit and loss—not a 2-week enterprise based on overseas charity.

Of great significance in medical missions is the matter of attitude and demeanor. Some mission hospitals are managed and sustained by outsiders who create an atmosphere that makes it difficult to attract locally trained medical personnel—particularly medical doctors. A hospital in Central Africa had five expatriate doctors on staff, but they could not get one locally trained medical doctor to join the staff. When local church leaders were asked about this, their reply was, "No local doctor in his right mind would work in that hospital." The five expatriates created an atmosphere that was too uncomfortable for a local medical doctor to feel at home. In this case, the outsiders brought in so many supplies and so much outside funding that they made themselves indispensable. Indispensable people can create an atmosphere that does not allow others to feel at ease in their own country.

What Can Be Done to Promote a Transfer to Local Ownership?

Every situation is different from every other. Therefore, it is not possible to prescribe one cure that is suitable for all. Having said that, the following are a few general suggestions:

The **first** step is to positively anticipate a change to local ownership. If you don't want it to happen, it is unlikely that it will.

Second, precipitate the change by doing things that will lead local people to discover the benefits of local ownership. This means proactively working toward change, not just wishing it would happen. Remember, however, that it may take considerable skill, creativity, and a great deal of patience. Not all efforts to precipitate change will be successful. But, if no attempts are made, little change can be expected. Most importantly, one must try to figure out how to precipitate change in a non-paternalistic way.

Third, learn all you can about how positive change takes place. Find out how Dr. Dan Fountain and his colleagues led Vanga Hospital in Congo to local ownership and effectiveness.[6] Also, on the World Mission Associates website (www.wmausa. org), there are scores of articles with suggestions about how to avoid or overcome unhealthy dependency. Of particular interest might be what I have written in Chap. 17 of *When Charity Destroys Dignity*, entitled "What Triggers the Move toward Self-Reliance?"

Fourth, be prepared to do serious restructuring, if necessary. There are two ways to balance a budget. One is to increase income. The other is to reduce expenses. Restructuring may be essential in order for the institution to become locally sustainable. Some programs created during the days of heavy outside subsidy may not be sustainable as an institution moves in the direction of local support. For example, decentralizing an institution can be done as portions of the workload are shared with smaller units at a distance such as village health clinics which have lower overhead costs than a hospital. This would be true of a move in the direction of village health clinics, something that was done at Vanga Hospital with great effectiveness. In this case, when the institution is decentralized, so is the expense budget, and that can be a major side benefit of the restructuring process.

Fifth, don't expect someone to hand you a ready-made solution that you put on like a glove. Such solutions will rarely be useful. But, with a willingness to learn and under the direction of the Holy Spirit, positive changes can occur.[7]

---

[6] Look in any good source of books for the writings of Dr. Dan Fountain, former missionary to Congo.

[7] For further information in this see a book by Ms Jean Johnson entitled *We are Not the Hero: A Missionary's Guide for Sharing Christ, not a Culture of Dependency* (Information in the bibliography).

Issues of Dependency in Relation to Preventive Healthcare

In recent years, there have been many reminders that curative healthcare has often received more attention than preventive care. Four names come to mind when I think about the trend toward preventive care. **One** is Dr. Dan Fountain who served at Vanga hospital in Northwestern Congo and turned it into a teaching facility training those who would live and work in rural villages. That was an effort to cut down the number of people who felt they had no option but to seek curative care.

A **second** name that comes to mind is Dr. David Hilton who worked in an area of Nigeria called Lardin Gabas for some years seeking to reduce the number of patients needing curative care in a hospital. This he did by becoming an educator in surrounding villages in attempt to lower the numbers of patients seeking curative care in a hospital. This was a merciful thing because villagers did not need to walk several days from where they lived to reach the hospital.

A **third** voice along this line is Dr. Arnold Gorske who has also been calling attention to improving healthcare through preventive measures among the general population. He favors linking up with such organizations as the World Health Organization (WHO) to raise awareness of not just curing, but preventing disease whenever and wherever possible. Remember, one way to reduce costs at a mission hospital is to improve the health of those who end up not needing to go to the hospital.

A **fourth** voice for the importance of preventive compared to curative care is Dr. Elvira Beracochea who serves with an organization called Realizing Global Health based in Fairfax, Virginia. She has written and spoken on these issues over the past several decades. Dr. Beracochea authored a book called *Health for All Now.* That title is similar to Dr. Fountain's book on Vanga Hospital. "Health for all by the year 2000" became a mantra for the WHO following a conference held in Alma-Ata, Ukraine, in September 1978.

These are only four examples among many others who have raised the banner for helping people to avoid sickness, not just helping them to get well after they become ill.

By now you must be wondering how this curative vs. preventive emphasis relates to sustainability or overcoming unhealthy dependency. Hopefully, you will see the relationship as I look at it from the perspective of local sustainability.

Working with Limited Resources

Decisions regarding healthcare often come down to the cost involved. There is limited funding available, and decisions often include who to help and who to leave unhelped, especially when there are many more seeking treatment than hospital staff can handle.

A first consideration is to simply look at the difference in cost between preventing illness compared to curing illness. Many attempts to prevent illness cost far less than the cost of curative healthcare. Look at one or two simple illustrations.

Dr. Fountain began to get a grasp of this when he saw the lack of sanitation in the villages surrounding Vanga Hospital. He began to see that the number of people visiting the hospital drop significantly when villagers took sanitation issues seriously. All of this is obvious and taken for granted by many people in the medical profession. But what does it take to help keep patients with bacteria borne diseases from reaching the hospitals? Think of it this way. Lower the cost of healthcare— moving toward sustainability—by helping the community at large to carry some responsibility for preventing illness. In order to get the best return on investment, it means that the "curer" should change his role to "educator" with a view to lowering the overall cost of healthcare.

Dr. Fountain has several illustrations of how important this is. I shall give one or two of his suggestions. On one occasion a young lad of 9 or 10 years of age was brought into Vanga Hospital with an obvious growing mass in his abdomen. Dr. Fountain proceeded to remove the mass in the operating theatre. It turned out to be a mass of worms the size of a base ball. Thankfully with that removed, and in a few days, the boy was dashing about ready to go back to his home.

About 6 months later, the same boy was back at Vanga with a similar growth and—you guessed it—another growth of worms. Dr. Fountain was again called to assist. His first reaction was that he was being asked to repeat the surgery because no one did anything about the reason why the boy was getting worms in the first place. So Dr. Fountain stayed in his home to reflect and pray about the situation before him and the young boy. As he prayed and meditated, the Lord seemed to say that he should go and lay hands on the boy—but the Spirit said "when you lay hands on the boy, be sure that you have a scalpel in your hand." He was to remove the mass again—yes—but also to do something about the cause or the boy would be back again after 6 more months because he continued to live in unsanitary conditions.

One thing led to another and Dr. Fountain began to visit the villages and advocate latrines as a way to cut down the exposure to such things as a recurring infection of worms. However, Dr. Fountain encountered resistance from villagers who simply did not believe in—or see the need for—latrines. As he traveled throughout these villages as an educator rather than a curer, he discovered that there was a resistance to the sanitation problem because many of them, as Christians, did not see the principle of latrines in scripture! This was not resolved until he showed them that indeed latrines were referred to in the Bible. He pointed them to Deuteronomy 23:12–13 which reminds them that they should take a hoe with them and cover their excrement. That was enough to convince the villagers that there was reason to believe what he was saying about sanitation.

My reason for bringing stories like this into the sustainability discussion is to show that it is far less costly for villagers to learn to prevent illness than to require sophisticated hospital equipment and surgical procedures.

Dr. Gorske in an unpublished article titled the *Quest for Shalom* brings to our attention the contrast between preventing and curing. He suggests that we should begin to look at the church as the greatest ally that the medical profession has in combating illness caused by human behavior. This set the wheels of my mind turning, and I began to wonder just how that would work. While Dr. Gorske sees the church as having the potential to improve the health of people in society, I began to think about society as a whole becoming involved in the promotion of good health. In short, what would happen if we began to think of every villager as a potential healthcare worker, promoting sanitation and a healthy diet? This would represent an unrealized local resource that could be mobilized for helping to resolve healthcare needs. All of a sudden one begins to see every villager as a potential unpaid volunteer—servants of the Church and its local community—helping to battle a problem in a way that costs little or no money. There will still be a place for expensive equipment in hospitals or clinics, but the number of people needing such costly equipment will be reduced considerably when villagers learn how to avoid illness.

The Medical Person as an Educator

Quite some years ago, I learned about the Lardin Gabas Rural Heath Programme in Nigeria. One of the things I learned was the conflict in the mind of a medical doctor who had to forcibly leave a crowded emergency room to go into the villages to show or tell people how not to become sick. That doctor told how difficult it was to walk away from people who may have walked a long distance to get to the hospital for treatment. But one question that comes out of all of this is how many of the people waiting in the halls of the hospital were there for preventable reasons. The most graphic description of this dilemma is told by Dr. Fountain in his book *Healing for All: The Vanga Story*.

> As I reflected on the situation of Kilamba, the boy with the intestinal obstruction due to ascaris worms, I did some simple mathematics. How often did the life of a seriously ill person coming to the hospital depend on me? Mr. Musiti and the other staff could handle common emergency procedures well ... However, certain conditions surpassed Paul Musiti's capabilities, and for these I was needed... How often did people come with these kinds of difficult situations? I calculated that we handled an average of one such acute emergency a week or fifty per year—fifty people whose lives depended on my presence and capabilities. This was a significant number, yet how many people whom we never saw died of preventable diseases out in the surrounding communities?
>
> The population the hospital served at that time was about 250,000 people with a birth rate of 40 per thousand, that meant 10,000 new-borns per year. Every baby or young child got measles in those days and the measles mortality rate was about 15 percent. That meant 1,500 infant deaths per year out there. In addition, malaria, malnutrition and other parasitic and intestinal infections took a frightful toll. The total number of uncared-for people dying in their communities certainly surpassed 5,000 per year or one hundred times the number of lives I would save by remaining only in the hospital. When people died in the hospital, we heard the wailing and had to help with the arrangements to return the body to the community for burial. But we heard nothing of the 5,000 people per year who died of preventable diseases in their communities. We did not hear the wailing or have to intervene in the burials. So we forgot them and ignored them. Yet these people's needs were as great as the needs of those who came to the hospital. The mathematics became compelling.[8]

---

[8] This is a quote from *Health for All: The Vanga Story*, pages 52–53.

Conclusion

The illustrations of transformed hospitals and curing vs. preventive healthcare which I gave above are evidence that it is worth the effort required to avoid or over-come unhealthy dependency. It is the way healthcare will reach many who are not now being served. Mobilization of local resources is the key. Think of it this way: If local resources are mobilized on a world-wide scale, there will be an immeasurable leap forward for global healthcare. If global healthcare remains heavily dependent on resources from western countries, many who are in need will not be served.

The world in which we live is desperate for available and improved healthcare. Consider the following statement made by a researcher at a large children's hospital in London, "Our greatest need is not for more research and technology. We already have more information than we are able to manage. The real need is for a new way of doing what we already know how to do."

Of course, this means being willing to adjust the paradigm on which we function. And such a shift is why new attitudes and procedures regarding sustainability are so important.

Bibliography

Beracochea, E. (2013). *Health for all now* (2nd ed.). Fairfax, VA: Realizing Global Health.

Corbett, S., & Fikkert, B. (2012). *When helping hurts: How to alleviate poverty without hurting the poor ... and yourself.* Chicago: Moody.

Fountain, D. (2014). *Health for all: The Vanga story.* Pasadena, CA: William Carey.

Gorske, A. (2014, September). *The Church, Shalom, and the "Slow Motion Disaster".* by Dr. Arnold Gorske.

Johnson, J. (2012). *We are not the hero: A Missionary's Guide for sharing Christ not a culture of dependency.* Sisters, OR: Deep River Books.

Little, C. (2005). *Mission in the way of Paul: Biblical mission for the Church in the twenty-first century.* New York: Peter Lang.

Reese, R. (2010). *Roots and remedies of the dependency syndrome in world missions.* Pasadena, CA: William Carey Library.

Schwartz, G. (2007). *When charity destroys dignity: Overcoming unhealthy dependency in the Christian movement.* Lancaster, PA: World Mission Associates.

Chapter 15
Aid Effectiveness: The Experience of Rwanda

Agnes Binagwaho

In 2002, when I began working with Rwanda's National AIDS Control Commission, there were fewer than 1,000 people in our country on antiretroviral therapy. Tens of thousands died uncounted each year, tearing families apart and leaving children orphaned. Twelve years later, we have more than 110,000 men, women, and children benefitting from this lifesaving treatment across Rwanda, and AIDS mortality rates have declined by more than 80 %. So I have lived through the dry spell, then seen the remarkable power of international solidarity and true partnership to transform the possibilities for alleviating suffering among the sick in developing countries. Access to effective healthcare has turned an HIV diagnosis from a death sentence into a manageable chronic illness, and it is upon this platform of chronic care that Rwanda has rebuilt its entire health sector and now aims to tackle chronic non-communicable diseases.

But throughout the last decade, Rwanda and our partners have learned that good intentions are not enough; we have made progress not only by mobilizing the necessary funding, but through a sustained and rigorous focus on implementation, quality improvement, national ownership, and true collaboration. Globally and in Rwanda, it has become clear that a major challenge to aid effectiveness in the health sector—and to improving health equity more generally—is a persistent gap between laudable charitable and real, measurable impact on the intended beneficiaries of development.

A. Binagwaho, M.D., M.(Ped.), Ph.D. (✉)
Rwanda, Ministry of Health, Kigali, Rwanda

Harvard Medical School, Department of Global Health
and Social Medicine, Boston, MA, USA

Adjunct Clinical Professor of Pediatrics, Geisel School of Medicine
at Dartmouth College, Hanover, NH, USA
e-mail: agnes_binagwaho@hms.harvard.edu

© Springer Science+Business Media New York 2015
E. Beracochea (ed.), *Improving Aid Effectiveness in Global Health*,
DOI 10.1007/978-1-4939-2721-0_15

This gap between what we know about addressing the greatest causes of preventable suffering and what we actually do is not insurmountable. In this chapter, I summarize key lessons on the pursuit of aid effectiveness in the health sector derived from Rwanda's experiences of the past decade.

Not All Aid Is Good

Aid should always aim to assist countries in their national development with the goal of allowing them to eventually become self-sufficient. While many involved in global health work agree with this sentiment in principle, it is often undermined in practice. One key lesson that we learned early on in Rwanda is that not all aid is good; in fact, there is such a thing as poison money. While this often occurs with financial disbursements that come with many strings attached, it can also be true of in-kind donations.

In early 2005, the Ministry of Health received a donation from an anonymous Canadian donor of dialysis machines through the Rwandan embassy in Canada. Facing a rising burden of renal complications due to long-term side-effects of many chronic diseases including HIV infection, we accepted the donation and agreed to pay for its transport to Kigali. Upon the machines' arrival, we were shocked to see that they had been labeled "not for human use!" Wanting to be resourceful, we allowed our colleagues in veterinary medicine to attempt to use it for animals that were suffering from renal insufficiency, but this was a failure. The Ministry of Health has thus been forced to store the machines for years, unable to destroy them without spending far more money to ship them elsewhere or properly dispose of them. Many of us cannot help but wonder if this entire venture might have been a clever waste disposal strategy on the part of our so-called generous donor rather than true aid.

Value Begins with Knowing Where the Money Goes

In Rwanda, we have long understood that aid effectiveness cannot be reduced to a simple equation; it is the result of a complex series of interacting factors over time. But making evidence-based decisions does require information about the outcomes achieved by financial inputs. Rwanda thus undertook two comprehensive studies of where specific streams of funding actually went: the 2010 National Orphans and Vulnerable Children Spending Account (NOVCSA) and the 2012 National AIDS Spending Assessment (NASA).

Rwanda's National AIDS Control Commission undertook the NOVCSA evaluation of its own accord in 2008—no such sector-wide assessments are currently required by donors or international policymaking bodies—in order to rectify the lack of systematic and reliable data on where money availed for serving orphans and vulnerable children (OVC) actually went. When we traced non-governmental organization (NGO) inputs, expenditures, and outputs through the assessment, we were shocked to find that in some cases, nearly 80 % of funds never reached the intended beneficiaries. The vast majority of OVC money that was included in international assessments as part of Rwanda's health sector spending was actually being spent on administrative overhead, travel expenses, and reports rather than the provision of services to meet the real needs of children and families. Equipping ourselves with this knowledge has allowed Rwanda's health sector to more effectively advocate for efficient coordination of aid, but many challenges still exist regarding the transparency of expenditures in other areas.

Building Systems, Not Only Projects

Rwanda's experiences rebuilding our health sector and attempting to accelerate widely shared economic growth have taught us that truly sustainable progress requires a focus on systems. The evolving debate in global health policy about the role of so-called "vertical" or disease-specific initiatives in contrast to "horizontal" or health systems-oriented efforts often poses a series of false choices. From the earliest days of the AIDS response in Rwanda, we have learned that urgency can be the enemy of the future, and that we do not have to choose between providing access to urgently needed treatment for HIV and investing in sustainable primary care infrastructure. By outlining a clear vision and coordinating the activities of all groups and stakeholders working in the health sector, we have been able to simultaneously address the current crisis while also investing in the future.

The same pregnant woman who wants to prevention of mother-to-child transmission (PMTCT) of HIV to her unborn child will also need a safe place to deliver her baby, and the same child who is born HIV-free will also need a full course of vaccinations. If that child falls ill with pneumonia or diarrhea, she will need high quality drugs provided in a timely manner by trained community health workers or health professionals, and the best way to guarantee these services to the child born HIV-free is to avail these services to all children. In early 2000, we understood this and focused on building a system instead of creating many fragmented vertical programs. This allowed us to move towards strengthening the entire health system based on geographic accessibility of affordable services so that it will benefit all without restriction. People living with HIV are also more vulnerable to many kinds of cancers, for which they require treatment and palliative care. In order to meet the needs of people living with and affected by HIV, we have thus conceived of our mission as fulfilling the right to health of each person over the entire course of their life.

In practice, this has meant that when the Ministry of Health has built capacity for HIV testing, we do so in such a way that the laboratory can be used for many other diseases and the technicians are trained in a broad array of technical procedures. When providing the infrastructure and supply chains to maintain a strong PMTCT of HIV program, we have built comprehensive antenatal clinics and delivery wards for all mothers in the area. In equipping health facilities to provide antiretroviral therapy, we have also invested in installing high-speed Internet connections in these facilities across the country and built reliable cold chains. This "horizontalization" of vertical aid has made effective use of resources, ensuring that the entire population benefits in addition to people living with HIV.

Rwanda's community-based health insurance scheme, known as *mutuelles de santé*, provides another example of the system-wide approach. *Mutuelles de santé* operates under a tiered enrollment fee structure ($12 per year per capita for the wealthiest 5 % of the population and $7 per year for the middle half of the population) and covers 90 % of healthcare costs for patients who are enrolled. The poorest quarter of the population, as assessed by a community-driven socioeconomic classification system called *ubudehe,* have their membership fees and co-payments subsidized by the government through the national budget and complemented by a grant from The Global Fund to Fight AIDS, Tuberculosis, and Malaria and President's Emergency Plan for AIDS Relief (PEPFAR). In July 2013, over 90 % of the population was enrolled in *mutuelles de santé*, with approximately 6 % of those remaining covered by public insurance for civil servants (RAMA) or private insurance plans.

Ensuring True Country Ownership

A key determinant of whether aid is used effectively is whether it is directed towards national priorities based on the needs of the population rather than the wishes of donors. Rwanda's approach to priority-setting has focused on ensuring that the country itself implements initiatives it is capable of overseeing. In the case of the AIDS response, this has required incrementally transitioning away from using foreign nationals to provide services with high overhead costs, as soon as we were able to do it, while keeping the quality. With the money saved by doing more with less, we have recruited university faculty member from USA. Rwanda now uses a large portion of funding available through the PEPFAR program to train Rwandan health professionals locally—who otherwise may not have had the opportunity to gain further medical training—through an initiative known as the Human Resources for Health (HRH) program, which was launched in 2012.

Through the HRH Program, we are leveraging the teaching expertise from 23 American universities to help build specialty training programs across a wide variety of clinical priority areas and increase the overall quality of our workforce. Over the course of 7 years, Rwandan health professionals will be better equipped to provide the long-term chronic care not only for complications of HIV disease, but also for other non-communicable conditions such as cardiovascular and lung diseases, cancer, and diabetes. Now that people living with HIV are increasingly burdened by these conditions, this program allows us to improve our local capacity to manage these chronic conditions among not only our HIV patient population, but also for all Rwandans who will benefit from a workforce trained with these disease management principles.

The HRH Program was made possible through the transition of PEPFAR funding to the Rwandan public sector, which marked the first time that the United States government had provided this type of direct budget support for health education to an African country. This has allowed the Ministry of Health to provide more services for the same amount of money, as it is far less costly for Rwandan nationals to operate programs in Rwanda than for foreigners to run them with their administrative overhead and travel expenses. This provides more health per dollar spent, dramatically increasing the value and variety of services rendered without compromising the quality of care provided.

Fostering International Accountability

Country ownership is often undermined by aid organizations headquartered in developed countries pursuing their own strategic directions, especially in cases when recipient countries have no opportunity to provide input regarding its actual needs. This leads to a lack of alignment between national priorities and some partner activities and decreases the chances that partners will supply accurate and timely reports to national health authorities. This lack of accountability among some development partners can be detrimental, and it often has been in Rwanda's recent history.

Accountability also goes both ways: the worst use of aid is the financing of corrupt governments. Also, the accumulation of overhead outside of the country and in the privileged pockets of the elites yields no benefit to the people who need this aid most. This is a well-known problem, but the world has reacted extremely softly and slowly in addressing it. Rwanda has taken the initiative to undertake third-party annual audits of all ministries, including the Ministry of Health. This important tool for ensuring transparency remains too rare across the world.

Looking to the Future

Aid that does not strengthen the public sector is essentially not sustainable. It may provide temporary services through NGOs, but undermines the future by failing to provide durability and the guarantee of continued service delivery to the poorest and most vulnerable over the long term. Only a strong, well-managed public sector can guarantee health to the vulnerable—not to mention many other social and economic needs—as a right. As the great American civil rights leader Martin Luther King Jr. said, "true compassion means more than flinging a coin to a beggar; it comes to see that an edifice which produces beggars needs restructuring." True partnership takes a long view of the right to health as a universal right, seeking to ensure aid effectiveness by changing the development conditions that place countries in a state of dependency and puts the poor at risk of premature mortality and preventable suffering.

Five Criteria of Effective Aid for the Health Sector

- Strengthen national institutions for evidence-based planning, monitoring and evaluation with clear targets as well as the strategies and policies to achieve them
- Assure that activities are supporting the national plan designed by the country, thinking about health as a piece of the overall development plan
- Assure rapid and high-quality transfer of capacity to local leaders
- Transfer funds through national channels when transparency and effectiveness have been guaranteed; where it is not, help the country to strengthen its systems
- Support sustainable development, taking a long view of the mission

Three Recommendations for Donors

- Immediately work on a legal framework for ethical engagement in development work in the respect of the Paris Declaration, Busan Declaration, Abuja Declaration, and Accra Call to Action
- Commit to supporting a country until it actually achieves an agreed upon goal, not simply to a timeframe
- Jointly monitor and evaluate the implementation of actions funded only in the respect of plans and targets agreed upon in advance, and without any other agenda than improving the welfare of the intended beneficiaries

Three Recommendations for Recipient Countries

- Conduct clear assessments of the needs across different sectors in order to reach targets determined with the participation of each constituency of the country
- Plan by taking into account the input of all constituencies (public, private, community, civil society)
- Insist upon transparency and accountability for all

Three Recommendations for Global Health Professionals

- Come and work with the goal of putting yourself out of work as soon as possible, and do not use humanitarian solutions as solely an income-generating activity
- Transparency and accountability both to those who fund you and to the country that you are working to assist
- Aim to proactively help the country you are working in to fill major implementation gaps by transferring capacity to make it happen

Further Reading

Binagwaho, A. (2010). Whose responsibility is it anyway? View 2. In J. Heymann, L. Sherr, & R. Kidman (Eds.), *Protecting childhood in the AIDS pandemic*. Oxford, England: Oxford University Press.

Binagwaho, A., Farmer, P., et al. (2014). Rwanda 20 years on: investing in life. *Lancet, 384*, 371–375. doi:10.1016/S0140-6736(14)60574-2.

Binagwaho, A., Kyamanywa, P., Farmer, P. E., Nuthulaganti, T., Umubyeyi, B., Nyemazi, J. P., Mugeni, S. D., Asiimwe, A., Ndagijimana, U., McPherson, H. L., Ngirabega, J., Sliney, A., Uwayezu, A., Rusanganwa, V., Wagner, C. M., Nutt, C. T., Eldon-Edington, M., Cancedda, C., Magaziner, I., & Goosby, E. (2013). The Human Resources for Health Program in Rwanda—A new partnership. *New England Journal of Medicine, 369*(21), 2054–2059.

Binagwaho, A., Ratnayake, N., & Smith Fawzi, M. C. (2008). Holding multilateral organizations accountable: The failure of WHO in regards to childhood malnutrition. *Health and Human Rights, 10*(2), 1–4.

Farmer, P. E., Nutt, C. T., Wagner, C. M., Karasi, J. C., Sekabaraga, C., Nuthulaganti, T., Habinshuti, T., Mugeni, S., & Drobac, P. (2013). Reduced premature mortality in Rwanda: Lessons from success. *The British Medical Journal, 346*, f65. doi:10.1136/bmj.f65.

Lu, C., Chin, B., Lewandowski, J. L., Basinga, P., Hirschhorn, L. R., Hill, K., Murray, M., & Binagwaho, A. (2012). Towards universal health coverage: An evaluation of Rwanda Mutuelles in its first eight years. *PLoS One, 7*(6), e39282.

Ministry of Health of Rwanda. (2012). Rwanda Human Resources for Health Program. Retrieved July 12, 2014, from http://hrhconsortium.moh.gov.rw/

Price, J. E., Leslie, J. A., Welsh, M., & Binagwaho, A. (2009). Integrating HIV clinical services into primary health care in Rwanda: A measure of quantitative effects. *AIDS Care, 21*(5), 608–614.

Chapter 16
How Local Organizations Increase Aid Effectiveness: The Experience of Peru

Pedro Jesús Mendoza-Arana

When we think of aid effectiveness in Peru, the first approach is to identify if objectives were met, both as evidenced by financial and non-financial indicators, and, if this was not so, sometimes we look into possible explanations. Very few times, however, this look goes deeper enough to generate an understanding of what really is underlying either success or failure of a project.

The main underlying factor in effectiveness is cooperation between organizations; thus, a better understanding of why and how organizations cooperate could orientate us to understand their dynamics at both sides and this understanding can guide us to increase aid effectiveness in a respectful and sustainable way.

In this paper we will focus in the organizational characteristics of local organizations, which can be in the government side (Ministry of Health), academia, or civil society Organizations (local NGOs, Universities, CBOs, and alike), using them as triggers for reflection on how to improve effectiveness based on Peruvian experiences.

Experiences in the Government

The Peruvian Ministry of Health—MINSA, has a history of strengthening the international cooperation area, by improving monitoring and evaluation efforts, as well as improving programming and negotiation capacities. This is embodied by the General Office for International Cooperation, whose Director reports to the Minister, and has a technical team composed of public servants with demonstrated experience in international development and cooperation.

P.J. Mendoza-Arana (✉)
Universidad Nacional Mayor de San, Marcos, Lima-Perú
e-mail: pedro.mendoza.arana@gmail.com

© Springer Science+Business Media New York 2015
E. Beracochea (ed.), *Improving Aid Effectiveness in Global Health*,
DOI 10.1007/978-1-4939-2721-0_16

In fact, shortly after the Paris Declaration Conference, MINSA called for a harmonization process to his counterparts. Although this call was more successful in some areas, such as Human Resources (Castro et al. 2008), MINSA has developed their strength in improving the effectiveness of cooperation programs and projects, and they have many articles and documents where they show their experience (Arosquipa et al. 2007; Castro et al. 2008).

Non-Government Experiences

In addition to the MINSA's experience, Peruvian organizations involved in cooperation ranges from grassroots organizations, local NGOs, and Universities; they all are very diverse, but having in common that are not linked to the government, and this means they are usually linked as well with non-government cooperation agencies; thus, we can examine their organizational characteristics in relation to a successful management of international cooperation projects, in order to point out some useful lessons that could be applied by others in order to increase aid effectiveness.

Organizational Key Factors for Success in Aid Effectiveness

I have identified five key factors for success at organizational level, to increase aid effectiveness:

1. *Personal relationships of key personnel*
   Having good personal relationships among stakeholders has been identified as a key factor for success, particularly in Non-Government cooperation. As one of my interviewees put it "you know, cooperation is ultimately a matter of personal trust." He was a priest, working in a small mission with people living with HIV and receiving a continuous flow of money coming from different supporting groups who, in his understanding, knew him and trust that he would make a good use of the funds. This seems to be the case more for Non-Official cooperation, which is an important channel in many countries and circumstances. This led to the need to create conditions for retention of skilled personnel, who not only know well the procedures that agencies require, but also have developed a sense of mission and identified themselves with the mission of development and have embodied it in their work.

   In the case of Universities, the positive result of having trust and good personal relationships was extremely clear (Mendoza 2007). One of the most important examples in Peru is the Natural History Museum. This Museum receive important funds for research, and one of the explanations is that professors working here achieved their master or doctoral degrees in different Universities oversea and were able to get ahead, thanks to their personal links with those who were before their research tutors, and now are their partners in research projects.

Another positive result is that permanence of these key personnel was highly valued by cooperation agencies, as a sign of stability and expertise. Although high-ranking officers can usually change with government management, intermediate officers who are permanent civil servants usually remain in their positions and they guard the institutional expertise and memory. We have found personnel with 15–20 years of experience in the International Cooperation Office at MINSA, or in some Universities or NGOs which are well known for their successful performance in international cooperation projects.

2. *Project management skills*
One lesson in this respect, painfully learned in Peru, is that project management skills are an absolute key factor for effective cooperation projects, and that "institutionalization does not mean administration" (Arosquipa et al. 2007). In the 1990s, some big projects operated in Peru through parallel administrations, with successful budgetary execution but unsustainable results. In the 2000s, the answer was to manage the funds through regular administrative offices, resulting in catastrophic execution due to heavy bureaucratic management rules. The lesson is that institutionalization means decision capacity, which can be ensured via directive boards, but that day-to-day management can be more effectively managed via specialized professionals.

Recent assessments of long-term projects also illustrates this point, such as the case of VIGIA Project, an USAID funded, 10 years-project, focused in supporting to the MOH in capacities to face emergent and re-emergent diseases. In an end of project external assessment, it was concluded that channeling the funds through MOH "builds up the MOH institutionally and reinforces its commitment to interventions and methodologies introduced by other Technical Assistance projects, so that it can draft work plans, carry out activities, and deliver services to a large number of people as a complement to other projects" (Terrell and Nelson 2010).

Likewise, an external evaluation by the Spanish Cooperation Agency (AECID) of his projects in Peru in the area of cultural patrimony concludes as a learned lesson that "structuring of management teams of the project into the regular structure of the local government is the main success of the project" (AECID 2011).

A particularly valuable project management skill is related to the development of measurements that make it possible for the organization to clearly manage the project activities and show the objectives of the project were accomplished. In their external evaluation of its projects, UNICEF (2004) pointed out the importance that operating organizations show a results-oriented management, focusing efforts in the proposed results and assuring the collection of data for proper baselines and final comparisons.

3. *Country comparative advantages*
Every country has characteristics that make it unique. It can be its historic background, cultural legacy, biodiversity, some endemic public health problem which it has been particularly successful in addressing. These characteristics can be turned into advantages.

Turning these characteristics into advantage that connect with priorities of a cooperation agency helps them to become a comparative advantage when you want to apply for funding from that cooperation agency. It is important that you understand which one is your advantage in order to increase your probability of success in the funding application.

This factor has also been identified by an UNDP report on south–south collaboration (UNDP 2008). It is interesting to note that speaking the same language as the cooperation partners, in general, is not considered a comparative advantage, because it is easy to solve by translators, which in turn takes us back to the very classic competitive advantage theory of Michael Porter, who said that a comparative advantage, in order to become a competitive advantage, was a feature that was not easy to copy or to resolve by the competitors, who would be always trying their best to equal any factor that they perceive as being responsible for your success. The "trick," then, is not only the identification of differences, but differences that can be sustained over time.

4. *Dedication of key personnel*

Many of our NGOs and Universities offer low salaries when compared to the salaries paid by cooperation agencies. Therefore, their staff is made of mainly by part time collaborators, professors, teachers, or field personnel. We have found a clear correlation between having dedicated (full time) personnel and the success of the institution in getting cooperation funds. Local organizations must build a core team for whom the fundraising and applying for grants from cooperation agencies is their basic duty, so they develop their expertise, devote the necessary time, and get the desired results.

5. *Ability to establish links with other organizations*

Experience shows that successful organizations are those who have learnt to establish discussion linkages with other organizations, namely cooperation networks, "roundtables" ("mesas" in Spanish), committees, or any other ways of adding value and expertise and sharing strengths in order to address issues as they arise and achieve more impact. This type of formal and informal communication helps cooperation parties to reduce transaction costs and to focus on the problem of achieving more from the aid process (Grupo Propuesta Ciudadana 2011). This seems to have been the rationale for the Global Fund Against HIV, TBC, and Malaria by establishing National Multisectoral Bodies, the "country coordinating mechanism" as the governing entity for the country applications for funds, and as such, it worked successfully in Peru.

A clear leadership role must be played by a public agency, as it is the case for the International Cooperation Agency in Peru (APCI). APCI is a government office reporting to the Prime Minister, with the mission of strategically orientate international cooperation funds, as well as to monitor NGOs and any organization, public or private, working with international cooperation funds. APCI existence is considered a plus in advancing development programs in Peru (Jaramillo 2012). However, this statement can also be challenged if the role is not clear, as we are going to see in paragraphs below.

Organizational Factors that Interfere with Aid Effectiveness

Similarly, I have identified four blocking factors that impede aid effectiveness at organizational level:

1. *Low priority for aid opportunities*

   Many institutions do not believe in looking for opportunities of getting cooperation funds, and this becomes a self-fulfilled prophecy. They do not believe they can access them, so they do not seek for the funds (do not allocate the personnel, or do not keep them, and so on), so they do not get funds.

   A variation on this factor is that the organization declares that taking advantage of cooperation opportunities is a priority, but this declaration is not backed up with resources that make it more than just lip-service. In the case of Peru, this was pointed out even for the national agency in charge of overseeing international cooperation (APCI), generating clear concerns among cooperation agencies because although the Agency exists, it does not provide a clear direction to the operating institutions about how to access funds, forcing them to assume strategic roles and making policy decisions that are actually a responsibility of a governing body (Grupo Propuesta Ciudadana 2011; AECID 2011).

2. *Deficient administration and reporting*

   Cooperation Agencies can be very philanthropic, but they are also accountable to someone else, sometimes a government, sometimes to a board, or others to the volunteers or individual donors they may have. So they need to have clear accounts, to show the money is being used for the purpose it was collected or allocated, and all this has to be done in a timely manner. If you work for a local organization and do not help them to report, you cannot expect them to help you.

   I have seen from very close, painful examples of cooperation programs that were not sustained because, in spite of high interest of the cooperation agency in the particular project, the reporting and accountability was too poor.

3. *Bureaucratic procedures*

   Many cooperation agencies get scared when talking about cooperation with public or government agencies because they are usually slow and bureaucratic in their administration. If you are in a public institution and want to get funds, you better streamline your procedures, in order to make it cooperation-friendly and demonstrate efficiency.

4. *Internal barriers to international cooperation*

   In many countries, there are ideological barriers deep inside local organizations, in many cases steaming from past history that make them to consider international cooperation as a form of imperialism or colonialism, which they struggled so hard to get rid of. In current times, international cooperation agencies subscribe policies of respect to country determination, and they are accountable for behaving in this manner too, so you could endorse the principles of the Paris Declaration and implement cooperation procedures that enforce the principles and overcome this kind of internal barrier.

Virtuous and Vicious Circles that influence on Aid Effectiveness

Next, I will elaborate more on these nine primary factors and how they are intertwined in two circles:

In the virtuous circle:

1. *Recruiting and retention mechanisms for key personnel*

   Having key personnel that embody development capacities that have been shown to be essential to both cooperating parties is essential to successfully execute the proposals and then later the projects. For example, in the evaluation of FEMME project (Seclen et al. 2006), Peruvian MOH concluded that "a Key Factor for Success was the participatory way in which the Emergency Care Guidelines were developed," because this participatory approach ensured acceptability and viability. If this is so, personnel with this ability to facilitate and develop participatory venues are key personnel, whose departure would affect the local organization. In sum, the Peruvian experience demonstrates that recruiting and retaining key competent professionals is crucial to the success of cooperation programs.

2. *Social prestige of the institution*

   We are not talking only about fame, but by social prestige, I mean the reputation and recognition that some institutions are really responsible and accountable for what they are doing. Everybody wants to become their partners in their initiatives, including cooperation agencies. The ultimate success in an initiative is also success for the cooperation agency.

3. *Opportunity-seeking attitude*

   International cooperation funds periodically change priorities. Having a proactive strategy and being alert of these changes, as well as the mechanisms that evolve (open bids, calls, partnerships, etc.), certainly is an attitude that some institutions have developed and that is highly effective. Being ready for the opportunities as they arise, local organizations can therefore be more effective in getting funding and in implementing programs effectively too.

   In the vicious circle:

1. *Fragmentation*

   Many Peruvian organizations are deeply fragmented, meaning that one Department does not know what other Departments within the same institution do; This lack of communication would not be so tragic, if it were not that this is replicated within the departments, where one unit does not know what its sibling unit does, and also replicated among teams in the same unit, and even between persons who are supposedly in the same supposed team.

   This has been identified in many instances; for example, when the national strategy for tuberculosis at the MOH was assessed, it was concluded that "compartimentalization in decision making probed to be deleterious" (Bonilla 2008). Open communication breeds transparency and collaboration which lead to more effective results.

2. *Bureaucratic culture*

The idea that status quo is the only way to be is another deleterious factor to effective cooperation programs. It undermines efforts for efficiency, for account-ability, and for results. Moreover, bureaucratic culture shifts the organizational focus away from results or social mission fulfillment, towards preservation of activism as a proof of social need. Although some analysts see this as the lack of a strong leadership in the institutions in the country, such as a national planning institute or a planning ministry (Grupo de Consulta Ciudadana 2011; Negron 2008), I think that the prevalent bureaucratic culture would, in the end, under-mine the operation of this very ministry or institute.

In other words, if organizations do not develop a strong sense of alignment of their operation to social needs, either self-identified, or proposed, or endorsed by government agencies, as it was the case for the Millennium Development Goals, the mission of such organizations will not benefit of collaborative and innovative partnerships with development cooperation agencies. In fact, in our perception, this lack of clarity on the mission is what some analysts, such as the Grupo de Consulta Ciudadana, state as the realization that, in spite of the existence of the National Center for Planning (CEPLAN), this institution has not been enough to orientate international cooperation flux.

Some international declarations seem to be in turn more successful than oth-ers in Peru, such as it has been the case for the Ottawa Chart for Health Promotion for organizations working in Health, but the analysis of effectiveness of national or international guidelines to convene institutional efforts is beyond the scope of this paper.

3. *Endogamy*

We have labeled so to a sense of many institutions, particularly when they are old, large, and traditional, that they believe that they are so good, that every other institution has to be less important than they are, and that they do not have any-thing to learn from others. I have coined a counter-endogamy slogan in Peru that goes like this: "There is no institution, no matter how small or how young, that cannot teach us something." With this slogan, we show we believe in network-ing, we believe in sharing, we believe in building, and we start to make effective development cooperation programs part of a new future, and real.

I hope these reflections, coming from my personal experience and my research, would unleash your own reflections. Years do not make us experts. Years give us the opportunity to develop expertise; in as much as we think permanently in ways to improve what we are doing.

I invite you, dear friend and colleague who read this, to seek in your own experi-ence, I am sure that you will have many more examples of good practices to follow and deleterious practices to avoid. Even more, you could ask yourself or to your fellows, which are your particular Key Factors for Success, those that you may already have, and you have to reinforce. And, although I do not like the term, per-haps we have to identify the Key Factor for Failure, and chop it down.

Any of them, please share it. We all will be happy to hear and learn from you.

References

AECID. (2011). External evaluation report on protects for cultural patrimony recovery 2007-2011.

Arosquipa, C., Pedroza, J., Cosentino, C., & Pardo, K. (2007). La ayuda oficial al desarrollo en el Peru. *Revista peruana de medicina experimental y salud publica, 24*(2), 163–178.

Bonilla, M. (Ed.). (2008). *Construyendo Alianzas Estratégicas para detener la Tuberculosis: La experiencia peruana*. Lima, Peru: MINSA.

Castro, J., Medina, J., Cosentino, C., & Castillo, O. (2008). La cooperación internacional en salud I: Tunupa o la arquitectura de los caminos de la solidaridad y el desarrollo. *Acta Médica Peruana, 25*(3), 181–186.

Grupo Propuesta Ciudadana. (2011). National consultation for the development of a proposal for the IV high level Forum in Busan, Lima, September 26 and 27.

Jaramillo, M. (2012). The changing role of international cooperation in developing countries (as they develop): A case study of skills development policies in Peru. *International Journal of Educational Development, 32*(1), 22–30.

Mendoza, P. (2007). *Gestión de la Cooperacion Internacional e Internacionalización de la Universidad Pública en el Perú. El caso de la Universidad Nacional Mayor de San Marcos*. Lima, Peru: ANR-UNMSM-Embajada de Francia.

Negron, F. (2008). *Partners or rivals? The relationship between Peruvian government and NGOs under Paris Declaration on Aid Effectiveness*. Tha Hague, The Netherlands: Institute for Social Studies.

Seclen, J., La Torre, E., & Roldan, R. (2006). *Evaluacion del impacto del proyecto FEMME en la reducción de la mortalidad materna y su importancia para la implementación de las políticas de salud en el Perú*. Lima, Peru: MINSA.

Terrell, S., & Nelson, D. (2010). *Assessment of three USAID/Peru health project implemented by the Ministry of Health: Vigia; coverage with quality; improved health for populations at high risk*. Retrieved December 5, 2012, from http://pdf.usaid.gov/pdf_docs/PDACR648.pdf

UNDP. (2008). Enhancing south-south and triangular cooperation. New York

UNICEF. (2004). Evaluación del Programa de Cooperación Perú-UNICEF.

Chapter 17
Food Aid Reform

Sarah Kalloch and Eric Munoz

The United States launched its food aid program in the 1950s at a time when federal
farm support programs were resulting in large surplus stocks of grain held in government warehouses. At the time it was conceived, the Food for Peace Program
served double-duty—it helped address humanitarian food needs while at the same
time reducing US domestic grain stocks. This approach to delivering aid to people
in need around the world has persisted despite the fact that farm support programs
in the US have fundamentally changed—the US government no longer holds grain
stocks in government warehouses—and new means of reaching people with emergency food are now available.

What Is Food Aid and How Does It Work?

Since its inception, the Food for Peace Program has fed millions of people. In Fiscal
Year 2011, the US spent $2.1 billion sending 1.91 million metric tons of food and
reaching 53 million people around the world.[1] The vast majority of this funding was
used to assist people impacted by man-made or natural disasters. In the aftermath of
such disasters, the ubiquitous image of bags of grain stamped with the words "From
the American People" makes the front pages of newspapers around the world, demonstrating US generosity to needs abroad.

The fundamentals of current food aid programs have not changed in the last five
decades. By law, food commodities (wheat, corn, and soybeans are some of the
most common food aid products) shipped as food aid must be purchased from
within the United States. At least half that aid must be transported on ships registered

---

[1] http://www.usaid.gov/sites/default/files/documents/1866/FY%202011%20IFAR%20FINAL.pdf

S. Kalloch (✉) • E. Munoz
Oxfam America, Boston, MA, USA
e-mail: sarahdaykalloch@gmail.com; emunoz@oxfamamerica.org

© Springer Science+Business Media New York 2015
E. Beracochea (ed.), *Improving Aid Effectiveness in Global Health*,
DOI 10.1007/978-1-4939-2721-0_17

in the United States and with US crew members (so-called US-flagged vessels). There are a number of food aid programs authorized in law. The largest program is called Title II. It accounted for approximately 77 % of the total food aid budget in 2011.

Most of the commodities are directly distributed in emergency situations. A smaller portion of US food aid is used for development activities such as maternal and child health and nutrition programs or agriculture development activities. To generate funds necessary to operate these programs, aid groups receiving US food aid often sell the food they receive in local markets. This process, called monetization, accounts for a majority of the development food aid under Title II. In Fiscal Year 2011, approximately $220 million in food aid was sold on local markets in developing countries.

In Congress, the historic ties to US farm policies means food aid programs are under the jurisdiction of the Agriculture Committees, though other foreign affairs matters fall under the authority of the Foreign Relations Committees. The fact that the Agriculture interests remain heavily involved in the oversight of US food aid programs underscores why the program has been so difficult to change.

What Is Wrong with US Food Aid Programs?

The complex web of rules and regulations that undergird the food aid program are no accident of Congress. In fact, the rules reflect the various interests who benefit from the program and make it difficult to change. In the past, for example, US farmers have looked to the food aid program as a tool to help buoy domestic prices and open new markets for US agriculture commodities abroad. The US maritime industry has similarly benefitted from the program since at least half of all food aid must be shipped on US-flag vessels.

These rules and regulations come with a cost both in terms of the speed of humanitarian response and the cost-effectiveness of the programs. Various studies on US food aid have been undertaken by the government's own auditing agency and by independent academics. The findings are largely consistent: US food aid takes longer to deliver and is more expensive than buying food closer to the region of need.

A 2009 study by the Government Accountability Office, for example, found that US food aid shipments, on average, take 4–6 months from time of procurement to final distribution.[2] This is an unacceptably slow response in the wake of natural disasters.

And the program is more costly than it needs to be. Local food aid sales often generate less cash than the cost of purchase, shipment, and storage. The result: approximately $93 million was lost in monetization in 1 year alone. If this money had not been lost, assistance could have reached thousands of additional people.

---

[2] http://www.gao.gov/new.items/d07560.pdf

As another example, the requirement that food aid must be shipped on US-flagged vessels adds unnecessary costs to the program. A study conducted by researchers at Cornell found that over just 1 year, the shipping requirement cost the government $140 million more than if the lowest cost ocean carrier had been used.[3]

Buying food closer to the region of need—so-called local and regional procurement (LRP)—is not permissible under the current law governing US food aid, but it should be. A program authorized in the 2008 Farm Bill allowed for the use of LRP on a pilot basis, and other countries have used this system for years.

Rather than a one-size-fits all approach, current US food aid programs need to be more flexible. In some instances, in-kind food assistance may be a beneficial and useful approach. In other instances buying food locally for distribution—or giving recipients cash or vouchers to buy food on local markets—provides important tools and mechanisms to get food quickly to people in need. Moreover, this approach can support local agriculture production, benefitting farmers and breaking the cycle of hunger.

For years, special interests have successfully kept Congress from reforming food aid programs. Going back to 2006, President Bush proposed allocating 25 % of the food aid budget for the US Agency for International Development (USAID) for local and regional purchase. This effort did not succeed. In his 2013 budget, President Obama similarly proposed retooling food aid also with the goal of increasing the use of LRP. What these proposals have in common is that they both seek to untie US food aid so it is no longer required that all US food donations be purchased from the US or shipped on US flag vessels. The Obama administration's proposal also would curb the use of monetization so that US food commodities no longer have to be sold in developing countries to generate cash for use in development programs. These reforms would dramatically increase the flexibility USAID has to design and deliver aid in the most efficient and effective ways possible.

Seven Reasons Why: Public Health, Economic, and Political Arguments for Food Aid Reform

This section outlines seven arguments for food aid reform that public health practitioners can take to their communities and Members of Congress.

#1 save more lives with the same amount of money: The number one reason to reform food aid: The US could save the lives of two to four million more people per year, with the same amount of money. Even with the majority of US food aid still being procured in the US, cutting unnecessary red-tape and regulations would mean that the US government can save up to $165 million, savings which translate into

---

[3] http://dyson.cornell.edu/faculty_sites/cbb2/Papers/Cargo%20Preference%2029%20June%20 2010.pdf

two to four million additional people reached with life-saving assistance.[4] And this is a conservative estimate. The Center for Global Development did a report in June 2013 that found the number of additional lives saved by reform could be as high as ten million.[5]

This is not an abstract figure: In 2011–2012, more than 9.5 million people in the Horn of Africa were severely impacted by a famine across Somalia, Kenya, Ethiopia, and Djibouti. Up to 260,000 people died, including 133,000 children. That famine has been followed by a food crisis across West Africa, by massive displace affecting millions of people in Syria, and by Typhoon Haiyan, among other humanitarian emergencies requiring food assistance. Countries in crisis look to the US for help, and by reforming food aid, we can help millions more moms and dads, kids and grandparents, and brothers and sisters get the food they need to survive.

#2 proof reform works: Independent evaluations by the United States and other development partners have shown local and regional purchase works. An independent evaluation of evaluating the US-funded LRP pilot program documented the value of this approach:

– Full procurement for LRP in emergencies was 45 days faster than the current US program.[6]
– For most commodities, except products that are highly processed such as vegetable oil, LRP was more cost-effective. For example, purchases of cereals such as corn and wheat were, on average, 53 % less expensive than the purchase of US-sourced commodities.[7]

The World Food Program, the largest provider of food aid in the world, has been sourcing food from developing countries since the 1970s and has extensively documented their success. Major bilateral donors such as Canada and the European Union have changed their food aid programs to follow this best practice. Ending poverty is complicated, and there is not always good data on what works. But LRP has a decade of experience and evidence demonstrating that it works.

#3 fight poverty and encourage local livelihoods: Food aid exists not to feed people forever, but to save lives in emergencies and build capacity for communities to feed themselves over the long-term. However, the current system has the potential to undermine agriculture in developing countries. For example, US rice imports to Haiti, both commercial and food aid donations, including in response to the earthquake 2010, undermined the livelihoods of small scale rice producers. Against subsidized imports, Haitian farmers simply could not compete, a fact President Clinton

---

[4] http://www.usaid.gov/sites/default/files/documents/1869/FoodAidReform_BehindtheNumbers.pdf

[5] http://www.cgdev.org/publication/food-aid-21st-century-saving-more-money-time-and-lives

[6] http://www.fas.usda.gov/info/LRP%20Report%2012-03-12%20TO%20PRINT.pdf

[7] http://dyson.cornell.edu/faculty_sites/cbb2/Papers/Lentz%20et%20al%20LRP%20time%20and%20cost%20Feb%202012.pdf

admitted to. "It was a mistake" Clinton testified at a hearing on Haiti's recovery efforts.[8]

On the other hand, LRP can support farmers and agriculture systems in developing countries by creating new markets and new demand. Critically, reform of US food aid programs would better also align our humanitarian efforts with the US government's Feed the Future program, which spends $1 billion per year empowering small farmers in low-income countries to increase their agricultural production. In 2013, Oxfam highlighted the success of Tanzanian farmer Emiliana Aligaesha, who won a contract with USAID to produce legumes for food aid and has since built a thriving business. Together with other local farmers, Emiliana formed a private company, Kaderes Peasants Development. USAID and the World Food Program are among their clients, buying beans for food aid distribution in the region.

Writes Oxfam of this LRP partnership, "This partnership with local farmers saves the money and time it might take to bring the same goods from the US, and, more importantly, ensures a market for hardworking and innovative farmers like Aligaesha. These purchases have a multiplier effect—as the group uses their profits to support other farmers with training, access to agricultural tools, and information on markets."[9]

Experts predict that farmers in developing countries will have to double their output over the next several decades in order to avoid global food insecurity on a massive scale. Meanwhile, growth in agriculture has been shown to be at least twice as effective in reducing poverty as growth in other sectors, as more than half of the 870 million people who are chronically hungry rely on agriculture for their livelihoods. Food aid reform will support that kind of transformation—with the end goal of ending food aid altogether.

#4 improve nutrition: In the first 1,000 days of a child's life, nutrition can make a major difference in mortality, morbidity, and lifetime health. LRP allows for more diverse, nutritious, and culturally acceptable food to be purchased and/or distributed, which can improve community health. Other kinds of food aid, like cash vouchers that can be used by families to buy food in local markets, also allows for more fruits, vegetables, and diverse nutritious food to make their way onto plates—not just big commodities like corn, wheat, soy, and vegetable oil.

Oxfam, which does not take US government funds, used vouchers in the Sahel food crisis of 2012, to great result. In Senegal, there was enough food in most markets to feed local communities, but many community members, who had experienced a failed harvest, did not have enough money to buy the food they needed. Oxfam's partner, FODDE, provided vouchers to families to buy food in markets, at the cost of $8 per person per month. Wrote Oxfam humanitarian advisor Elizabeth Stevens, who spent time in Senegal doing the voucher disbursement to document the program:

---

[8] http://www.foreign.senate.gov/hearings/hearing/?id=3f546a93-d363-da0b-b25f-f1c5d096ddb1
[9] http://www.oxfamamerica.org/files/emiliana-aligaesha-brief.pdf-1

"Cash payments quickly go to work in the local markets, benefiting not only the people who receive the money directly but also the local farmers and vendors they buy from. And cash provides flexibility. A food distribution might involve fixed rations of beans and grain—the non-perishables that can travel long distances—but people who receive cash can buy a variety of foods, including eggs, fresh fruit, and vegetables. Furthermore, those who have pressing medical concerns can make the choice to spend some of their money on doctors and medicines."[10] Indeed, good nutrition is not just about food, but also the access to basic medical care to treat illness that sap strength and rob children of the nutrients they need. Cash programs can help tackle the multi-dimensional problem of malnutrition by empowering people with the resources they need to ensure food security.

The US LRP pilot program evaluation cited several examples of LRP programs that allowed communities to access more diverse and nutritious foods. Three school feeding projects were able to buy nutrient-rich foods like canned fish, fortified cereal bars, and in Nicaragua, eggs, dairy, fruits, and vegetables. Based on the six vouchers programs that were part of the LRP pilot, the independent evaluators concluded that "vouchers have been a relatively low-cost option for procurement; vouchers also give beneficiaries the ability to choose between foods in a way that best meets their households' needs and to personally select the quality of food they want."[11]

#5 gradual changes and flexibility: Food aid reform proposals represent a slow evolution, not a revolution, in food aid. Allowing for more regional and local purchase will not end US food shipments abroad. The key provision of food aid reform is flexibility. Every emergency is different, and US should be able to use any and every system at its disposal to bring aid. The US food aid system is now dominated by rigid rules which dictate where the US can buy food and how it is shipped. Adding some flexibility to the system is an acknowledgment that what is most effective in Afghanistan may not be what is most effective in the Philippines, and that what is needed in a famine may be different than what is needed during a natural disaster or conflict.

#6 bipartisan support: In one of the most divided Congresses on record, Republicans and Democrats have found something in common—food aid reform. In one of the rare occasions on which US food aid policy was directly debated and voted on, it received strong bipartisan support, though it came just short of passage. In 2013, Republican Congressman Ed Royce and Democrat Elliot Engel proposed sweeping reform of food aid as part of the reauthorization of the US Farm Bill. The House vote on the Royce-Engel Amendment on food aid reform in the Farm Bill in June 2013 split Democrats and Republicans right down the middle: 98 Democrats voted for reform, and 94 against, and 105 Republicans voted for reform, and 126 against. The end vote: 203 for and 220 against, a loss by just 9 votes. Many Republicans and Democrats from farm and port states voted against food aid reform,

---

[10] http://www.oxfamamerica.org/articles/sahel-food-crisis-201cnow-i-have-peace201d
[11] http://www.fas.usda.gov/info/LRP%20Report%2012-03-12%20TO%20PRINT.pdf

and both liberals and fiscal hawks voted in support—including House Minority Leader Nancy Pelosi and House Majority Leader Eric Cantor.

#7 everyone else is doing it—why aren't we?: The US is the only major donor country that continues to rely solely on sending food to humanitarian crisis spots, rather than buying food close to the region of need. Since 1988, the percentage of food sourced directly from donor countries has fallen from 92 to just 44 %. The European Union passed legislation in 2005 that dramatically overhauled their own food aid program, untying aid and allowing for increased use of LRP. In 2006, after the devastating tsunami in Southeast Asia, Canada realized how much more rice it could buy directly from Sri Lanka, for Sri Lankans, and changed its food aid procurement policy to allow for LRP, a move that was supported by Canadian farmers. In 2011, over 87 % of all countries providing food aid used some combination of LRP, almost double the figure from 1988.

Opponents: And Why Their Arguments Don't Work

Despite the overwhelming evidence that food aid reform will save lives and money, there remains small but powerful opposition to reform. The strongest opponents are special interests representing the agribusiness lobby and major maritime firms. This section will dissect their arguments against food aid reform and provide public health professionals with data to refute the claims that reform will hurt American jobs, American leadership, and national security.

American farmers: Agribusiness has argued that food aid reform will hurt American farmers and cost US jobs. This is simply not true. When the food aid system was founded, the US government was holding large stocks of US agriculture commodities, and providing aid was one way to do some good with this grain. Sixty year on, the landscape has radically changed. Demand for food is growing globally, and 2009–2012 marked the four most lucrative years in history for US agriculture, with over $478 billion in exports.[12]

Food aid makes up a minuscule percentage of that booming agricultural market. Food aid made up just 0.86 % of US agricultural exports FY2002–2011, and in FY2011, accounted for just 0.56 % of US farm profits.[13] Even the American Farm Bureau, which has come out against this reform, has said "Exports via food aid are a small drop in the market."[14]

Given strong demand for commodities, driven by an emerging global middle class, population growth, and an explosion in demand for biofuels, farmers have enjoyed several years of historically high food prices, demonstrating there are

---

[12] http://www.usaid.gov/foodaidreform/us-farmers
[13] Ibid.
[14] http://www.reuters.com/article/2013/05/01/usa-foodaid-lobbying-idUSL2N0D21F420130501

plenty of market opportunities beside food aid.[15] In June, both Cargill and the National Farmers Union came out in support of food aid reform. In fact, most US farmers are not part of the food aid system at all.

The American Farm Bureau spokesperson quoted above stated, "Our concern is less about decreasing an important revenue stream for US agriculture. It's more about the loss of a sense of pride." As Oxfam Director of Policy Gawain Kripke pointed out, US agribusiness should "step aside and let Congress and our leaders improve the (food aid) program... Doing so might actually help feed an additional four million people worldwide, which is truly something of which Americans could be proud."[16]

Shipping industry: The US shipping industry has been at the forefront of advocacy against food aid reform. They claim that decreasing the amount of food aid shipped on US-flagged carriers will destroy American jobs and undermine the nation's shipping industry. In June 2013, the food aid reform vote failed in Congress in part because of the engagement of unions in anti-reform advocacy: one Hill staffer told Oxfam that for many Democrats, it was like watching mommy and daddy fight, with unions on one side and anti-poverty activists on the other, both stalwarts of the liberal movement.

The Transportation Trades Department of the AFL-CIO wrote a letter to Congress on June 18th, the day before the vote on the Royce-Engle food aid amendment in the House, claiming food aid reform would undermine the nation's maritime industry and cost seafaring jobs.[17]

The problem with their argument is that they conflated the entire US cargo preference program with the food aid portion, which is in truth very small. Food aid makes up a minuscule percentage of US cargo—just 1.5 million tons out of the 1 billion tons of freight moved by the US cargo preference program in 2011—or 0.15 %.[18]

The real scandal here is that food aid has been used to subsidize the US shipping industry—to the cost of American taxpayers and communities in crisis around the world. USA Maritime, a lobbying group for the shipping industry, told Congress that 33,000 American jobs depend on the transportation of US food aid.[19] Professor Chris Barrett and his team at Cornell found that number to be significantly smaller— and very costly to taxpayers. Wrote Barrett, "The cost of maintaining this untapped pool of roughly 1,400 mariners on ACP vessels in FY2006 amounted to approximately $99,300 per mariner."[20]

---

[15] http://www.fao.org/worldfoodsituation/foodpricesindex/en/

[16] http://politicsofpoverty.oxfamamerica.org/2013/05/01/reforming-food-aid-can-save-millions-but-pride-a-deadly-sin/

[17] https://www.documentcloud.org/documents/814076-afl-transportation-trades-department-letter.html

[18] http://www.usaid.gov/foodaidreform/frequently-asked-questions-food-aid-reform

[19] http://usamaritime.org/wp-content/uploads/2013/06/USA_Maritime_FARRM_Bill.pdf

[20] http://dyson.cornell.edu/faculty_sites/cbb2/Papers/ACP_-_policy_brief_Nov_2010_Final.pdf

Indeed, the "buy American" flavor of cargo preference is something of a chimera itself. Many US flagged ships are in fact owned by foreign companies, like shipping giant Maersk who, in a nod to America, has named some of its carriers after US states. The Maersk Alabama, famously hijacked by Somali pirates in 2009, was in fact carrying US food aid. Professor Barrett estimates that at least 40 % of ships involved in cargo preference programs are owned by foreign companies. Maersk, which is Danish, has been one of the fiercest proponents of cargo preference and spent $650,000 in lobbyist fees in 2011 alone.[21]

Maersk was not alone. According to the Center for Public Integrity, the Marine Engineers Beneficial Association, the AFL Transportation Trades Department, and USA Maritime together contributed more than $750,000 to Members of House of Representatives in 2012. And it worked. 107 Congress people received contributions from these groups: 83 votes no on food aid reform, 29 votes yes, and 5 abstained—a 77.4 % success rate for the maritime industry.[22]

National Security

The US food aid program emerged after World War II as a way to keep the peace. George Marshall said, "Hunger and insecurity are the worst enemies of peace" and the Marshall Plan put food at the center of rebuilding Europe. The Marshall plan's food aid programming became the basis for our modern food aid infrastructure. But arguments that food aid reforms will make America less safe are specious at best.

This argument has been made by shipping interests including USA Maritime and the AFL-CIO, and by Members of Congress—many of whom have received significant donations from these organizations, as noted above. In April 2013, Congressmen Elijah E. Cummings (D-MD), Ranking Member of the House Committee on Oversight and Government Reform, and Duncan Hunter (R-CA), Chairman of the House Coast Guard and Maritime Transportation Subcommittee spearheaded a letter to President Obama, signed by 28 Members of Congress, claiming food aid reforms "threaten our national security preparedness by reducing the domestic sealift capacity on which our US military depends."[23]

Sounds dire, right? Not according to the experts on military preparedness, the Department of Defense. In June 2013, DOD Under Secretary of Defense for Acquisition, Technology, and Logistics Frank Kendall sent a letter to Congressmen Royce and Engle, stating reform "will not impact US maritime readiness and

---

[21] http://www.bostonglobe.com/opinion/2012/12/11/better-feed-starving-people-stop-serving-lobbyists/Q9BY29FNG4eztYFwji7bnO/story.html

[22] http://www.publicintegrity.org/2013/11/06/13687/how-shipping-unions-sunk-food-aid-reform

[23] http://cummings.house.gov/press-release/cummings-bipartisan-house-members-urge-president-obama-continue-food-peace-program

national security," and that reforms would have no bearing on any militarily useful vessels. [24]

This is backed up by a seminal Government Accountability Office Study now almost 20 years old that was tasked with finding out if, in fact, the food aid cargo preference law met its stated national security objective. The GAO found that the food aid-related cargo preference law did not "significantly contribute to meeting the intended objectives of helping to maintain US-flag ships as a naval and military auxiliary in time of war or national emergency or for purposes of domestic or foreign commerce." The report found the Department of Defense did not consider the cargo ships used to haul food aid as militarily useful. In terms of manpower, while the ships crews could be a pipeline for the Ready Reserves Forces, DoD did "not believe that applying cargo preference to food aid programs is a cost-effective means of providing for crews."[25]

Professor Barrett has come to similar conclusion, finding, "Contrary to the national security objectives of cargo preference laws, 70 % of US-flag vessels eligible to carry food aid in 2006 failed to qualify as militarily useful under MARAD criteria. Indeed, the priority system used to award bids under ACP directly disadvantages the most militarily useful US flag vessels."[26]

In an excellent article from Foreign Policy, John Norris called food aid cargo preference "a six-decade entitlement for US shippers with zero military value."[27] Over the past 60 years, the nature of warfare has changed dramatically, from the Vietnam War fought deep in jungles to today's war on terrorism being fought by drones. Over six diverse decades of warfare, continued Norris, "There has been no documented call-up of citizen mariners for national security purposes from agricultural cargo preference vessels since the program began. If we did not need this capacity in such major land wars as Vietnam, Iraq, or Afghanistan, it is frankly impossible to imagine when we would."[28]

The impact of food and hunger on global security can't be underestimated. In fact, saving more lives through food aid reform may have a positive national security benefit unto itself. Josette Sheeran, former head of the World Food Program, has said that hungry people have three options: "They revolt, they migrate or they die."[29] If the US is able to speed aid to two to four million more people per year, this increased aid may help stabilize regions in conflict and bring about faster peace.

Myths and realities: In addition to these arguments against food aid reform, two myths persist—that reforms will open aid to corruption and that reform will dampen American goodwill and leadership. Neither is true.

---

[24] Letter on file with the author.

[25] GAO cargo report.

[26] http://dyson.cornell.edu/faculty_sites/cbb2/Papers/ACP_-_policy_brief_Nov_2010_Final.pdf

[27] http://www.foreignpolicy.com/articles/2013/05/21/ship_storm_food_aid:reform?page=full

[28] Ibid.

[29] http://www.theglobeandmail.com/report-on-business/careers/careers-leadership/josette-sheeran-wages-the-ultimate-food-fight/article598360/

Corruption: Members of Congress have expressed concern that regional and local purchase, including cash/voucher systems, are more open to corruption than sending direct food aid. Members have argued that it is a lot harder to steal 50 t of food aid than it is to steal bags of money. In fact, USAID has strong systems in place to discourage corruption and track all forms of food aid.[30]

The key here is both strong accountability mechanisms and flexibility. Not all food aid systems will work in every country and crisis context. There may be a crisis where corruption is a real threat: if USAID has the full complement of aid options available, it can determine which will be most appropriate for that situation and the increased risk of corruption.

US leadership: America's food aid programs were founded to save lives—and to promote American good will and global leadership. When President John F. Kennedy renamed existing food aid programs "Food for Peace" in 1961, he said, "Food is strength, and food is peace, and food is freedom, and food is a helping (hand) to people around the world whose good will and friendship we want."

Food aid reform will maintain the critical public relations and diplomacy components of Food for Peace and other aid programs—and may even build on them. How will recipients know the grain grown in Tanzania is from the American people? Simple: where appropriate, food purchases via LRP will still be delivered to recipients in the iconic US-branded packaging.

But RLP has the power to do even more to build American good will. Hungry people appreciate receiving food from the US—but many communities are more interested in trade than aid and the long-term impacts economic partnerships can have on ending poverty. If the US can boost local farmers and local economics, that good will could be even more powerful to US-global relations. Tanzanian farmer Emiliana is a critical ambassador for US food aid—not as a recipient but as a business partner. The best kind of PR is partnerships, and that is what regional and local purchase offers—a twenty-first century vision of US leadership and goodwill.

State of play: Momentum is building for food aid reform. 2013 saw the first up or down vote on reform in the House of Representatives, and it lost by the narrowest of margins during a deeply contentious Farm Bill debate. There are several avenues for food aid reform. The Farm bill is reauthorized every 5 years, giving an opportunity to re-examine food aid programs and make changes. The President has also used his annual budget request as a platform to seek changes to the program. Last year, President Obama tried to reform food aid through this process and there is anticipation he will include reform in future budgets. Congress has shown an interest in reforming the program and there is always the opportunity for stand-alone legislation.

Role of health professionals in food aid reform: Public health professionals have a significant role to play in food aid reform. As advocates, they can counter the arguments of special interests with the talking points above. The day before the only up

---

[30] http://www.usaid.gov/foodaidreform/frequently-asked-questions-food-aid-reform

or down vote on food aid reform ever, there was a flurry of activity by these lobby groups—we need a hurricane from the health community to force Members of Congress to be accountable for their votes. If your Members of Congress voted yes on food aid reform, thank them and encourage them to become champions of this bi-partisan approach to saving lives. If they voted no, call their office or schedule a meeting to help dispel any myths they may have about food aid reform.[31] Engage state and national public health associations and other professional organizations in similar advocacy.

As Boston Globe columnist Farrah Stockman notes, food aid "benefits are big enough for a small group to fight for, but small enough for the rest of us to ignore." The public health community can help turn the tide with targeted advocacy by bolstering Congressional supporters and holding the 203 Members of Congress who voted against food aid reform accountable.

As program managers, public health practitioners should consider LRP and cash/voucher systems when constructing food aid programming. Public health leaders can continue to add to the literature on the efficacy of LRP and cash/voucher programs and increase our understanding of how food aid can improve nutritional outcomes for communities in crisis.

Typhoon Haiyan has reignited the debate on food aid reform. After the storm hit, the US was able to use $7.75 million to buy food close to the region of need, emergency airlift 55 t of food, and then ship over 1,000 t of food from a US rice supply stored in Sri Lanka for such emergencies. Even with US rice waiting in neighboring Sri Lanka, that shipment was not set to reach the Philippines for a month—far too long for communities in crisis.[32]

What do several former Secretaries of Agriculture, politicians on both sides of aisle, aid groups like Oxfam and Care, Cargill and the National Farmers Union, and think tanks from the Heritage Foundation and CATO to Brookings and the Center for American Progress, have in common?[33] Food aid reform. It is quite possible these groups have never agreed on anything, but they agree on this. Food aid reform is a public health priority that can save lives without another penny of US taxpayer money. It is high time for the US Congress to act.

---

[31] The final result of this vote can be found at: http://clerk.house.gov/evs/2013/roll262.xml.

[32] http://www.brookings.edu/blogs/up-front/posts/2013/11/18-typhoon-yolanda-haiyan-food-aid-ingram

[33] http://www.oxfamamerica.org/campaigns/food-justice/we-agree-food-aid-is-ripe-for-reform

Part IV
What Can Be Done to Achieve More in Global Health?

Chapter 18
The International Health Partnership: Monitoring Transparency and Accountability

Tim Shorten and Shaun Conway

The primary mechanism by which the IHP+ promotes mutual accountability is through an intervention (called IHP+Results[1]) to monitor IHP+ partners' individual and collective progress in implementing the commitments set out in the IHP+ Global Compact. Initially starting with a results framework as the basis for monitoring (see below), the experience of trying to monitor progress since 2009 led to the negotiation of an agreed

---

During the process of compiling IHP+Results performance reports, the IHP+Results team was initially occupied with liaising with representatives from each of the participating IHP+ signatories (36 out of 56 in 2012) to collect data. In some cases this can be fairly straightforward, in others it is very time consuming—largely depending factors that are specific to participating partners—for example, whether they work in sectors other than health, whether they have internal reporting systems in place to report progress. Once we had the data we needed, we spent a lot of time cleaning it (ensuring consistency of interpretation as far as possible, making sure it would not be rejected by our database), and then we produced an IHP+Results performance scorecard for each participating signatory. This is the 'special sauce' of the process. The scorecards enable to be identified issues for discussion, quickly and simply. In Nigeria, presentation of the scorecard to a senate committee on aid helped the Senate know more about how external aid was being used—and a senate fund was set up to support transparency and accountability; in Mozambique, partners decided to use some of the indicators to broaden the data available on the delivery of aid. At the fourth IHP+ country health sector team meeting in Nairobi (Dec 2012), over 200 delegates used the scorecards to cut to the chase on issues that were pressing and in need of attention. It's the potential for enhancing accountability dialogues that makes the scorecards interesting.
Tim Shorten, IHP+Results Programme Manager

[1] The IHP+Results Consortium is led by Re-Action! UK (recently renamed Results LAB) in cooperation with the London School of Hygiene & Tropical Medicine, Oxfam GB, and country researchers in the participating IHP+ countries. See www.ihpresults.net [accessed 25 March 2013] for more details. http://www.internationalhealthpartnership.net/en/results-evidence/results-of-past-monitoring-of-ihp-commitments/

T. Shorten (✉)
Independent Consultant
e-mail: tjshorten@gmail.com

S. Conway
e-mail: shaun@9needs.net

© Springer Science+Business Media New York 2015
E. Beracochea (ed.), *Improving Aid Effectiveness in Global Health*,
DOI 10.1007/978-1-4939-2721-0_18

monitoring framework which has been successfully implemented in three rounds of
monitoring (2010, 2012 and 2014). Key features of this monitoring framework include:

* Agreed by the IHP+ Mutual Accountability Working Group, and by the IHP+
  Scaling Up Reference Group (SuRG).[2]
* Including an agreed set of standard performance measures (12 for Development
  Partners (DPs), 10 for IHP+ country governments) drawn from the Paris
  Declaration indicators applied to the health sector.
* Presenting findings using Partner- and Country Scorecards (see examples below).

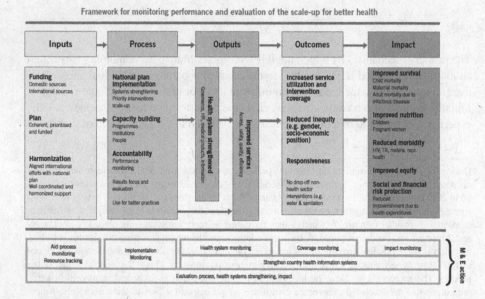

Framework for monitoring performance and evaluation of the scale-up for better health

The Results Framework Used by the IHP+

In 2012 this monitoring framework was implemented on a voluntary basis. Data
was collected from a sub-set of 36 IHP+ signatories[3] that chose to participate (up
from 25 that opted to participate during the 2010 process). Each agency self-reported

---

[2] The SuRG was a key part of IHP+ global governance structures at the time that the monitoring
framework was agreed.

[3] Nineteen IHP+ country governments: Benin, Burkina Faso, Burundi, Djibouti, DRC, Ethiopia, El
Salvador, Mali, Mauritania, Mozambique, Nepal, Niger, Nigeria, Rwanda, Senegal, Sierra Leone,
Sudan, Togo, and Uganda. Seventeen Development Partners: AusAID, AfDB, Belgium, EC, GAVI,
Germany, the Global Fund, Netherlands, Norway, Spain, Sweden, UK, UNAIDS, UNFPA,
UNICEF, WHO, and World Bank.

data for the set of Standard Performance Measures (listed below). A structured survey tool[4] was completed by the representatives of Partner Country governments and Development Partners over the period February to April 2012. The overall development partner response rate was 75 %. IHP+Results clarified data gaps and issues, analyzed the findings, and calculated the performance scorecards using transparent criteria.

IHP+Results Standard Performance Measures

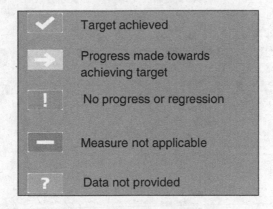

[4] The survey tool was available in English, French, and Spanish both in MS Excel format and as an online tool (which was a new development in the 2012 monitoring process).

IHP+ Governments		IHP+ Development Partners		
Standard Performance Measures	Target	Standard Performance Measures	Target	Link to Paris Target
1G: IHP+ Compact or equivalent mutual agreement in place.	An IHP+ Compact or equivalent mutual agreement is in place.	1DP: Proportion of IHP+ countries in which the partner has signed commitment to (or documented support for) the IHP+ Country Compact, or equivalent agreement.	100% of IHP+ countries where the signatory operates have support for/commitment to the IHP+ compact (or equivalent) mutually agreed and documented.	
2Ga: National Health Sector Plans/Strategy in place with current targets & budgets that have been jointly assessed.	A National Health Sector Plan/Strategy is in place with current targets & budgets that have been jointly assessed.	2DPa: Percent of aid flows to the health sector that is reported on national health sector budgets.	Halve the proportion of aid flows to the health sector not reported on government's budget(s) (with ≥ 85% reported on budget).	**PD3** Aid flows are aligned on national priorities
2Gb: Costed and evidence-based HRH plan in place that is integrated with the national health plan.	A costed, comprehensive national HRH plan (integrated with the health plan) is being implemented or developed.	2DPb: Percent of current capacity-development support provided through coordinated programmes consistent with national plans/strategies for the health sector.	50% or more of capacity development support to each IHP+ country in which the signatory operates are based on national health sector plans/ strategies	**PD4** Strengthen capacity by co-ordinated support
		2DPc: Percent of health sector aid provided as programme based approaches.	66% of health sector aid flows are provided in the context of programme based approaches.	**PD9** Use of common arrangements or procedures
3G: Proportion of public funding allocated to health.	15% (or an equivalent published target) of the national budget is allocated to health.	3DP: Percent of health sector aid provided through multi-year commitments.	90% (or an equivalent published target) of health sector funding provided through multi-year commitments (min. 3 years).	
4G: Proportion of health sector funding disbursed against the approved annual budget.	Halve the proportion of health sector funding not disbursed against the approved annual budget.	4DP: Percent of health sector aid disbursements released according to agreed schedules in annual or multi-year frameworks.	71% of health sector aid disbursed within the fiscal year for which it was scheduled.	**PD7** Aid is more predictable
5Ga: Country public financial management either (a) adhere to broadly accepted good practices or (b) have a reform programme in place to achieve these.	Improvement of at least one measure (ie 0.5 points) on the PFM/CPIA scale of performance.	5DPa: Percent of health sector aid that uses public financial management systems.	Reduce by one-third the aid not using public financial management systems (with ≥ 80% using country systems).	**PD5a** Use of country public financial management (PFM) systems
5Gb: Country procurement systems either (a) adhere to broadly accepted good practices or (b) have a reform programme in place to achieve these.	Improvement of at least one measure on the four-point scale used to assess performance for this sector.	5DPa: Percent of health sector aid that uses country procurement systems.	Reduce by one-third the aid not using procurement systems (with ≥ 80% using country systems).	**PD5b** Use of country procurement systems
		5DPc: Number of parallel Project Implementation Units (PIUs) per country.	Reduce by two-thirds the stock of parallel project implementation units (PIUs).	
6G: An agreed transparent and monitorable performance assessment framework is being used to assess progress in the health sector.	A transparent and monitorable performance assessment framework is in place to assess progress in the health sector.	6DP: Proportion of countries in which agreed, transparent and monitorable performance assessment frameworks are being used to assess progress in the health sector.	Single national performance assessment frameworks are used, where they exist, as the primary basis to assess progress in all countries where the signatory operates.	**PD11** Results-oriented frameworks
7G: Mutual assessments, such as joint annual health sector reviews, have been made of progress implementing commitments in the health sector, including on aid effectiveness.	Mutual assessments (such as a joint annual health sector review) are being made of progress implementing commitments in the health sector, including on aid effectiveness.	7DP: Proportion of countries where mutual assessments have been made of progress implementing commitments in the health sector, including on aid effectiveness.	Annual mutual assessment of progress in implementing health sector commitments & agreements (such as the IHP+ country compact and on aid effectiveness in the health sector) is being made in all the countries where the signatory operates.	**PD12** Mutual accountability
8G: Evidence that civil society is actively represented in health sector policy processes - including health sector planning, coordination & review mechanisms.	At least 10% of seats in the country's health sector coordination mechanisms are allocated to civil society representatives.	8DP: Evidence of support for Civil Society to be actively represented in health sector policy processes - including health sector planning, coordination & review mechanisms.	All signatories can provide some evidence of supporting active civil society engagement.	

Critical Assumptions and Qualifiers

A number of limitations exist with the agreed monitoring framework, in some cases inherited from limitations in the Paris Declaration indicator set. They key limitations of the IHP+ framework are:

- *Limited scope of reporting framework.* It is possible that the IHP+ made progress in areas that were not tracked through the agreed reporting framework used by IHP+Results. Efforts were made to draw on additional data, but this was not the primary focus of our efforts.
- *Self-reported data.* The IHP+Results process allowed limited opportunity for triangulation of the data provided by participating IHP+ signatories. Some triangulation efforts were considered—including comparison with other aid effectiveness analyses, structured discussions at country level, and an informal peer review of Development Partner scorecards. In practice these proved challenging to systematically and meaningfully execute within available time and resources.
- *Limited data set.* There are still some notable omissions from the participants list, including the Bill & Melinda Gates Foundation. And whilst they are not IHP+ signatories, the lack of data on US Government performance means that the country data sets represent a picture of IHP+ signatories performance, not overall Development Partner performance[5]. The number of participants does not allow for rigorous statistical analysis. There is also a relatively small time series, albeit growing.
- *Lack of qualitative and interpretive data provided by participating signatories.* The development and agreement of IHP+Results monitoring framework was heavily influenced by concerns about the transaction costs of reporting. As a result both DPs and Partner Country governments were not asked to provide mandatory qualitative data. This limits IHP+Results' ability to fully understand points of complexity and nuance, and to explore how and why results have been achieved.
- *Weaknesses in specific indicators.* In particular, the indicators for the strength of country systems and DP use of these systems are not as specific and sensitive as necessary to form strong conclusions. As a result, firm conclusions on the use of national Procurement Systems are hard to draw.

The framework does though provide the basis for credible findings and robust conclusions and recommendations as the basis of discussions on how to improve the effectiveness of future aid.

---

[5] USAID became a member of the IHP+ in May 2013 and participated in the 2014 round of IHP+ monitoring.

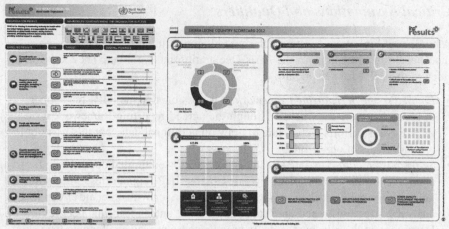

IHP+Results Partner Scorecard   IHP+Results Country Scorecard

Is the Quality of Health Sector Aid Improving?

The following findings are from IHP+Results 2012 Annual Performance Report, available at www.ihpresults.net.

> On current performance, Development Partners will not meet the Busan targets that have been renewed from the Paris framework for delivering more effective aid (in the health sector).
> IHP+Results 2012 Annual Performance Report

There has been progress on some aid effectiveness indicators
Partner Country governments strengthened leadership and aid governance...
Of the 19 Partner Countries and 17 Development Partners that participated in this review:

- 18 Partner Countries had national health plans (of which 11 have been jointly assessed), 11 had compacts, and 10 Partner Countries had both
- 13 Partner Countries had a performance framework in place
- 14 Partner Countries had a Mutual Assessment process in 2011
- 14 Partner Countries were engaging civil society in national planning and review processes

... they strengthened country financial management systems, and some increased financing for health ...

- 13 Partner Countries met the target for improving Public Financial Management systems
- 10 Partner Countries had Public Financial Management systems that were rated as being adequate for Development Partners to channel funding through

- 3 Partner Countries (Burkina Faso, El Salvador and Rwanda) allocated more than 15 % of their government budget to health, and a further 8 were moving towards the 15 % target
- 10 Partner Countries had improved the disbursement of their national health budget

Country Public Financial Management Systems

PARTICIPANTS IN 2010 & 2012

PARTICIPANTS ONLY IN 2012

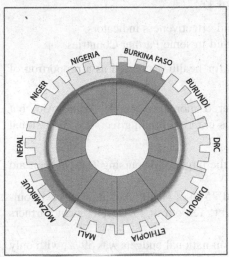

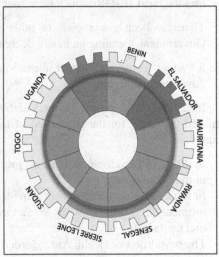

Development Partners are supporting country leadership ...

- Development Partners with a country presence mostly supported compacts, used National Results Frameworks, and participated in mutual assessment exercises
- All Development Partners supported civil society, mostly with financial support or advocacy to engage them in health planning processes

... and they are providing better coordinated support.

- Development Partners exceeded the target for providing coordinated capacity building support (at baseline and in 2011).
- 81 % of Health Aid was programme aid (rather than projects) in 2011, and 8 Development Partners met the target of 66 % of their aid being programme aid.

Five Partner Countries that signed the IHP+ in 2007 appear to have received more effective aid

- Ethiopia, Mali, Mozambique, and Nepal had national plans, compacts, results frameworks, and mutual accountability process. Burundi had all except Mutual Accountability process.
- All five Partner Countries received more aid recorded on national budget and through country Public Financial Management systems in 2011 than in 2007.
- Most received more long-term commitments and predictable aid.
- Uganda and Mali (nine) met the most IHP+Results targets (out of ten) and five other Partner Countries met eight targets.
- Germany (11), AusAID, the Netherlands, and the World Health Organization (9) met the most IHP+Results targets (out of 12).

There has been less progress on other aid effectiveness indicators. Government spending on health decreased in some Partner Countries.

- 5 Partner Countries' budget allocation for health decreased as a proportion of government budget

In 2011, Development Partners delivered more predictable Health Aid, but missed the target for the proportion of this external funding recorded on national budgets ...

- In 2011, 16 Development Partners met the target of disbursing 71 % of their aid in the planned year
- In total, Development Partners provided 75 % of Health Aid in multi-year commitments in 2011, below the 90 % target. Ten out of 17 Development Partners met the target
- The proportion of Health Aid recorded on national budgets was 59 %, with only nine Development Partners meeting the 85 % target

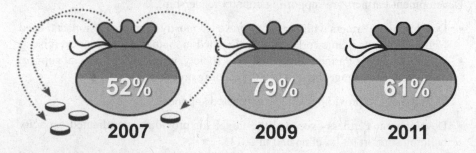

...Development Partners did not increase the proportion of aid delivered through country systems...

- The overall proportion of Health Aid using country Public Financial Management systems was 58 % in 2011, far short of the 80 % target.

- Only five Development Partners (Norway, Netherlands, EC, UK, and World Bank) met the target of 80 % of aid flowing through country Public Financial Management systems, although two more were close.
- Only two Development Partners (World Bank and Belgium) met the target of using national procurement systems for 80 % of procurement funding.
- The number of parallel implementation units fell (from 64 to 39) between the baseline year and 2011.[6]

What Does the Future Hold for the IHP+?

Whilst the findings summarized above are drawn from IHP+Results 2012 monitoring process, this was the fourth separate report that had been complied on IHP+ implementation.[7] The experience of producing these reports provides important lessons that should be considered in future adaptations to IHP+ activities, including monitoring.

Independent Reports on IHP+ Implementation (2008–2012)[8]

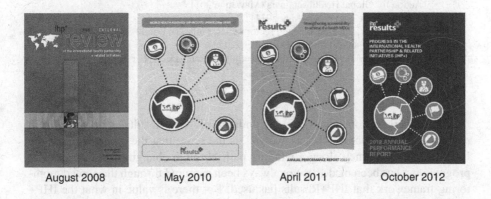

| August 2008 | May 2010 | April 2011 | October 2012 |

The first round of IHP+Results monitoring (conducted during 2009, presented at the World Health Assembly in May 2010) provided insights into the state of preparedness of IHP+ signatories to meet their commitments to accountability as set out in

---

[6] Ensuring that only the same Development Partners and same Partner Countries were counted in both baseline and latest year data.

[7] A further round of IHP+ monitoring was undertaken in 2014, after this chapter had been finalised.

[8] Copies of these reports are available at www.internationalhealthpartnership.net.

the Global Compact, it also enabled learning on how to conduct sector level monitoring of aid effectiveness implementation. This experience underlined the importance of gaining commitment from IHP+ signatories to an agreed monitoring framework, which was in turn critical to ownership and participation in subsequent monitoring rounds (2010, 2012 and 2014). This kind of learning has characterized IHP+ monitoring efforts—the process has evolved through adaptations: with each round of monitoring there has been growing support and participation, and growing confidence in findings. The existence of an independent advisory group to oversee the development and implementation of IHP+Results methodology proved invaluable in reinforcing confidence in the credibility of the findings that the methodology produced.

Perhaps most importantly, enabling the transparent availability of data on health sector implementation of aid effectiveness commitments has enabled a different type of conversation, and growing ownership of IHP+ processes by country governments. Other groups have drawn on IHP+Results data to conduct related analyses,[9] and there are a growing number of examples where IHP+Results findings have been discussed in national and international forums.

Examples of Use of IHP+Results Findings
- Annual side events at World Health Assembly (2010, 2011, 2012)
- Action for Global Health seminars (May/June 2011)
- Nigeria senate committee (May 2011)
- Mozambique joint annual health sector review (July 2011 and Feb/March 2012)
- Burundi joint annual review (December 2012)
- IHP+ Country Health Sector Team meeting, Nairobi (December 2014)

What emerges from reviewing the findings of IHP+Results' work, and from reflecting on the process as it has evolved, is the sense that the progress under the IHP+ reflects a journey along a winding path, through changing landscapes. The progress that has been made has not always been captured through the agreed monitoring framework that IHP+Results has used. But there is value in what the IHP+ offers, providing it continues to learn and adapt.

---

[9] See the Center for Global Development's Quality of Official Development Assistance for Health index (Health Quoda): http://www.cgdev.org/files/1426169_file_QuODA_LJ_SF1.pdf [accessed 7 December 2012].

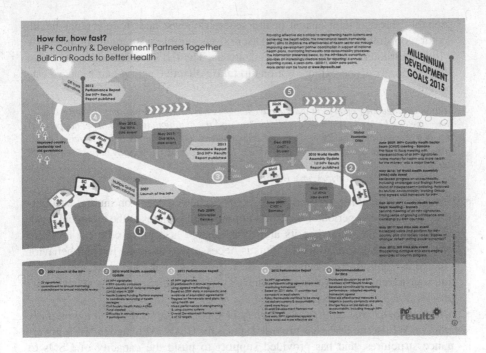

How can Progress be Accelerated?

Consistent with the OECD reporting on the implementation of the Paris Declaration,[10] it is clear that health sector progress on health sector aid effectiveness is not fast enough. IHP+Results made recommendations for how progress can be accelerated. Reflecting on these and other work that has happened within the IHP+,[11] the following issues are important for the IHP+ to assimilate in its future strategies and operations.

- *Stronger focus on delivery of aid.* It is important that IHP+ partners continue to put effort into strengthening leadership, putting in place the policies and plans that provide a framework for coordinated support to improving health outcomes, and strengthening country systems. But more attention is needed on the delivery of aid. Development Partners should ensure that their aid is recorded on budget, more predictable and channeled through national systems.
- *Stronger focus on mutual accountability.* IHP+ partners need to discuss their individual and collective performance, and make explicit commitments to address areas of slowest progress—this will give true credibility to IHP+ efforts on mutual accountability. Discussions should happen at the country level—

---

[10] Aid effectiveness 2005–2010: progress in implementing the Paris Declaration (OECD), pp. 18.
[11] Options for the future strategic direction of the International Health Partnership+: the findings of a consultation with stakeholders (Devillé and Taylor 2011).

probably through joint annual health sector reviews, and more regular health sector coordination mechanisms. Discussions should also happen internally within multilateral and bilateral organizations. The IHP+ should address areas of slowest progress and explore options to take collective action and to accelerate progress.

The anticipated step change in aid effectiveness has not been achieved, but IHP+Results reporting can be used to promote accountability, and the finding that this is not yet happening is a missed opportunity to drive aid effectiveness. Opportunities must be seized to improve mutual accountability and civil society have a critical role to play in pushing this agenda.
   IHP+Results 2012 Performance Report

- *Stronger political mechanisms.* As part of a renewed focus on mutual accountability, and after a period of focusing on plans and policies at the technical level, the IHP+ should strengthen its ability to engage at a more political level (to complement its technical work). This is necessary as a means for real behavior change as some of the changes that are required to make aid more predictable and transparent and flow through country systems require decisions at headquarters level and changes to policies.

- *Stronger focus on support Civil Society Organizations (CSOs) to meaningfully engage.* Whilst the IHP+ has provided space for CSOs to engage in IHP+ governance structures, and has provided support to build the capacity of CSOs to engage in policy dialogue at country level,[12] further support is needed. Civil Society has a critical role to play at all stages of the health policy, planning, implementation, and review process. Its involvement can help ensure that national plans reflect country priorities (not just government priorities); with the right capacity CSOs can enable the triangulation of self-reported performance data and can play an important voice in demanding accountability for results. Better means (measures and processes) to assess and monitor the meaningful engagement of CSOs in health policy and planning processes.

- *Further adaptation to monitoring efforts.* At the end of 2012, the IHP+ partners agreed to continue their monitoring efforts. Monitoring is likely to adapt in line with plans to monitor the implementation of the Busan Partnership for Effective Development Co-operation[13] (see box below). In the same way IHP+ monitoring will maintain a limited set of standardized indicators which could be incorporated into existing country processes, and reviewed in joint annual health sector reviews. Any global reporting on IHP+ progress will pick up available data from countries, rather than conducting new data collection exercises.

Post-Busan monitoring arrangements

---

[12] See http://www.healthpolicyactionfund.org/ for more details [accessed 7 December 2012].

[13] http://www.aideffectiveness.org/busanhlf4/about/global-partnership.html [accessed 7 December 2012].

The agreed monitoring arrangements for the Global Partnership for Effective Development Co-operation maintain six of the indicators used to monitor the Paris Declaration with some additional ones[14]; but they emphasize country data collection processes over global surveys—any global reporting will gather data that is available at the time of reporting, rather than conducting new data collection exercises.

- *Continued, strengthened support to country-level efforts.* The direction of travel on monitoring is in line with broader agreement to maintain the IHP+ focus on supporting country-level planning and implementation.[15] This may happen through the development of tools and guidance, such as the Joint Assessment of National Strategies.[16]
- *Continued international level platform.* Whilst IHP+ will continue its main focus at country level, there is also an acknowledgement of the importance of the global level and that this should continue in some form.

Whether and how the IHP+ assimilates these issues as it continues to evolve remains to be seen. Whether political momentum and support is maintained on the aid effectiveness agenda is likely to have a central role in any considerations on IHP+ future. The role of countries in articulating their needs and demands for more effective aid (and more broadly for development effectiveness) is critical. And with the likelihood that the global health architecture will continue to change—this is one of the key questions about the Post-2015 Development Agenda[17]—the need for the IHP+ as a driver and facilitator of better coordination and more effective joint working will be stronger. It is our hope that the need for donors to attribute results to their specific support (in order to maintain support for aid budgets) does not crowd out the need to support countries to deliver their own priorities and to manage external support effectively and efficiently to achieve this.

---

[14] http://www.aideffectiveness.org/busanhlf4/images/stories/Indicators_targets_and_process_for_global_monitoring.pdf [accessed 7 December 2012].

[15] Options for the future strategic direction of the International Health Partnership+: the findings of a consultation with stakeholders (Devillé and Taylor 2011), pp. 3.

[16] http://www.internationalhealthpartnership.net/en/tools/jans-tool-and-guidelines/ [accessed 25 March 2013].

[17] http://www.worldwewant2015.org/health [accessed 25 March 2013].

Chapter 19
Social Media and Aid Effectiveness

Eckhard F. Kleinau

Many readers will already be very familiar with social media and their personal or professional use, while others may not yet have seen their value or taken to it because of technology barriers. The objective of this chapter is to highlight the use of social media in the context of international development and aid effectiveness. The services, technologies, and examples presented throughout this chapter are meant to illustrate the utility of social media in this context but not to give an exhaustive review or recommend that readers adopt certain media over others. Far too many options for each type of social media exist to mention them all. Moreover, the landscape of social media providers changes rapidly and new media emerge every few years. Everybody using social media makes choices based on personal preferences and strikes a balance between the value of information and time invested to track or publish different social media. Such considerations apply to individuals subscribing to social media as well as organizations deciding on which social media to maintain a presence.

Social media are omnipresent today—not only in high-income countries. Access to the Internet and mobile phones in developing countries has increased exponentially over the last 15 years and with it access to social media such as social networks, blogs, and tweets. In Africa Internet users increased from 4.5 million in the year 2000 to almost 170 million in 2012,[1] and mobile phone subscriptions jumped from fewer than 20 million in 2000 to almost 650 million in 2012, more than in the USA or the European Union (Yonazi et al. 2012). Close to 100 million of the mobile phones in Africa have at least rudimentary Internet capabilities, with mobiles

---

[1] Internet usage information reported at http://www.internetworldstats.com/stats.htm (accessed 12/22/2012) and comes from data published by Nielsen Online, by the International Telecommunications Union, by GfK, local ICT Regulators, and other reliable sources.

E.F. Kleinau, M.D., Dr.P.H., M.S. (✉)
GRM Futures Group, Washington, DC, USA
e-mail: ekleinau@futuresgroup.com

© Springer Science+Business Media New York 2015
E. Beracochea (ed.), *Improving Aid Effectiveness in Global Health*,
DOI 10.1007/978-1-4939-2721-0_19

expected to surpass computers for accessing the Internet within a few years. Why does it matter that a manager of a development program, for example, in Nairobi, Kenya, has access to social media?

I am going to use a personal experience to answer this question. Much of our work in international development requires specific expertise, for example, in impact evaluations, health systems strengthening, or organizational learning and knowledge management. A constant challenge is finding people with the right expertise, often at a moment's notice. Recently, my company was seeking a proposal writer with grants management experience and instructional designers with human resource management experience for an eLearning contract, both in a specific geographic area. Traditionally, we advertise and search large online recruitment databases such as monster.com or Devex's jobs and career services. Unfortunately, our inquiries did not yield any resumes that met all the necessary technical and geographic criteria as well as years of experience. Does this sound familiar? We were lucky, though, thanks to the world's largest professional network on the Internet, LinkedIn. My personal network on LinkedIn included several people with the background we were looking for.

How can a social network help finding experts whether in Washington, Nairobi, or many other towns or rural communities worldwide? Networks like LinkedIn not only connect us to colleagues around the world with whom we keep personally in touch, although most of us start with a small group of people we know well, but also reach many times more through these existing connections. As our personal network grows, we identify more and more professionals not only in our main line of work but also in many associated and new areas.

Data, data Everywhere, but no Information to be Any Wiser[2]

Hiring the right consultant for a job is certainly important for development programs, which contributes to aid effectiveness in a small way. Today, social media play a much larger role in international development by narrowing the gap between data richness and information poverty in some sectors such as health and economic growth. Social media have also become vital for reducing the information imbalance by gathering data in sectors notoriously difficult to assess such as governance and politics and therefore allowing greater civil society involvement in development activities.

While the above adaptation of an old mariner's rime may exaggerate the state of international development, who has not felt on occasion that the sheer amount of data such as the world development indicators is overwhelming; yet we feel we are missing crucial knowledge. Data are often at a macro (country or groups of countries) level and lag by several years, which do not help practitioners in finding program relevant information. On the other hand, we get detailed accounts of processes from periodic project reports that meet administrative requirements, but that tell us

---

[2] "Water, water everywhere nor any drop to drink" is a quote from "The Rime of the Ancient Mariner" by Samuel Taylor Coleridge, 1797–1798.

little about whether programs make a true difference in the lives of people and how they were able to do so.

Transparency and accountability requires that organizations share information and that people have the means to access it. Aid effectiveness depends on information in two ways. Firstly, information is crucial for implementers to improve program performance and aid effectiveness. Implementers of development assistance and aid beneficiaries such as frontline health workers or farmers can be more productive when they have access to vital technical, process, and market information. Secondly, governments, donors, and stakeholders depend on information for knowing whether foreign aid is effective in reaching those in greatest need and meeting its intended objectives. Aid should also be delivered efficiently by achieving the best results with the least amount of funding, which depends on competent management, good governance and accurate information.

Unfortunately, information is often hard to obtain. Donors and aid recipients alike provide information that is incomplete, fragmented, and, in the absence of standardized measures, difficult to compare against common benchmarks. Importantly, feedback from beneficiaries and technically rigorous impact evaluations are rare. With few exceptions, we know even less about the costs of delivering aid and whether alternative approaches could have resulted in better outcomes with fewer resources. Donors and aid recipients have made progress by sharing more data especially through the Internet, for example, the Millennium Challenge Corporation. However, information still needs to be much more detailed, comprehensive, and timely to learn from experience, avoid duplication of efforts, and focus on results as well as improve transparency and accountability towards civil society and other stakeholders in donor countries and abroad.

Donors' and aid recipients' efforts of sharing information clearly leave much unanswered about aid effectiveness. What other means do civil society organizations, citizens, and other stakeholders have to become informed and engage in advocacy and actions? Social media—using Web 2.0 technologies[3]—have become an increasingly important source of information about aid and governance and have greatly facilitated coordination and collaboration among stakeholders and citizens. The use of social media in developing countries has risen dramatically with the rapid expansion of mobile telephony and especially the affordability of smartphones. "Often governments are less informed than the people because of the social media revolution," said Brookings Institution's Daniel Kaufmann at a discussion in 2012.[4] The discussion of aid has long since moved from special interest groups to public forums.

---

[3] Web 2.0 is the term given to describe a second generation of the World Wide Web that is focused on the ability for people to collaborate and share information online. Web 2.0 basically refers to the transition from static HTML Web pages to a more dynamic Web that is more organized and is based on serving Web applications to users. (Quoted from http://www.webopedia.com/TERM/W/Web_2_point_0.html; accessed 12/22/2012.) Web 2.0 refers to technologies that make the web faster, more accessible, easier to publish to, and a better tool to connect with friends and colleagues. Social media are built on these technologies.

[4] Can Media Development Make Aid More Effective? http://cima.ned.org/events/can-media-development-make-aid-more-effective; accessed 11/25/2012.

What do an Earthquake in China and Election Violence in Kenya have in Common? The Role of Social Media in International Development Today

The Internet features an innumerable number of blogs about aid, many managed by well-known organizations, such as The Guardian's Global Development Blogosphere[5]; individuals with an interest in foreign aid drive many others such as Laurie Garrett's blog.[6] Events where aid is discussed can be followed through a—sometimes over-powering—number of tweets such as @aids2012[7] with thousands of followers. For example, during the Arab Spring, which began in late 2010, and in Papua New Guinea in 2012, social media such as Facebook, tweets, and blogs greatly facilitated civil society engagement in the practice of politics and were used to voice and organize political protest.

The role of social media may be easier to illustrate by looking at each type of media and how they improve transparency, accountability, and good governance and, hopefully, aid effectiveness. The big three social media services—Facebook, Twitter, and YouTube—combined with independent blogging do not require any special computer skills and allow anybody to share information and reach vast audiences from their home or as an eyewitness in Cairo's Tahrir Square by simply using a mobile phone with a camera. All these social media integrate seamlessly with each other; a YouTube video incorporates easily into a Facebook page or a blog that also feature Twitter feeds.

Social media have given aid recipients a voice during elections, natural disasters, and conflict situation; however, this is not yet the case—with a few exceptions—in the daily business of global development. Efforts to give ordinary citizens in developing countries a say in how aid is perceived and whether it is managed fairly and transparently do not lack but have not yet had the success its advocates have hoped for. While technical barriers have lessened substantially with the spread of mobile phones, cultural and political barriers and economic hardships facing poor and marginal populations need to be overcome for these citizens to voice their opinions and concerns through social media. For example, in 2010 the Tanzania-based NGO Daraja initiated the Maji Matone (Raising the Water Pressure) program and asked villagers to report outages in their water systems via Short Message Service (SMS). These citizens' reports were used to put pressure on local government to address problems with rural water supplies. Unfortunately, the uptake by the population was negligible and the program halted over a year later. However, there is good news that comes with the bad. Daraja was very upfront about the failure and wrote in their blog about the reasons.[8] This is an example where social

---

[5] http://www.guardian.co.uk/global-development/series/global-development-blogosphere
[6] http://www.lauriegarrett.com/index.php/en/blog/#&panel1-1
[7] https://twitter.com/aids2012
[8] http://blog.daraja.org/2011/12/maji-matone-hasnt-delivered-time-to.html, accessed 12/22/2012.

Table 19.1 Popular social media: features and common uses

Social media	Features	Common uses
Facebook	Social network for connecting with friends, share personal updates, photos, videos, links, etc.	Individuals and aid organizations engaging on a social level, making global development more approachable, fund raising
LinkedIn	Professional network for sharing resumes and experiences, acting as references, recommending colleagues	Individuals looking for professional connections and seeking job opportunities, aid organizations recruiting personnel
YouTube/Flickr	Sharing videos and photographs	Aid organization and individuals sharing field experience, speeches, training, etc.
Twitter	Broadcast short messages to followers	News flashes about latest events in global development, sharing links to new, interesting, or innovative information
Web-integrated Short Message Service (SMS)	Sharing or receiving information on a mobile phone integrated with social media-type websites	Crowdmapping of events and services, sharing business and educational information with phone subscribers, collecting data from the field
WordPress, Blogger, Blog	Publishing on the Internet and incorporating photos and videos	Sharing opinions, summarizing and linking to interesting stories, articles, and events about global development and aid effectiveness
Wikipedia	User-maintained Internet encyclopedia	Sharing facts about global development and aid effectiveness

media foster global transparency and learning. Daraja's case is featured in FAILfare, a resource for "Learning from #FAILs in ICT and Mobiles for Development."[9] While aid organizations and governments may not yet have reached a full partnership with aid recipients today, social media will play an important role in reaching this goal.

While the social media mentioned in this chapter are the most popular, many alternatives exist, often offering additional and innovative features. Readers can find these services easily through Internet search engines like Google. A comparison of popular social media may help readers decide which media to subscribe to or to adopt for their place of work. Table 19.1 highlights their key features and common uses.

Social and Professional Networks

The best-known social network is probably *Facebook*, which was launched in February 2004 and counted over one billion active users in 2012. Facebook allows its members to make connections, share interests and news, communicate frequently

---

[9] http://failfaire.org/, accessed 12/22/2012.

with each other, and join groups. Beside its role in civil movements (Safranek 2012) mentioned above, donors and aid organizations make their presence known on Facebook, for example, the US Agency for International Development (USAID), the UK Department for International Development (DfID), Save the Children, CARE International or Futures Group,[10] sharing information about current initiatives, inviting the public to comment and tag items they like and share them with other readers.

LinkedIn, founded in 2002, is the largest social networking website for people in professional occupations with more than 175 million registered users in 2012 in more than 200 countries and territories. It allows registered users to maintain a list of contacts, called "connections." Users can invite anyone (whether a LinkedIn member or not) to connect as long as there is mutual interest in establishing a connection. From personal experience, many of our readers can attest to how powerful such a professional network can be, which goes far beyond traditional networks that only rely on interpersonal relationships. LinkedIn connections become a known and trusted resource with shared interests by following the simple rule of only inviting connections who we would recommend to other colleagues and only accepting invitations from people who we know or who share detailed professional profiles. Recommendations from clients and colleagues further enhance people's profiles on LinkedIn as do endorsements—a feature added more recently. With endorsements people in your network acknowledge the specific skills of a LinkedIn member. Lastly, members can join special interest groups on LinkedIn such as Economic Development Specialists or Global Public Health.

While Facebook has by far the largest membership readers may want to check out other networking tools such as Google+, Ning, MySpace, Friendster, FriendFeed, Diaspora, Bebo, and others. They all offer the basic functionality of messaging, commenting, and connecting to friends and colleagues. In addition they also offer different features that my appeal to people's goals such as engagement, communication, fundraising, and others.

Video and Picture Sharing

YouTube

YouTube is a video-sharing website, founded in 2005, where users can upload, view, rate, and share videos. Visitors can find videos on many development topics here that show how programs operate in the field telling a more compelling story than many written reports. Algezeera's video about the sanitation crisis in India had almost 68,000 views; and Plan's video about Community Led Total Sanitation

---

[10] http://www.facebook.com/USAID; https://www.facebook.com/ukdfid; https://www.facebook.com/savethechildren; https://www.facebook.com/carefans; https://www.facebook.com/FuturesGroup

(CLTS) was watched 12,000 times.[11] Such interest may be surprising given the subject matter, but this is also an indication that people across the world have become aware about the great need for better sanitation in many parts of the developing world. These two examples were not even the most watched videos on this subject matter, others attracted several times as many views. Visitors can find videos on any program supported by public and private donor aid, including soy bean production, child nutrition, small and medium enterprise development, microcredits, and good governance. Aid effectiveness and an obstacle to achieving it, corruption, feature in several videos. Girls' education in Africa is the subject of many videos such as Plan Canada's "Shewmantu's story—The power of girls' education," which was viewed over 20,000 times.[12]

With the rapid spread of mobile phones with still photo and video capabilities, YouTube has become the site where eyewitnesses can post their videos of tragic events almost as soon as they happen. Videos from the 2010 earthquake in Haiti were seen by hundreds of thousands of viewers and have raised funds for the victims, especially when involving celebrity spokespersons. Social media in general and YouTube specifically have become important tools for fundraising by organizations providing humanitarian assistance, especially when they attract a huge number of views, sometimes exceeding one billion, which is called videos gone viral (Dixon and Keyes 2012).

Flickr

Flickr is an image and video hosting website and online community that was created by Ludicorp in 2004 and acquired by Yahoo! in 2005. It is a popular website for users to share and embed personal photographs, many related to global development. Flickr is widely used by bloggers to host images that they embed in blogs and other social media.

Microblogging (e.g., Tweeting)

Microblogging is a broadcast medium in the form of blogging but limited to a short line of text, 140 characters in the case of tweets (Twitter). Many social network sites provide microblogging services, including Facebook and Google+ where they may be called "status updates." A widely known service is provided by Twitter, which launched in 2006, in the form of tweets. Other providers include Cif2.net, Jaiku, Plurk, and Tumblr. In the 2012 elections in Ghana voters at polling stations would tweet about an incident at their station. These tweets and several other social media

---

[11] http://www.youtube.com/watch?v=orIFs72HGmM;http://www.youtube.com/watch?v=TnRPsUwCT30
[12] http://www.youtube.com/watch?v=BGiF96dzt6Q

were used immediately by the Social Media Tracking Centre, which was set up by the African Election Project (@Penplusbytes) with support from DFID (@DFID_ UK). The Centre then alerted key elections stakeholders such the National Elections Security Task Force (NESTF), Electoral Commission of Ghana, civil society organizations, and the media about serious election irregularities for necessary action (allAfrica 2012). For example, tweets about issues with biometric verification systems for voter registration were reported by @ghanaelections. This is only one of innumerable examples of the use of tweets for the benefit of civil and social causes in developing countries.

For those readers not used to tweeting, a brief description of how Twitter works follows. Users who want to tweet need to set up a free Twitter account and username. The username begins with the "@" sign followed a unique name such as @Calestous referring to Prof. Calestous Juma from the Harvard University Kennedy School of Government. To just follow a tweeter no Twitter account is required, only an Internet browser or dedicated software on a mobile phone or computer is needed to receive tweets. Twitter usernames are often referenced in a tweet pointing to other tweeters. Another common element in a tweet is a word preceded by a "#," which is called a "hashtag." Hashtags indicate trending topics such as #malaria; they instruct Twitter to find all tweets with the same hashtag regardless of the author. Any tweeter can create a hashtag; but new hashtags should be used sparingly, especially if similar ones exist already. When a tweet begins with the letters "RT" this indicates a "re-tweet" of someone else's tweet who is identified by "@usename" in the tweet. Lastly, tweets often contain a hyperlink with what looks like a random collection of letters and numbers. These are abbreviated links to websites using a so-called URL shortener such as bit.ly, ow.ly, goo.gl, and tr.im; they are easy and free to use. For example, "ow.ly/ghTty" takes tweet followers of @InnoInHealth to a World Health Organization (WHO) press release from December 2012 about the World Malaria Report 2012, which signals a slowdown in the fight against malaria. The actual web address for this press release is 77 characters long.[13] Most web addresses need to be shortened in tweets because they are too long and would either take up most of the 140 characters or exceed this limit.

Web-Integrated Short Message Service

SMS is a text messaging service component of phone, web, or mobile communication systems that begun implementation in 1992. SMS have become a predominant means of mobile-to-mobile communication in developing countries, because of the much lower costs compared to voice calls. Although technically not a social media, SMS has much in common with microblogs, which together with other social media seem to have slowed SMS growth according to recent usage statistics (Om Malik 2012). Initially, SMS messages had to be 160 characters or less due to the signal

---

[13] http://www.who.int/mediacentre/news/releases/2012/malaria_20121217/en/index.html

formats used for telephone networks; however, due to advances in messaging technology, today's messages can be longer. Photos can be easily attached to SMS communications, which is often referred to as Multimedia Messaging or MMS. Messages are increasingly integrated with social media sites, including Facebook. SMS have played an important role in organizing civil movements in Arab countries and elsewhere. The following three examples illustrate how the use of SMS can provide important global health solutions; they are just a few of many applications that use SMS alone or in combination with websites and social media.

Authenticity of Medicines

Counterfeit drugs have become a serious public health threat in many developing countries (Schenker 2008). They not only deny patients effective treatment, but also require more expensive medical treatment as an illness is allowed to progress unchecked and may even result in patients' death. SMS has become a tool in the fight against fake drugs.

Dr. Ashifi Gogo witnessed firsthand the effects of counterfeit medications in his native Ghana and co-founded the mPedigree Network in 1997 striving to establish an "Electronic Resource System" for Africa's consumers to query the origin of their medicine. He founded Sproxil in 2009, which developed the Mobile Product Authentication (MPA) application. MPA places a scratch-off label with a unique, random code on products. Purchasers of drugs send this code via SMS to a toll-free phone number in their country and receive a reply almost instantly indicating whether the product is genuine or not before even leaving the pharmacy. If a fake product is found, a consumer is given a hotline number to call in order to report the fake product, and the hotline operators then report it to the appropriate authorities in the country. Using SMS for authenticating vital medicines has become feasible in most countries in Africa, Asia, and elsewhere. For example, Ghana's high rate of mobile penetration—over 70 % in 2010 according to the World Bank—put this technology in the hands of most consumers.

Mobile Alliance for Maternal Action

The Mobile Alliance for Maternal Action (MAMA) is engaging an innovative global community to deliver vital health information to expectant and new mothers through mobile phones. MAMA is a public–private partnership launched in May 2011 by founding partners USAID and Johnson & Johnson with supporting partners—the United Nations Foundation, mHealth Alliance, and BabyCenter. MAMA is delivering mobile health information services in Bangladesh, India, and South Africa—countries with elevated maternal and infant mortality and morbidity and high use of mobile phones. In total, 35 countries used MAMA services by the end of 2012.[14]

MAMA services include up to three text (SMS) messages a week during pregnancy and the first year of the baby's life. These regular messages build on each other throughout pregnancy and babyhood. In addition, there are audio scripts about critical health indicators and suggested actions for the mother to take. SMS messages and audio scripts are delivered according to the pregnancy timeline of each mother and also suggest services such as prenatal care, tetanus toxoid vaccinations, and well-child care that should be obtained at certain times during pregnancy and after birth. Mothers are reminded repeatedly about upcoming service appointments.

FrontlineSMS and Ushahidi ("Testimony" in Swahili)

Ushahidi.com is an Internet platform created in the aftermath of Kenya's disputed 2007 presidential election that collected eyewitness reports of violence sent in by e-mail and SMS text message and displayed them on a Google map. It became a combination of social activism, citizen journalism, and geospatial information services. The Ushahidi platform was developed as a "rapid prototype" model that enabled individuals, as well as members of NGOs, to submit reports via SMS or e-mail detailing acts of violence and trouble spots. Kenyans could send an incident report with location details to a short code number. The messages were received by an administrator who would attempt to verify the information with the original sender. If the report proved credible, it was uploaded onto Google Maps in as close to real time as possible. What resulted was a map populated with aggregated reports of incidents of violence and looting and the identification of places in need of aid relief. The platform helped to fill a void left by the mainstream media and provided Kenyans with information vital to their safety and peace of mind.

An analysis by the Kennedy School of Government found that Ushahidi was better overall at reporting acts of violence as they began. The data collected by Ushahidi was superior to that reported by the mainstream media in Kenya at the time. The service was also better at reporting nonfatal violence as well as information coming in from rural areas (Shirky 2010).

On a technical note, SMS messages are routed through FrontlineSMS and synchronized with Ushahidi. FrontlineSMS allows mobile phone users to text messages to large groups of people anywhere there is a mobile signal. It is used in over 80 countries not just for election monitoring but also for improving health and education services. Since its initial design, Ushahidi became a web and mobile platform that allows users to analyze large amounts of text data and create and visualize and share stories on a map, which is also called Crowdmapping. In addition, Ushahidi

---

[14] MAMA website accessed on 12/22/2012 at http://healthunbound.org/mama/what-is-mama

allows individuals to share their stories on their own terms using the tools they already have. FrontlineSMS and Ushahidi are free to download by anybody and are likely to be used again in Kenya's 2013 elections.

Blogs

There exists such a large number of blogs, and they have become so much part of our professional (and personal) life, that mentioning any to our readers seems pointless. For those inclined to continue reading, here are some "fun" facts. Historically, blogs originated in some form in the early 1990s and were termed weblogs in 1997. The short form "blog" was adopted in 1999. Blogs are discussion or informational websites consisting of discrete entries ("posts") typically listed in reverse chronological order. Until 2009 blogs were usually the work of a single individual sharing stories, opinions, interesting facts and news from other sources. Blogs are often focused on special interest topics such as global climate change,[15] which is managed by a group of writers. Other blogs such as SocioLingo Africa[16] or Chris Blattman,[17] Yale University, are maintained by one person and cover many different issues and news from African music to anarchist's views of international development to International Monetary Fund (IMF) investments. "Multi-author blogs" (MABs) have become more common, with posts written by large numbers of authors and professionally edited. This includes blogs form the Center for Global Development and the Guardian's Poverty Matters development blog.[18] Who can start a blog? Everybody—and for free! Blog hosting services such as WordPress, Blogger, and Blog offer all the tools necessary online. They are intuitive and require no technical knowledge of publishing on the Internet. Once a prospective blogger has set up a free account the first blog can be up on the World Wide Web within minutes.

Wiki

Wikis are websites for knowledge management and Internet encyclopedias and exist since 1994. Best known is *Wikipedia*, which was launched in 2001. A wiki allows its users to add, modify, or delete its content via a web browser. Many wikis allow users to contribute to a wiki, others restrict access to editing functions. However, most wikis are managed to prevent inappropriate content to be posted to a wiki website. Ward Cunningham, developer of the first wiki, and co-author Bo

---

[15] http://www.realclimate.org/ with over 17 million total visits, accessed 12/31/2012.

[16] http://www.sociolingo.com/ with over 3,000 visits per month.

[17] http://chrisblattman.com/ with over 17,000 followers; accessed 12/31/2012.

[18] http://blogs.cgdev.org/globaldevelopment/; www.guardian.co.uk/global-development/poverty-matters

Leuf, in their book The Wiki Way: Quick Collaboration on the Web, describe the essence of the Wiki concept as follows:

- A wiki invites all users to edit any page or to create new pages within the wiki Web site, using only a plain-vanilla Web browser without any extra add-ons.
- Wiki promotes meaningful topic associations between different pages by making page link creation almost intuitively easy and showing whether an intended target page exists or not.
- A wiki is not a carefully crafted site for casual visitors. Instead, it seeks to involve the visitor in an ongoing process of creation and collaboration that constantly changes the Web site landscape.

What content do wikis address? A better question is actually "what can you not find on Wikipedia?" Readers seeking information about "Long-acting reversible contraception" will find a concise description of intrauterine devices, hormonal implants and injections.[19] The topic of this book, aid effectiveness, is covered in detail on its own Wikipedia page.[20] Readers can check the fact that wiki pages are efforts of a global community on the revision history for each page.[21] There is no limit for users to create a page on a new topic.

To Tweet or Not To Tweet...

In conclusion, while readers decide themselves whether social media can help or hinder in their global development work and promote aid effectiveness, some recommendations and conventional wisdoms may help in this decision.

- Time is a scarce commodity: social media require time to read, to write, or both. Thousands of new posts appear every day on social media sites, even on topics such as global development, but not everything is worthwhile reading. Readers will easily find the media that provide the most value.
- The fellowship of the blog: readers interested in becoming a voice in global development and aid effectiveness could start a blog, tweet, networking group, or other social media very easily. However, large readerships only develop when new posts are made frequently and, of cause, the content is appealing to a large audience.
- Less can be more: most users of social media prefer short and to the point contributions. There exist many other sources for scholarly articles and elaborate opinion pieces.

---

[19] http://en.wikipedia.org/wiki/Long-acting_reversible_contraception, accessed 12/22/2012.
[20] http://en.wikipedia.org/wiki/Aid_effectiveness, accessed 12/22/2012.
[21] http://en.wikipedia.org/w/index.php?title=Aid_effectiveness&action=history, accessed 12/22/2012.

- Share and share alike: making friends on social networks works best when everybody is willing to share information about themselves—but within limits to prevent identity theft.
- An open secret: social media content is usually visible to the world and not the place to share company secrets or information not meant for public consumption.
- Rules of engagement: the tone on social media should be collegial and never personal or insulting. Harassment is not tolerated in the workplace and there is no place for it on the Internet.

Social media can be stimulating and entertaining, if used wisely. They can give a voice and rise to fame for anybody who cares about global development and aid effectiveness.

References

allAfrica. (2012, December). Ghana: African Elections Project deploys SMTC for Ghana's 2012 Elections. Press Release. Retrieved from http://allafrica.com/stories/201212040694.html

Dixon, J., & Keyes, D. (2012). The permanent disruption of social media. *Stanford Social Innovation Review*. Winter 2013. Retrieved from http://www.ssireview.org/articles/entry/the_permanent_disruption_of_social_media

Om Malik. (2012). Mobile data is growing, but voice & sms slowing. Gigaom. Retrieved December 22, 2012, from http://gigaom.com/mobile/as-mobile-data-zooms-voice-sms-revenues-slow/

Safranek. (March, 2012). Social media & regime change. *ProQuest Discovery Guides*. Retrieved from http://www.csa.com/discoveryguides/discoveryguides-main.php

Schenker, J. L. (2008). MPedigree's Rx for counterfeit drugs. *Bloomberg Businessweek, Global Economics*. Retrieved December 22, 2012, from http://www.businessweek.com/stories/2008-12-03/mpedigrees-rx-for-counterfeit-drugsbusinessweek-business-news-stock-market-and-financial-advice

Shirky, C. (2010). *Cognitive surplus: Creativity and generosity in a connected age* (p. 16). New York: Penguin Press.

Yonazi, E., Kelly, T., Halewood, N., & Blackman, C. (2012). *eTransform Africa: The transformational use of information and communication technologies in Africa*. Washington, DC: The World Bank, the African Development Bank.

Chapter 20
Advocating for Results

Sam Daley-Harris

One can address the question of aid effectiveness from many different angles. This chapter will address an issue to which very little attention is paid, the role of citizen advocacy for aid effectiveness, especially deep advocacy. By deep advocacy we mean the kind of interactions with the media, members of Congress, and other community leaders that will create champions for effective aid as distinguished from the more familiar mouse-click advocacy or call campaigns to leave messages at a Congressional switchboard. Advocacy that creates champions for effective aid can be a critical ingredient to successfully addressing the unnecessary poverty and ill health faced by more than a billion people around the world. Of course, the lack of such champions can retard progress and move the world backward.

We saw a sad but clear example of this in late 2011. On World AIDS day, just as leading advocates were announcing that the end of AIDS was in sight, the Global Fund to Fight AIDS, Tuberculosis and Malaria (Global Fund) was announcing that there would be no funding provided over a 2-year period. The tremendous effort that allowed the Global Fund to come into existence and which then helped propel dramatic progress on AIDS and other pressing health issues is now put in jeopardy as support is withdrawn. This is a story that is not over yet, but it is a challenge that mouse-clicks alone are not likely to solve.

S. Daley-Harris (✉)
RESULTS, Microcredit Summit Campaign, and Center for Citizen Empowerment
and Transformation, Princeton, NJ, USA
e-mail: sam@empoweringcitizens365.org

© Springer Science+Business Media New York 2015
E. Beracochea (ed.), *Improving Aid Effectiveness in Global Health*,
DOI 10.1007/978-1-4939-2721-0_20

Seeing the World with New Eyes and New Questions

Let me tell the story of one citizen advocate whose inspiring actions as a volunteer 25 years ago are now being replicated in his work as a staff member of the Citizen Climate Lobby. After starting 50 chapters of RESULTS, the citizen lobby on ending global poverty, I moved to Washington, DC in 1985 as its first staff member and attended a breakfast briefing with the President of the International Fund for Agricultural Development (IFAD), a small UN agency based in Rome. IFAD's funding was being threatened by a funding squabble between the US and OPEC. We began to lobby on behalf of IFAD and they sent us videos of three programs in which they had invested; one was a Dutch documentary about a little bank in Bangladesh that gave microloans to 42,000 borrowers called the Grameen Bank. We were moved by the unleashing of the human spirit, by redemption—people's honor and worth being restored—and by people being set free from poverty.

During 1985 the 50 RESULTS chapters would watch the video on Grameen Bank and then write their members of Congress on behalf of IFAD. The next year we prepared to have legislation introduced on microenterprise development, as it was called at the time, and in 1987 the legislation was introduced.

Over a 1-year period between November 1986 and November 1987 the volunteers in RESULTS generated 100 editorials on the microenterprise legislation, not letters to the editor or op-ed pieces (there were more of those), but 100 editorials written by the newspapers themselves. That same year more than 200 members of Congress cosponsored the legislation. These are impressive numbers in any context, but all the more so because it was 1987 and virtually no one outside of Bangladesh had heard of microcredit, Muhammad Yunus, or Grameen Bank.

It is difficult to describe the levels of hopelessness and cynicism that must be overcome for ordinary citizens to reach out to members of Congress or to get through to editorial writers who are more prone to speak to experts and often find difficulty writing about an obscure issue that isn't in the news. This, however, is part of the work that must be done if we are to seriously address aid effectiveness and ultimately issues like ending global poverty and ensuring a stable climate.

Political Transformation Begins with Personal Transformation

The following story describes this process of moving from hopelessness to action. The activist I will introduce to you had experience with the media which was far greater than most RESULTS volunteers, but I am sharing this story because of the process his group had to go through to reach out to a conservative member of Congress. Steve Valk, a long-time RESULTS volunteer, is now a member of the staff of the Citizens Climate Lobby, a RESULTS-styled citizen lobby focused on resolving climate issues. Until recently Steve had worked for decades designing features sections at the *Atlanta Journal-Constitution* newspapers. Here is how Steve described his route into RESULTS.

....There has always been within me a deep desire for social justice, to make what was wrong in the world right. I couldn't go by a crooked picture without straightening it out and I couldn't go by a problem without wanting to fix it.

....In 1984 I was an angry young man who wanted to change the world but couldn't see how. I was getting more involved in music and songwriting and wasn't particularly interested in some lobbying group that my friend Sara was involved with that was trying to do something about ending hunger. I thought it was nice that she was trying to do something, but I didn't want to waste my time on a hopeless cause. I would take her to her meetings and then pick her up afterwards. It wasn't until six months later that my curiosity got the better of me and I decided to go to a RESULTS meeting.

Being a journalist I'm inclined to approach most things with a skeptical nature. Being a journalist, I was also not sure how deeply to get involved with political causes, but I couldn't just leave that crooked picture alone, and when I realized that nobody else was going to straighten it out, I took a deep breath and dove in. Over the years I have come to terms with this because my position at the newspaper is one where I have absolutely no influence about what goes into the paper or how it is written. I design pages for the features sections, but it's somebody else who assigns and edits the stories and it's somebody else who writes the stories and takes the pictures. As I began to get involved with RESULTS I saw myself as a link between people who had important information that could save lives and the media that could make that information available to the public.

....I started believing I could make a difference. I've always been the kind of person who likes to 'get involved' with causes, but until RESULTS my involvement always seemed to have a Don Quixote-like quality. I dreamed the impossible dream only to be rudely awakened at some point.

Valk was able to generate a wire story in 1985 on the funding squabble between the USA and OPEC that had the potential to kill IFAD and Sara, the woman who would eventually become his wife, was able to generate an editorial in the newspaper. He was elated with his ability to get the right information to the right people, but he considered his greatest breakthrough with RESULTS to be the conversion of Congressman Pat Swindall, a conservative Republican from Georgia.

Within weeks of Pat being sworn into office [in January 1985], four RESULTS volunteers, myself included, met with the Congressman to request that he co-sponsor and vote for the Famine Relief in Ethiopia bill that had just been introduced in Congress. One of the volunteers who did not meet with us for a breakfast practice session before the meeting, wound up being a loose cannon of sorts, insisting that we cut military spending to feed the hungry, putting the conservative Swindall in a defensive, so to speak, posture. Swindall made it clear that he didn't think the government should be involved in humanitarian aid and it was something best left to the churches and private sector to take care of. A few weeks later Pat was one of only 15 or so Congresspersons out of more than 400, who ended up voting against the famine relief bill and he made headlines giving a big speech about it on the floor of the House.

Valk describes the shame he felt about his Representative's vote.

Have you ever seen the fans of a very bad sports team who sit in the stands with bags over their heads because they are ashamed to be seen rooting for such losers? If politics were a sport and we were sitting in the stands watching our Congressman playing on the field, we would be wearing those bags on our heads over the shame we felt having Pat Swindall as a representative. Our thoughts and discussions about him were very negative, and we pretty much wrote him off figuring our best chance was that maybe he would be defeated in two years.

But at the suggestion of RESULTS staff, we began to shift our thinking on Pat. There was this prayer that Newton Hightower had written to his member of Congress [in Houston, TX], Rep. Bill Archer, someone he had similar difficulties with two years before. We adapted it to Swindall. We added Swindall's name and it went:

Thank you God for Pat Swindall. We know that he is a good man who wants to do right in the world. We know that he struggles with the same problems we do: closing our hearts to those who don't agree with us. There are no thoughts or feelings that he has had that we haven't had and vice versa. We pray for all of us to have compassion for people in our country and far away, for rich and poor. We pray that Pat and we will be less frightened of each other. We pray our focus will me more to love and appreciate him and less to change him. Help us to remember that sharing love with the world is the highest contribution we can make and will lead to children being fed and the planet surviving. Forgive our righteousness and anger. Open our hearts and minds to find the next expression of love for Pat that he can receive.

Valk describes his group's breakthrough with Congressman Swindall, a breakthrough that that was 2 years in the making. In order to have these breakthroughs we must expand systems of volunteer support that allow citizens to be this persistent and committed to breakthroughs.

We eventually let go of our negative attitude toward Pat. Instead, we began to see him as a human being who, just like us, did not want to see people dying in the world from hunger and disease. All he needed was a little education. We began to show up at "Chat with Pat" sessions around the district. There were other people with other issues in the Congressional district who had bones to pick wit Pat (we jokingly called the sessions "Spat with Pat"), and whenever they did, they didn't get anywhere. If anything, he stiffened his resolve and defended his position. When he got around to us he was visibly relieved to see us greeting him with a handshake and a smile instead of a scowl and a sharp tongue. Then we would give him a two-minute briefing on an issue such as IFAD. And when we started talking about enabling a farmer to grow a ton of wheat for a year for the same amount of money it would cost to send a ton of wheat one time, well, he started listening a little closer. Gradually a relationship of trust and respect was built.

In the Spring of 1987 RESULTS launched its microenterprise legislation with the Self-Sufficiency for the Poor Act. We decided it was time for an office visit with Pat, and four of us took off time from work to go see him. It was late afternoon and we must have been a sight sitting in his waiting room with a TV and VCR to show him the Grameen Bank video. Earlier in the day, feeling very confident, I told Sara that after Pat agreed to cosponsor the legislation I would ask him if we could write an op-ed piece in support of the bill to appear under his name.

'I don't know Stephen, I think you'd be pushing it,' Sara responded.

But I figured once he's committed to the bill, what did I have to lose?

The four of us piled into a small office and set up the TV and tape. We all took a deep breath and the Congressman joined us. Everyone spoke brilliantly in the meeting. As we were showing the video, Pat was sitting on a desk, knees drawn under his chin, staring intently at the screen. We told him about the tremendous opportunity of the Self-Sufficiency for the Poor Act and asked him to become a cosponsor.

'I'd be delighted to be a cosponsor,' he said.

Sensing we were on a roll, I began to ask about the op-ed, but before the words were even formed in my mouth the Congressman spoke.

'You know,' he said, 'I think it's important on an issue like this that we try to build public support in the media. I have a column that appears in the local paper and I'm thinking maybe you can write a piece about this bill, and we can run it in my column. Do you think you could do something like that?

I glanced over at Sara with a smile so wide it hurt. 'Pat I'd be more than happy to do it.' I was now ghostwriting for a man who two years earlier voted against famine aid for Ethiopia.

That experience changed me. I now see that everyone has the potential to do the right thing if given the opportunity. It's refreshing to see people as possibilities rather than obstacles.

Steve Valk's story was one of hundreds as more than 200 members of the House and Senate cosponsored the legislation and more than 100 editorials were generated, two-thirds of them mentioning Grameen Bank. This laid the groundwork for the expansion of microfinance globally.

Just as there are people in the world who are hungry for food and desperate to get an education for themselves and their children, Americans are hungry to have more meaning in their lives—to live lives that truly matter. All Americans want this, but only a small number are awake to this desire. Many of those who know they want to make a difference in the world are already donors to major aid organizations. They truly would like to light up their members of Congress and inspire their local media on the issues these organizations care about.

But they are thwarted by two major impediments: (1) feelings of hopelessness and inadequacy about making a difference as an advocate and (2) an inability to find a structure of support that will help them through their despair and truly empower them to make a difference, a structure of support that can coach them through transformations like these: from "I don't make a difference" to "I do make a difference," from "I can't fight city hall" to "I am city hall".

Steve Valk had access to such a structure of support. He and the others in RESULTS were on nationwide telephone conference calls each month with guest speakers to help deepen their understanding and inspiration. They were on weekly coaching calls for group leaders. They were given packets to take to their editorial writers. They received monthly action sheets to prioritize and focus their action.

Steve and others have brought these methods to Citizens Climate Lobby (CCL). CCL's first chapters were started in September 2007. In 2014 CCL had grown to more than 225 chapters in the USA and Canada. In 2010 CCL volunteers had 106 meetings with members of Congress or their staff. In 2014 there were 1,086 such meetings. In 2010 CCL volunteers had 36 letters to the editor published. In 2014, 2,253 letters to the editor were published.

Citizens must demand from the groups they care about the kind of support that allows these achievements and those organizations must find ways to provide it.

Soul of a Citizen author Paul Loeb has said that messages sent in an e-mail campaign are counted, but they are also discounted. We must train citizens to become deep advocates for effective aid, advocacy that cannot be discounted.

Portions of this essay are taken from the twentieth anniversary edition of Reclaiming Our Democracy: Healing the Break between People and Government *Copyright 2013 by Sam Daley-Harris and published by Camino Books, Inc., Philadelphia, PA. Used by permission of the publisher. All rights reserved.*

Sam Daley-Harris is Founder of RESULTS, the citizen lobby focused on ending global poverty and founder of the Microcredit Summit Campaign. Currently he heads the Center for Citizen Empowerment and Transformation which he launched in 2012.

Chapter 21
Effectiveness of the Census-Based Impact Oriented Approach

Henry B. Perry and Thomas P. Davis

Introduction

In the rural highlands of Guatemala, a community health worker made a routine home visit and encountered a severely malnourished child who had been having repeated bouts of diarrhea and pneumonia. By providing education to the mother to improve the child's nutritional status, by improving the hygienic situation in the home, and by providing appropriate antibiotic treatment for episodes of pneumonia, the child returned to good nutrition and health. Without this kind of outreach and support, this child would very likely have died. We have seen and heard about many similar cases in which health programs using the framework we will be describing in this chapter have been able to prevent deaths of children and save the lives of mothers with complications related to pregnancy.

Over the course of our respective careers of more than six decades (combined) of experience in planning, managing, and evaluating programs for mothers and children in high-mortality, resource-constrained settings in more than 40 countries around the world, we have found that a framework for program implementation that involves maintaining contact with every household on a frequent basis and delivering evidence-based interventions at the community and household levels is essential for identifying those in greatest need and ensuring the interventions reach those who need them. Such approaches are essential for achieving high levels of coverage, and high levels of coverage are essential for saving as many lives as possible in resource-constrained settings. In addition, it is important to use locally acquired information

H.B. Perry (✉)
Department of International Health, Johns Hopkins Bloomberg
School of Public Health, Baltimore, MD, USA
e-mail: hperry2@jhu.edu

T.P. Davis
Feed the Children, Oklahomo City, DC, USA
e-mail: tdavis@feedthechildren.org

© Springer Science+Business Media New York 2015
E. Beracochea (ed.), *Improving Aid Effectiveness in Global Health*,
DOI 10.1007/978-1-4939-2721-0_21

regarding what the leading causes of death are in the program area. This enables to most appropriate interventions to be delivered to the program population. In order for such a framework to function, it is essential for the program staff members to develop a relationship with the community that is as bidirectional as possible, since community members often need to volunteer to carry out many of the required activities, and the program staff members are interacting with families in their homes.

Programs that are based at facilities—whether they are hospitals, health centers, or health posts—are unlikely (at least in priority areas of low-income countries) to be numerous enough to be readily accessible to everyone in the population. And there is a very high likelihood that those who live furthest away from the health facilities are those in greatest need of services and are least likely to use them. In 1966, Dr. Larimer Mellon had been running a hospital in rural Haiti for a decade and came to the conclusion that he was never going to make any progress in improving the health of the people served through hospital services alone. He and those who worked with him then developed community-level services that reached every household. The results achieved in the 1970s through this approach set a new standard for what can be achieved through community-based integrated programs (Berggren et al. 1981).

Another reason that facility-based programs alone with little community outreach are inadequate is that—to achieve many of the United Nations Millennium Development Goals (MDGs) for health—household-level behavior change must occur. Deutschman (2007) cites three necessary ingredients for successful behavior change: (1) the person forms a *new, emotional relationship* with a person or community that inspires and sustains *hope*; (2) the new relationship helps the person learn, practice, and master *new habits and skills* that he/she will need; and (3) the new relationship helps the person to learn *new ways of thinking* about his/her situation and how he/she can improve it. To this list, we would add that barriers to adopting healthy behaviors need to be reduced, and this often requires investigation in the program setting of what these barriers actually are. Therefore, what we call formative research is a priority. The amount and quality of contact between project staff and community members to develop the relationships, skills, hope, and new thinking are often not possible when health promotion is principally done by overworked clinical staff working within health facilities.

Unfortunately, since the mid-1980s, the global health agenda has been driven by short-term, top-down, vertical disease-oriented approaches and programs that do not foster community participation and that do not emphasize extension of services—including health promotion—to the household level. Prior to that time—during the 1970s and early 1980s—there was broad and widespread enthusiasm for primary health care as defined at the International Conference on Primary Health Care at Alma Ata, Kazakhstan, in 1978, with its emphasis on integration, addressing the social determinants of health, inter-sectoral approaches to health improvement, equity, and maximizing community and individual self-reliance and participation (World Health Organization and UNICEF 1978). The concept of primary health care as a comprehensive approach to providing basic health services in partnership with communities (while at the same time addressing epidemiological priorities in the local population) lost favor in the 1980s, in part due to the lack of demonstrated cost-effectiveness and health impact shown by more selective approaches (Walsh and Warren 1979).

The limitations of highly "verticalized" (top-down), selective approaches to health improvement—whether they are focused on child survival, reduction of maternal mortality, or control of HIV/AIDS, tuberculosis, and malaria—are now becoming increasingly apparent. They are heavily dependent on external donors, and long-term financial support becomes difficult to sustain from in-country resources. They can have destructive effects on health systems by creating distortions in funding and draining human resources and programming capability from other programs in the health sector. Finally, and perhaps most importantly, they lead to disempowerment of communities since building partnerships between health programs and communities is not prioritized and because such programs tend to be highly technically oriented and driven from higher levels in the health system.

The need for a "middle way" that can bring back the vision and broad appeal of primary health care inspired by Alma Ata in 1978 while at the same time producing measurable results in health improvement has been recognized by many (Mosley 1988). Some have expressed this as a need for "diagonal" approaches that are neither wholly vertical nor wholly horizontal (i.e., comprehensive programs, with a balanced emphasis that includes top-down, selective elements as well as comprehensive elements) (Sepulveda et al. 2006). Although some have claimed that "we are all 'diagonalists' now," there has not yet emerged a compelling set of principles or overarching framework which fills this need.

The purpose of this chapter is to describe a framework—the census-based, impact-oriented (CBIO) approach—that we believe fulfills this need. Although the CBIO framework can be usefully applied in any setting, we think it is most effective for the most difficult and challenging communities where mortality levels are quite high, where health systems are quite weak, and where resources for providing health services are severely constrained. We will describe what the CBIO approach is, its history, its evolution over the past two decades, examples of CBIO projects and programs (including examples from field programs where CBIO principles have contributed to program effectiveness), and tools that are available to facilitate implementation of CBIO principles.

The Principles of the Census-Based, Impact-Oriented Approach

Goals

The overarching goal of the CBIO approach is health improvement (broadly defined) at the population level. Specific goals are to improve the health of a geographically defined population (a community, set of communities, or larger population) and to demonstrate whether an improvement in health has in fact been achieved through partnership with the community. The term "census-based" is meant to convey the notion that program-related activities are geared to a population that is enumerated and that includes every person within a defined geographic area. The term "impact-oriented" is meant to convey the notion that program-related activities are oriented toward measurable health improvement. Inherent in the CBIO approach is the idea that health and health behavior within a population will be defined at various points in time, a set of actors will be dedicated to obtaining these measurements, and these actors will be guiding health-related program activities toward health improvement based on these measurements.

Community partnerships are an essential element of the CBIO approach. The scientific evidence base arising from programming for health in high-mortality, resource-constrained settings is quite clear: that effective implementation of "proven" interventions requires community-based programming, community partnerships, and behavior change at the household level. Therefore, if programs are to achieve optimal impact in health improvement, working in partnership with communities is essential. Effective partnerships between programs embracing CBIO and communities involve developing activities that both respond to the perceived health needs of communities and address epidemiological priorities with interventions that have been shown to be effective. Without responding to perceived health needs, it is difficult to develop community partnerships. Epidemiological priorities, which are the most frequent, serious, readily preventable or treatable conditions in the community, set of communities, or otherwise geographically defined population, are usually also community-perceived priorities but not always.

A relationship of trust is essential to develop an effective partnership between the health program and the community. Developing trust requires time and experience in responding to community priorities and in demonstrating success in improving health. Thus, implied in the CBIO approach is a long-term relationship between the health practitioner and the community.

Guiding Principles

To improve the health of the community, it will be necessary for the health practitioner to make a "diagnosis" of what we refer to as the epidemiological priorities. Just as in the practice of the medical care individual patients, the more accurate the diagnosis, the more likely the prescribed "treatment" is likely to improve the health of the population. A community diagnosis needs to be determined at various points in time—every 3–5 years—since epidemiological priorities and the availability of effective interventions change over time.

Locally acquired surveillance data are the best source of information about the epidemiological priorities in the community. Although relatively accurate data are often available at the national and subnational levels (e.g., province, region, or state), there is nonetheless considerable variation in health conditions from one area of the country to another. Therefore, local data should be obtained if possible through partnership with the community. The best way to obtain accurate local surveillance data is through routine systematic visitation of all homes to register vital events, identify disabilities and serious illness, measure baseline levels of health (as defined by rates of mortality, serious illness, and disability), and measure changes over time. Alternative approaches to achieving this goal involve periodic surveys within the community. The advantage of routine systematic visitation of all homes is that it also enables the practitioner to develop a relationship of trust with all members of the community and to provide essential health-related services at the time of the home visit, such as health promotion, provision of basic commodities (e.g., micronutrients, family planning supplies, and insecticide-treated bed nets), identification of malnourished children (e.g., through the use of mid-upper-arm circumference measurement), identification of patients needing acute illness care (e.g., community-based management of childhood pneumonia, diarrhea, or malaria), and referral for facility-based care. Finally, routine visitation of all homes is an effective way of determining what the community's health priorities are. These data can be complemented by small-sample survey data (e.g., knowledge, practice, and coverage surveys) to identify patterns and changes in behaviors and behavioral determinants.

Another advantage of routine systematic visitation of all households for surveillance purposes is its greater ability to identify high-risk groups. When surveillance is carried out through sampling households, high-risk subgroups are harder to identify. From the public health standpoint, identifying high-risk subgroups and focusing programmatic attention on them are a critical strategy for improving the health of populations. One of the most important aspects of surveillance is identifying deaths that occur—and the age and sex of the person who died and, using standard verbal autopsy techniques developed for children, making as accurate a diagnosis of cause of death as possible. And by asking about deaths in the recent past as well as registering births and deaths over time, it becomes possible to establish baseline mortality rates in the program area and observe changes in these rates over time.

Identifying and responding to community health priorities is essential for building a partnership between the community and the health practitioner and for establishing a relationship of trust. Such a relationship is essential for effective health programming and long-term health improvement. In addition to the methods already mentioned, focus group discussions, key informant interviews, and other qualitative methods can be used to assess perceptions of community members regarding their health priorities.

Another important part of this initial diagnosis that has been added more recently is formative research around the determinants of key health behaviors. These are described in the CBIO tools section. This formative research is helpful in designing program interventions that are carefully tailored to the local context.

Initial Steps (in a Pilot area)

The health practitioner needs to establish trust with the community to begin a partnership. As this relationship forms and matures, it will then be possible for the community, working with the health practitioner, to define the community in terms of its geographic boundaries, begin surveillance, determine the epidemiological priorities, and the community's perceived health priorities (which may be very different from the epidemiological priorities). Most likely, the community's health priorities are going to revolve around a perceived need for improving the availability of medical care for acute illness. Responding effectively early on to community perceived health priorities is an important means of establishing a partnership of trust between the health practitioner and the community.

Through this emerging relationship, the health practitioner and the community work together to define the community (or communities) of interest, their geographic boundaries, and details about inhabitants and their location. Then, exploratory activities can be undertaken for appropriate methods to determine health problems in the population area and to address them, followed by a pilot project.

Definitive Steps

On the basis of the experience from the initial steps, a definitive community diagnosis can be made. This involves in part determining the epidemiological priorities (defined earlier), determining their underlying causes through formative research (including determinants of key behaviors), and identifying those persons at greatest risk. This is best done by visiting every household, although it could be done through repeated visits to a sample of households to reduce costs. The community diagnosis also involves determining what the community perceives its priorities to be. Again, this can be obtained by visiting every household, a sample of households, or through standard qualitative research methods (e.g., focus group discussions and key informant interviews).

On the basis of the epidemiologically based and community-perceived priorities, a final set of program priorities is created based on a blending of these two categories of priorities. Following that, a determination of the available resources needs to be carried out. These are not only financial resources but also human and physical resources that are available for program implementation. (Community volunteers have been widely used in many projects based on CBIO principles, as will be described later.) With the available resources in mind, it becomes possible to develop a plan for program implementation.

After a period of time—say 3–5 years—there is a need to evaluate the program and repeat the steps necessary to make a community re-diagnosis, redefine the resources available, plan for the next period of implementation, and implement the modified plan (Table 21.1).

Table 21.1 Basic elements of the census-based, impact-oriented approach

Overarching goal	1. Health improvement at the population level
Specific goals	1. Improvement of health in a specific, geographically defined population
	2. Intermittent measurement of population health, with orientation of program priorities toward health improvement
	3. Building partnerships between communities and the health-oriented program(s) is essential for achieving maximal success in health improvement
Guiding principles	1. Diagnosis of epidemiological priorities is essential in order for the health practitioner to "prescribe" an effective "treatment" (and the diagnosis and the prescribed treatment may change over time as health conditions change over time and as effective treatments change over time)
	2. Locally acquired surveillance data (best obtained through visitation of all households or a sample of households) is the most desirable approach to defining epidemiological priorities and to measuring changes in the level of health in the population over time
	3. Choosing the right interventions and strategies for implementing these interventions (especially those that involve behavior change) can be aided by formative research techniques such as focus group discussions, key informant interviews, barrier analysis, and positive deviance inquiry. These techniques are also useful in identifying community-perceived health priorities
	4. Identifying and responding to community health priorities is essential for building a partnership and trust
Initial steps (in a pilot area)	1. Develop a relationship of trust between the health practitioner and the community
	2. Define the community (geographic boundaries, number and location of inhabitants)
	3. Carry out exploratory and then pilot planning and program implementation
	4. Define community priorities
Definitive steps (in the complete program area)	1. Determine the most frequent, serious, readily preventable or treatable causes of sickness, disability, and death, their underlying causes (through formative research), and those persons at greatest risk
	2. Determine the health priorities as defined by the community members themselves
	3. Establish program priorities based on epidemiologically defined and community-defined priorities
	4. Develop a work plan based on the program priorities and the resources available
	5. Implement the program
	6. Evaluate the program and carry out a community re-diagnosis (after 3–5 years)

Historical Antecedents of the CBIO Approach

Epidemographic surveillance of all households is an approach that dates back to the 1930s, when Dr. John Gordon, then working at the Rockefeller Foundation, directed a study in Romania to detect an outbreak of scarlet fever in a small town. At that time, he set up a system to visit every family twice a week and to swab the throats of all the children to detect the first and subsequent cases of scarlet fever. It was the first epidemic ever studied from beginning to end. This was made possible by carrying out routine visitation of all households to identify the first case and then to follow the epidemic to the last case (Wyon 2001). The approach of visitation of all households for surveillance purposes was later implemented in a variety of settings, including in the Ding Xian program in China (the forerunner of the Barefoot Doctor Program in China) (Taylor-Ide and Taylor 2002) and later in the Khanna Study in north India in the 1950s and 1960s (Wyon and Gordon 1971) and in the Narangwal Project (Kielmann et al. 1983; Taylor et al. 1983), also in North India, in the 1960s and 1970s, where provision of services at the time of home visits was added to surveillance during home visits. The concept of epidemographic surveillance through home visitation was proposed back in 1971 as a means of guiding field programs where conventional health services fail to reach the bulk of the population (Frederickson 1971).

The Narangwal Project added the dimension of community participation and community partnerships to routine systematic home visitation. These concepts were further developed in the Jamkhed Project in central India in the 1970s and 1980s (Arole and Arole 1994), where visitation of all homes and community participation were further extended by engaging marginalized groups (outcaste women who were rehabilitated from life-threatening illnesses such as tuberculosis) in the provision of health services at the village level and by addressing the social determinants of health (e.g., lack of food and water).

In the 1970s, these concepts were also applied in communities around the Hospital Albert Schweitzer (HAS) in Haiti (Berggren et al. 1981) and in the 1980s and 1990s in communities in rural Bolivia (Perry et al. 1998, 2003). CBIO as an approach arose out of the experience in Bolivia and through support from those previously involved in similar activities, most notably John Wyon (in the Khanna Study and through his support to the Berggrens) and Warren and Gretchen Berggren (through their work at the HAS and in Petit Goave in Haiti). Although previous projects and programs had developed many of these principles and implemented them, they were not identified and consolidated as a specific framework and a unified approach prior to that time.

Through a long-term and close professional relationship that the senior author had with John Wyon, the ideas and principles that came to form CBIO slowly came into being during the 1980s and early 1990s through the programmatic experience of field staff in Bolivia and the technical support provided by the senior author with the guidance of John Wyon.

Implementation of the CBIO Approach over the Past Two Decades

In 1993, an Expert Panel reviewed the CBIO approach as it was developed and implemented by Andean Rural Health Care (ARHC) in Bolivia in the 1980s and early 1990s. The Panel—composed of distinguished and experienced leaders in international health at that time, including faculty from the Johns Hopkins and Harvard schools of public health, senior staff members at UNICEF and other leading NGOs, and senior technical staff at USAID—concluded that the approach was promising and should be tried out in other locales in developing countries and should undergo further evaluation of its potential. However, no funding was ever identified to make this possible.

ARHC, the NGO that established the CBIO approach, continued to use CBIO to guide its programs in Bolivia. ARHC eventually changed its name to Curamericas Global as it gradually expanded its programs to Guatemala, Mexico, Haiti, and Liberia. In all locations, curamericas has continued to rely on CBIO as its guiding framework for program implementation.

CBIO never seemed to gain any traction among international donors, mostly because of its holistic approach, the higher costs per beneficiary compared to narrower selective approaches, and its long-term time frame. Donors were looking to fund projects that were more narrowly focused for shorter periods of time. However, child survival programming did fit nicely within the CBIO framework because it gradually became increasingly apparent that success in child survival programming depends on reaching all households with health promotion to bring about behavior change, and these principles were embedded within the CBIO framework. Thus, Curamericas was able to continue to receive funding from the USAID Child Survival and Health Grants Program for its activities in Bolivia, Guatemala, Haiti, and Liberia.

Over time, NGOs involved in child survival programming around the world have gradually begun to implement certain aspects of CBIO, most notably mapping of all households, taking a census, using verbal autopsies to estimate as best as possible causes of child deaths, and developing a process for reaching every home periodically with a community health volunteer.

During the past decade, a new approach to maternal, neonatal, and child health programming has emerged that builds on CBIO principles. This is the Care Group model. In this model, a program develops an outreach strategy in which a low-level paid staff member (usually called a Promotor) meets every 2–4 weeks with a group of 6–15 female volunteers (called a Care Group) who each take responsibility for approximately 10–15 households. After each meeting, each of the Care Group Volunteers visits the 10–15 households for which she is responsible and delivers a health promotion message. A number of these projects include vital events registration by the Care Group Volunteers.

In some Care Group projects, a baseline retrospective mortality study and qualitative methods are used to identify the community-defined and epidemiological priorities and patterns in the project area. Some projects also use verbal autopsies (conducted by the Promoter) over the life of the project to identify trends in child mortality patterns.

So, although all the CBIO steps are not followed in the Care Group model, a number of CBIO elements are definitely present. Curamericas Global now combines Care Groups with all of its programs. The Care Group model has shown impressive results as demonstrated in publications (Edward et al. 2007; Perry et al. 2010) and as demonstrated by the outstanding results achieved by a number of NGOs in terms of rapid gain in population coverage of key child survival interventions.

Two pioneering health programs in the developing world are in India, and both have developed and utilized CBIO principles even though they do not actually use the term CBIO to describe their approach to programming. The Jamkhed Comprehensive Rural Health Project (Jamkhed Comprehensive Rural Health Project 2012) in Ahmednagar District of Maharashtra State and SEARCH (Society for Education, Action, and Research in Community Health) in Gadchiroli District of Maharashtra State establish a community diagnosis using CBIO principles and implement a program derived from that diagnosis (SEARCH, 2015). They have both built relationships of trust with the communities they serve, use vital events registration and routine contact with all households to determine epidemiological and community-perceived priorities and to deliver essential services, and both have been global leaders in making progress in achieving the MDGs—not only in maternal and child health but also in women's empowerment, poverty reduction, and control of tuberculosis (Arole and Arole 1994; McCord et al. 2001; Mann et al. 2010; Bang et al. 1990, 2005b).

The HAS in Haiti began implementing many CBIO principles beginning with the work of Drs. Warren and Gretchen Berggren under the mentorship of Dr. John Wyon in 1967. Routine systematic home visitation by Community Health Workers and attention to epidemiologically as well as community-defined priorities have been a part of the HAS primary health care programs for more than a half-century now, with marked reductions in under-five mortality compared to the rest of rural Haiti (Perry et al. 2007).

Finally, the NGO BRAC in Bangladesh has developed a pioneering maternal, neonatal and child health project in the slums of urban Bangladesh reaching 6.9 million people that maps all households and uses CHWs to routinely visit all households; identifies pregnant women; ensures that all receive prenatal care; provides appropriate birthing support in a local birth hut staffed by trained attendants who are former traditional midwives; and provides home-based neonatal care and community case management of serious childhood illness (A. Kaosar, personal communication, 2012). Staff from two organizations in Nicaragua learned about CBIO on their own and chose to use it for program implementation: AMOS Health and Hope program in 27 rural communities dispersed throughout Nicaragua (AMOS Health and Hope 2012) and the Village-based Community Health Promotion Program in the Bilwaskarma/Waspan area of the Autonomous North Atlantic Region (P. Haupert, personal communication, 2012). In both community-based programs, the vital events surveillance registration system has indicated that the infant mortality rates have declined to 0 during the last few years (P. Haupert, personal communication, 2012; L. Parajon, personal communication, 2012).

ARHC's CBIO Primary Health Program in Montero, Bolivia, has an outstanding track record of reduction in infant and maternal mortality and identification and successful treatment of patients with tuberculosis (Mosham 2011). There has not been a maternal death in this population in more than a decade, the infant mortality rate is 7 deaths per 1,000 live births (compared to 6 in the USA), and the program has been a national leader in its TB control program.[1] Importantly, the Montero Primary Health Care Program in Montero is fully funded now from long-term sustainable sources—most notably from the municipal government, the ministry of health, and locally generated income. It has been in operation now for more than two decades, and thus it has been able to achieve what CBIO was originally intended—namely providing a framework for long-term programming.

Usefulness of the CBIO Approach for Accelerating Progress in Achieving the Millennium Development Goals for Health

By its very nature, organizations implementing CBIO are working with communities to undertake a continuous surveillance of the major health problems in the communities and to address together the epidemiological priorities identified through surveillance and the health priorities as defined by community members. The MDGs were adopted in the year 2000 by the United Nations for the purpose of focusing global efforts on challenging but achievable development targets, including goals mentioned in the next section for health and nutrition (United Nations 2000). What evidence is there that the CBIO approach has been useful in accelerating progress in achieving the health-related MDGs?

Goal 1: Eradicate Extreme Poverty and Hunger

This goal calls for halving the proportion of people who suffer from hunger between 1990 and 2015. Numerous projects that have utilized CBIO principles have demonstrated improvements in the nutritional status of children as measured by anthropometry and as measured by improvement in the population coverage of the micronutrient vitamin A. Perhaps the most important of these was a Care Group project implemented by Food for the Hungry in Sofala Province in Mozambique between 2005 and 2010 in a population of 1.1 million people (Davis et al. 2015). The level of undernutrition (defined as weight for age) declined by from 26 to 18 % in approximately one-half of the project area where the project worked from the outset and

---

[1] The work in Bolivia established by Andean Rural Health Care is now directed by a Bolivia NGO, *Consejo de Salud Rural Andino* (2012).

from 27 to 16 % in the other half of the project area where the project worked for the final 2 years of the project. The rate of decline in malnutrition was more than four times the rate for Mozambique as a whole during the same period. Many changes in nutrition-related behaviors (e.g., exclusive breastfeeding) were seen concurrently.

Goal 4: Reduce Child Mortality

This goal calls for reducing the under-five mortality rate by two-thirds between 1990 and 2015. As mentioned above, implementation of CBIO in Bolivia led to a reduction of the under-five mortality rate by half of that for a comparison area (Perry et al. 1998, 2003). The Jamkhed Comprehensive Rural Health Project, using CBIO principles, demonstrated a marked decline in its infant mortality rate from 170 deaths per 1,000 live births in 1972 to 52 only 4 years later (Arole and Arole 1994) while declines in other rural areas in the state of Maharashtra (where the project did not operate) were much smaller. A more recent independent study comparing under-five mortality in the Jamkhed project area with that of surrounding villages found that the 1–59-month mortality area during the 15-year period from 1992 to 2007 (after which most of the decline in under-five mortality had already been achieved) was still 30 % less than in surrounding villages (Mann et al. 2010). The CBIO approach used at SEARCH in Jamkhed has led to a 30 % decline in under-five mortality through the introduction of community-case management of pneumonia (Bang et al. 1990) and a 70 % decline in neonatal mortality through the introduction of home-based neonatal care (Bang et al. 2005a). As a result of this pioneering work and confirmation of the effectiveness of community case management of pneumonia and home-based neonatal care, these interventions are being scaled up in high-mortality, resource-constrained settings at present in India and throughout the world. But, unfortunately, broader CBIO principles are not being embraced at the same time.

The HAS program in Haiti achieved the longest sustained impact on under-five mortality reported in the scientific literature to date, with an under-five mortality rate in the year 2000 that was still less than half that for rural Haiti (Perry et al. 2006). BRAC's Manoshi Project for maternal, neonatal, and child health in urban slums in Bangladesh is demonstrating that—after 5 years of implementation—the neonatal mortality rate is only one-half of the national rate (A. Kaosar, personal communication, 2012).

The achievement of an infant mortality of 7 deaths per 1,000 live births in a low-income, peri-urban setting in Montero, Bolivia, is a major achievement, especially considering that nationally the infant mortality rate is 42 (UNICEF 2012) and recent estimates of infant mortality for infants born to mothers with no more than a primary level of education, which is the educational level served by the Montero program, are in the range of 56–72 (Instituto Nacional de Estadística (Bolivia) and DHS+/ORC Macro 2004). Figure 21.1 demonstrates the markedly greater rate of decline of the infant mortality rate in Montero compared to that for national, departmental, and urban rates.

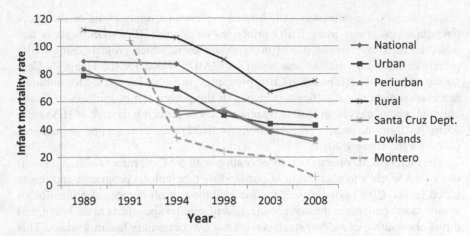

Fig. 21.1 Decline in infant mortality in the Montero Primary Health Care Project in comparison to National, Departmental, and Urban Changes, 1989–2008. *Sources*: (Instituto Nacional de Estatística (Bolivia) and DHS+/ORC Macro 2004; Montero Primary Health Care Program 2011)

Goal 5: Improve Maternal Health

MDG 5 calls for reducing by the maternal mortality ratio by three-fourths between 1990 and 2015. Programs and projects that use CBIO principles have demonstrated marked increases in the coverage of antenatal care and marked increases in the percentage of births attended by persons with formal training. This presumably has led to a reduction in the maternal mortality ratio, although few of them have reliable statistics for computing changes in the maternal mortality ratio.

The Jamkhed Comprehensive Rural Health Project reported a maternal mortality ratio of 70 per 100,000 live births at a time when 85 % of births occurred in the home and the national maternal mortality ratio was more than 230 (McCord et al. 2001; UNICEF 2008). BRAC's Manoshi Project for maternal, neonatal and child health in urban slums in Bangladesh is demonstrating that, after 5 years of implementation, the maternal mortality ratio is two-thirds of the national level (A. Kaosar, personal communication, 2012). And, as mentioned previously, in the Montero, Bolivia, CBIO project, no maternal deaths have been identified in this program area in a decade.

Goal 6: Combat HIV/AIDS, Malaria, and Other Diseases

MDG 6 calls for halting and beginning to reverse the spread of HIV/AIDS by 2015; achieving by 2010 universal access to treatment for HIV/AIDS for all who need it; and halting by 2015 and beginning to reverse the incidence of malaria, and other major diseases. Unfortunately, only limited evidence currently exists on the effectiveness of programs using CBIO principles to control HIV/AIDS, malaria and other diseases. But, to cite one of many examples in which projects using CBIO principles have raised awareness about HIV/AIDS, Food for the Hungry's Care Group project (which is based on CBIO principles) in Sofala Province, Mozambique, achieved statistically significant increases in the percentage of mothers of young children who could cite at least two known ways of reducing the risk of HIV: from 35 to 76 % in one project area and from 44 to 72 % in their second project area (Food for the Hungry 2010).

The NGO BRAC operates (in collaboration with the Government of Bangladesh) one of the world's largest and most outstanding tuberculosis programs, and this is based on the CBIO principles of routine visitation of all homes, identification of symptomatic patients in the home, collection of sputum specimens in the home, and direct observation of treatment, all carried out by community health workers. This program, which now reaches more than 50 million, has reported a prevalence of tuberculosis in the districts where BRAC is working to be only half that in districts where BRAC is not working (Chowdhury et al. 1997). As mentioned earlier, the Montero Primary Health Care Program in Bolivia has received numerous national awards for its outstanding tuberculosis program. Unfortunately, to our knowledge no evidence exists regarding the effectiveness of programs using CBIO principles in controlling HIV transmission or malaria.

The above evidence, derived from many projects and programs using CBIO principles, suggests quite strongly that the CBIO approach is effective in addressing global health goals and, if implemented broadly, could help to accelerate achievement of the MDGs for health.

Examples from Field Programs Which Have Utilized Local Surveillance Data to Enhance Program Effectiveness

One of the early striking findings from applying CBIO in Bolivia in the 1980s was the marked contrast in the epidemiological priorities in the program area in the highlands (on the Northern Altiplano, where communities were situated at 12,500 ft above sea level or height) and in the lowlands, with its tropical climate (in the peri-urban communities of Montero). Through home-based surveillance, we were able to document that leading causes of death in the highlands were respiratory problems occurring during the first 2 months of life while in the lowlands it was diarrhea and malnutrition occurring during the 6–18-month age group (Perry 1993). This led to markedly different program interventions. In Montero, the program focused on hygiene, clean water, nutrition education, and preparation and use of oral rehydration solution. On the Northern Altiplano, it led to more frequent home visits to newborns and early referral for treatment for respiratory infections.

In one program in Gaza Province, Mozambique, malaria was found to be far and away the leading cause of under-five mortality (World Relief 2009) while in another program in Sofala Province, Mozambique, diarrhea and neonatal causes were dominant (Food for the Hungry 2010). In the rural highlands of Guatemala, implementing CBIO made it possible to determine that pneumonia was far and away the leading cause of child death (Curamericas 2007). In rural Haiti, an evaluation revealed that the under-five mortality rate was twice as great in the rural mountainous area of the program as it was in the more central plains (Perry et al. 2006). In central India in the 1980s, SEARCH used the findings from its surveillance to determine that childhood pneumonia was the epidemiological priority and then set out to develop a program for expanding access to proper treatment provided by Community Health Workers in the home (Bang et al. 1990, 2005a). Then, in the 1990s, SEARCH determined that neonatal mortality had become the epidemiological priority and then set out to expand access to improved neonatal care by again using Community Health Workers to provide home-based neonatal care.

The potential of using surveillance findings based on routine home visits for strengthening the community diagnosis is apparent in these examples, as is the power of community-based workers well known to families in delivering interventions to the home when they are well trained and appropriately supervised.

The CBIO Approach in the Current Global Health Context

There is now a need for fresh new approaches that enable health programs in high-mortality, resource-constrained settings to be able to not only accelerate progress in achieving the MDGs for health but also serve in the long term to more effectively improve the health of the populations that they serve. Short-term vertical approaches are not the long-term answer. In fact, the authors of the now famous 1979 Walsh and Warren article that led to many of these more vertical approaches considered selective primary health care to be an interim solution. The actual title of their article is "Selective primary health care: an interim strategy for disease control in developing countries." Before his death, John Wyon wrote in 2001 in an unpublished document the following: "I have come to believe that, through the CBIO approach, the public health profession has unique contributions to make to problems of both excess births and excess deaths" (Wyon 2001).

Tools for Implementing the CBIO Approach

A manual for implementing CBIO is available for download from the CORE Group Web site (Shanklin and Sillan 2005). The Care Group model, utilizing many CBIO principles, is also readily available on the Internet as well (Laughlin 2004), as is a Web site devoted to Care Groups (Care Group Working Group 2012). A recent manual for prospective vital events registration through routine home visitation has just been prepared and is also available on the CORE Group Web site (Purdy et al. 2012).

A CBIO principle is to use locally acquired data to guide programming. Several tools related to formative research and qualitative assessment are useful adjuncts when using the CBIO framework. One of these is Barrier Analysis, which assesses the importance of determinants from the Health Belief and Theory of Reasoned Action models of behavioral change (Davis 2004, 2012).[2] Another tool is positive deviance analysis, which can help to identify currently successful strategies in place that might be applied more systematically to improve program performance (The Positive Deviance Initiative 2012). Positive deviance analysis was first applied to identify practices of mothers who had normally nourished children in settings where childhood undernutrition is common. This is referred to as the Hearth Model. However, the approach has now been applied to many areas of health programming.[3]

Conclusion

The CBIO approach describes a framework for public health practitioners and communities to come together to respond to both epidemiological and community-perceived priorities in a way that builds partnerships, utilizes principles of epidemiological surveillance, and capitalizes on the increasingly powerful evidence that interventions delivered in the community outside of facilities can achieve high levels of coverage and demonstrate notable improvements in population coverage of key interventions and reduce the mortality of mothers and children. Given the increasingly urgent need to accelerate progress toward achieving the health-related MDGs in countries with a high disease burden—especially in Africa—and given the strong evidence so far regarding the effectiveness of the CBIO approach, there should be increasing efforts to scale up programs using the CBIO approach, to rigorously monitor the effectiveness of scaled-up applications of the CBIO approach, and to modify implementation strategies based on these assessments. The CBIO approach has an important contribution to make in achieving the MDGs for health in settings where progress to date has lagged.

---

[2] For an online tutorial on the method, see http://barrieranalysis.fhi.net. For a narrated presentation on this method, see http://www.caregroupinfo.org/vids/BAVidIpad/story.html.

[3] One type of positive deviance study which focuses on nutritional status is the Local Determinants of Malnutrition Study methodology. For a narrated presentation on this approach, see http://www.caregroupinfo.org/vids/LDMVidiPad/story.html.

References

AMOS Health and Hope. Available from April 26, 2015, from http://www.amoshealth.org/

Arole, M., & Arole, R. (1994). *Jamkhed—A comprehensive rural health project*. London: Macmillan Press.

Bang, A. T., et al. (1990). Reduction in pneumonia mortality and total childhood mortality by means of community-based intervention trial in Gadchiroli, India. *Lancet, 336*(8709), 201–206.

Bang, A. T., Bang, R. A., & Reddy, H. M. (2005a). Home-based neonatal care: Summary and applications of the field trial in rural Gadchiroli, India (1993 to 2003). *Journal of Perinatology, 25*(Suppl 1), S108–S122.

Bang, A. T., et al. (2005b). Neonatal and infant mortality in the ten years (1993 to 2003) of the Gadchiroli field trial: Effect of home-based neonatal care. *Journal of Perinatology, 25*(Suppl 1), S92–S107.

Berggren, W. L., Ewbank, D. C., & Berggren, G. G. (1981). Reduction of mortality in rural Haiti through a primary-health-care program. *The New England Journal of Medicine, 304*(22), 1324–1330.

Care Group Working Group. (2012). *Care group web page*. Retrieved April 26, 2015, from www.CareGroupInfo.org

Chowdhury, A. M., et al. (1997). Control of tuberculosis by community health workers in Bangladesh. *Lancet, 350*(9072), 169–172.

Consejo de Salud Rural Andino. Retrieved April 26, 2015, from http://www.csra-bolivia.org/intro.php

Curamericas (2007). *Census-based, impact-oriented child survival project in the Department of Huehuetenango, Guatemala: Final evaluation (2002-2007)*. Raleigh, NC: Curamericas.

Davis, T. (2004). *Barrier Analysis Facilitator's Guide: A tool for improving behavior change communication in child survival and community development programs*. Retrieved April 26, 2015, from http://barrieranalysis.fhi.net/annex/Barrier_Analysis_Facilitator_Guide.pdf

Davis, T. (2012). *Designing for behavior change*. Retrieved April 26, 2015, from http://www.caregroup.org/storage/Tools/DBC_Curriculum11113.pdf

Davis, T., et al. (2015). Reducing child global undernutrition at scale in Sofala Province, Mozambique, using care group volunteers to contact mothers frequently with health messages. *Global Health: Science and Practice, 1*(1), 35–51.

Deutschman, A. (2007). *Change or die: The three keys to change at work and in life*. New York: Regan/HarperCollins Books.

Edward, A., et al. (2007). Examining the evidence of under-five mortality reduction in a community-based programme in Gaza, Mozambique. *Transactions of the Royal Society of Tropical Medicine and Hygiene, 101*(8), 814–822.

Food for the Hungry. (2010). *Expanded impact child survival program, final evaluation report, Gaza Province, Mozambique (2005-2010)*. Phoenix, AZ: Food for the Hungry International.

Frederickson, H. (1971). Epidemographic surveillance—Introduction. In H. Frederickson & F. L. Dunn (Eds.), *Epidemographic Surveillance—A Symposium* (pp. 1–28). Chapel Hill, NC: Carolina Population Center.

Instituto Nacional de Estadística (Bolivia), & MEASURE DHS+/ORC Macro (2004). *Encuesta Nacional de Demografia y Salud*. Instituto Nacional de Estadística (Bolivia), La Paz, Bolivia.

Jamkhed Comprehensive Rural Health Project. (2012). *Comprehensive Rural Health Project Impact*. Retrieved April 26, 2015, from http://www.jamkhed.org/impact/impact

Kielmann, A. A., et al. (1983). *Child and maternal health services in rural India: The Narangwal Experiment. Integrated nutrition and health care* (Vol. 1). Baltimore: Johns Hopkins University Press.

Laughlin, M. (2004). *The care group difference: A guide to mobilizing community-based volunteer health educators*. Baltimore: World Relief and the Child Survival Collaborations and Resources (CORE) Group.

Mann, V., et al. (2010). Retrospective comparative evaluation of the lasting impact of a community-based primary health care programme on under-5 mortality in villages around Jamkhed, India. *The Bulletin of the World Health Organization, 88*(10), 727–736.

McCord, C., et al. (2001). Efficient and effective emergency obstetric care in a rural Indian community where most deliveries are at home. *International Journal of Gynaecology and Obstetrics, 75*(3), 297–307; discussion 308–309.

Montero Primary Health Care Program. (2011). *Health Information System*. Montero, Bolivia: Consejo de Salud Rural Andino/Montero.

Mosham, H. (2011). Description and impact evaluation of a model community-based primary health care program in Montero, Bolivia. *Hubert Department of Global Health*. Emory University, Atlanta, GA.

Mosley, W. H. (1988). Is there a middle way? Categorical programs for PHC. *Social Science & Medicine, 26*(9), 907–908.

Perry, H. B. (1993). *The census-based, impact-oriented approach and its application by Andean Rural Health Care in Bolivia, South America*. Lake Junaluska, NC: Andean Rural Health Care.

Perry, H., et al. (1998). The census-based, impact-oriented approach: Its effectiveness in promoting child health in Bolivia. *Health Policy and Planning, 13*(2),·140–151.

Perry, H. B., Shanklin, D. S., & Schroeder, D. G. (2003). Impact of a community-based comprehensive primary healthcare programme on infant and child mortality in Bolivia. *Journal of Health, Population, and Nutrition, 21*(4), 383–395.

Perry, H., et al. (2006). Reducing under-five mortality through Hopital Albert Schweitzer's integrated system in Haiti. *Health Policy and Planning, 21*(3), 217–230.

Perry, H., et al. (2007). Long-term reductions in mortality among children under age 5 in rural Haiti: Effects of a comprehensive health system in an impoverished setting. *American Journal of Public Health, 97*(2), 240–246.

Perry, H., et al. (2010). Averting childhood deaths in resource-constrained settings through engagement with the community: An example from Cambodia. In J. Gofin & R. Gofin (Eds.), *Essentials of community health* (pp. 169–174). Sudbury, MA: Jones and Bartlett.

Purdy, C., Weiss, W., & Perry, H. (2012). *The Mortality Impact Assessment System: An NGO field manual for registering vital events and assessing child survival impact using the Care Group Model*. Washington, DC: The CORE Group.

SEARCH (2015). Society for Education Action and Research in Community Health. Retrieved April 26, 2015, from http://www.Searchgadchilsoli.org

Sepulveda, J., et al. (2006). Improvement of child survival in Mexico: The diagonal approach. *Lancet, 368*(9551), 2017–2027.

Shanklin, D., & Sillan, D. (2005). *The census-based, impact-oriented methodology: A resource guide for equitable and effective primary health care*. Curamericas and the CORE Group.

Taylor, C. E., et al. (1983). *Child and maternal health services in rural India: The Narangwal Experiment. Integrated Family Planning and Health Care* (Vol. 2). Baltimore: The Johns Hopkins University Press.

Taylor-Ide, D., & Taylor, C. (2002). *Just and lasting change: When communities own their futures* (pp. 93–101). Baltimore: Johns Hopkins University Press.

The Positive Deviance Initiative. (2012). *The positive deviance initiative*. Retrieved April 26, 2015, from http://www.positivedeviance.org/

UNICEF. (2008). *UNICEF statistics for India* [cited December 20, 2012].

UNICEF, & WHO. (2012). *Countdown to 2015. Maternal, newborn and child survival. Accountability for maternal, newborn and child survival: An update on progress in priority countries*. Geneva, Switzerland: World Health Organization.

United Nations. (2000). *Resolution55/2 adopted by the General Assembly: United Nations Millennium Declaration*.

Walsh, J. A., & Warren, K. S. (1979). Selective primary health care: An interim strategy for disease control in developing countries. *The New England Journal of Medicine, 301*(18), 967–974.

World Health Organization, & UNICEF. (1978). Declaration of Alma-Ata: International conference on primary health care. In *International conference on primary health care, Alma-Ata, USSR*.

World Relief. (2009). *Expanded impact child survival program, final evaluation report, Gaza Province, Mozambique*. World Relief, Baltimore.

Wyon, J. (2001). *The evolution of John Wyon's ideas leading to the census-based, impact-oriented approach to primary health care* (Unpublished).

Wyon, J. B., & Gordon, J. E. (1971). *The Khanna study: Population problems in the rural Punjab*. Cambridge, MA: Harvard University Press.

Chapter 22
Effective Advocacy for Aid Effectiveness

Smita Baruah

Introduction

Advocacy is strongly supporting an idea or a cause and the process of influencing decision makers about that idea or cause. In international development, advocacy is targeted towards political institutions to ensure that their policies are responsive to people's needs. Advocates often raise an issue or identify gaps in policies and propose solutions.

Therefore, advocates are already engaged in making policies more effective. International development advocates have long been calling for more effective aid even before the term was formalized. As an advocate, one wants to affect change so that the world is a better place to live. When one is a member of Amnesty International or took part in Model U.N. or signed up to receive action alerts from the ONE campaign, that person is trying to make the world a better place to live.

I was one of those individuals who led a human rights club in college, who became a member of Amnesty International, and who joined numerous listservs that promoted gender rights, addressed antipoverty across the globe, or messaged against child labor. And it was because of this desire to change that I came to Washington to study and work in international development and eventually spent my entire career advocating for more effective programs.

This chapter will discuss the important role that advocacy plays in making aid more effective. Most of the examples used in this chapter are based on my experience in working with various coalitions and issues.

S. Baruah (✉)
Global Health Policy and Advocacy Save the Children USA, Washington, DC, USA
e-mail: baruahsmita@gmail.com; SBaruah@savechildren.org

© Springer Science+Business Media New York 2015
E. Beracochea (ed.), *Improving Aid Effectiveness in Global Health*,
DOI 10.1007/978-1-4939-2721-0_22

Aid Effectiveness

Over the last decade there has been increased recognition that international aid must be more harmonized and more effective. This means better coordination among donors so that they are not duplicating efforts at the country level, greater alignment with a country's needs and priorities, and sending the aid directly to local organizations and institutions to build sustainability. For civil society organizations this also means that international aid must be accountable to the people, promote gender equality, transparency, and empowerment.

Nongovernmental organizations or civil society organizations are development actors themselves. As key players in the implementing field they are also working towards making aid more effective on the ground. However, civil society organizations are not only engaged in aid effectiveness through improved implementation but also heavily engaged in the policy dialogue.

There is a strong connection between a government's policies and programs on the ground. Policies or guidelines can sometimes cause international aid to be ineffective. It can sometimes hinder the ability to reach the most in need.

Therefore, strong policy dialogue at national level, including international development partners, is needed to increase aid flows and their effectiveness and to better align donor approaches and activities with country priorities and existing processes.

Civil society advocacy organizations play a key role in engaging in this policy dialogue and fostering necessary changes at the policy level which eventually can have an impact on programs that are being implemented on the ground.

This chapter will focus on the role of civil society in improving policy to thereby foster effective international assistance. It will summarize the process of influencing policy and how improved policies can lead to improved implementation of health programs.

Effective Policies for Effective Aid

In academic terms "aid effectiveness" often refers to creating more alignment and harmonization among donors and with country governments. It refers to the effort to avoid duplication of activities and maximize a donors' reach in a country or a community. For example, if a country identifies the prevalence of HIV as a priority as well as the need to immunize children, resources from donor countries should ensure that they are addressing both needs. However, when HIV funding was at its peak, donor governments would all invest in HIV treatment. At times, they would all be in the same communities at the same time.

From an advocate's point of view, "aid effectiveness" is not only about harmonization and reducing duplication of efforts but also ensuring that donor and country policies do not serve as an obstacle to improving people's lives. For example, some countries' policies do not allow nurses to administer an antiretroviral drug or treat a patient for other diseases. They must defer to a doctor for those services. However, there are a limited number of well-trained qualified doctors in rural communities. Nurses can ably take on some of the duties of a full time physician. Due to country policies on task shifting, nurses' roles are limited. A country's policies on what is known as "task shifting" (e.g., shifting a portion of physicians' duties to nurses) can have an impact on the ground as fewer patients in the community are able to receive the necessary HIV treatment and care in many countries due to the nurses limited functions.

"Effective Aid" also means following through on written policies. For example, the USA has signed 27 Global Health Initiative country strategies. Each strategy includes specific objectives and targets for improving health outcomes. For example the Kenya country strategy states that the USA will focus on integrating maternal and child health programs into existing health programs, focus on increasing access to family planning, and focus on reducing the burden of neglected tropical diseases. Beneath these overall objectives, it lays out several sub-objectives. An advocate would review the implementation of these policies which includes gathering evidence from the field on whether or not maternal and child health programs are indeed being integrated into existing health systems. If not, the advocate will engage in a dialogue with the US government.

Effective Advocacy for Effective Policies

How does one ensure that the right policies are being promoted and followed through upon? Good advocacy is usually based on evidence. An advocate first identifies the gaps between policy and implementation, usually based on stories from the field. For example, 2 years ago the Office of the Global AIDS Coordinator released new policy guidance for reaching men having sex with men and injecting drug users with HIV treatment, prevention, and care services. The new policies were designed to enable organizations to integrate more services into their IDU programming and reach more drug users. However, up until last year, these new policies were still not being integrated into country operational plan guidances or other technical documents. Implementing agencies were still operating under the old policies as the old policy language was still being used in the operational plans which limited their ability to reach a great population in need and expand its services. This represented a gap between the written policy and actual implementation.

An advocate uses such evidence to engage in a policy dialogue with OGAC to ensure that new country operational plans reflect the new guidance on reaching MSM and IDUs through expanded HIV prevention, treatment, and care services which would thereby result in more effective programming which result in more IDUs being treated for HIV and reducing the number of HIV infections.

Illustration of Effective Advocacy

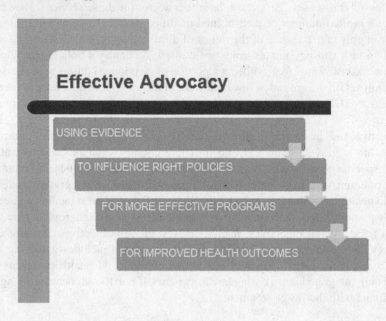

Another example is Save the Children International's EveryOne Campaign. Save the Children International, an organization devoted to improving the lives of children around the world, identified three major gaps in countries' ability to address child health. These were number and capacity of health workers, addressing malnutrition and increasing access to vaccines. In spite of the progress made towards reducing child mortality, 6.9 million children were continuing to die from preventable diseases at the launch of this campaign. What else was required to reverse this trend? Based on its own field experience, Save the Children recognized that communities lacked health professionals to treat children for diarrhea or pneumonia or counsel new mothers about the importance of breastfeeding. Based on this evidence, it launched a specific campaign called the *Every One* campaign to advocate with donor and country governments to work towards narrowing the gap in quantity and quality of health workers and to increase a child's access to nutrition (www.everyone.org). This campaign is now being implemented in various ways in select country members such as Save the Children USA.

The Cycle of Influencing Policy

The ability to change policy does not occur overnight. It happens over time through sometimes a long drawn out process. It took 22 years since the discovery of HIV/AIDS for the US government to launch a major effort to curb the global spread of

HIV. Identifying the gaps between policy and implementation is only the first step towards fostering effective policy for effective aid.

The common cycle of influencing policy is:

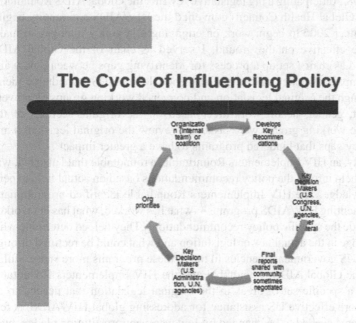

Once an advocacy organization identifies the gaps, it develops key recommendations for improving policy. Policy can be affected in a variety of ways. Advocates target key legislation that might be in play in the US Congress that could have an influence on the Administration's policies. Advocates also target key Administration documents such as the HIV Treatment and Prevention Guidance for IDUs or a five-year strategy on maternal and child health.

Once it develops its core set of recommendations and the vehicle through which to push it, advocates begin to engage in a dialogue with key stakeholders. That includes key congressional staff or representatives in various US government agencies and outside stakeholders who could have an influence on key US government representatives. The next section will illustrate a specific case study on how this cycle of influencing policy works in practice.

The Cycle of Influencing Policy for Promoting More Effective HIV/AIDS Policies

In 2008, then President George W. Bush enacted into law P.L. 110-293 Tom Lantos & Henry Hyde US Global Leadership Against AIDS, Tuberculosis, and Malaria Reauthorization Act of 2008. This bill extended the President's Emergency Plan for

AIDS Relief (PEPFAR) for another 5 years. The first bill launching this initiative was passed and enacted into law in 2003. The 2003 legislation that established the President's Emergency Program for AIDS Relief (PEPFAR) was set to expire in September 2008. Anticipating a big legislative rewrite, the Global AIDS Roundtable (housed at the Global Health Council) convened the HIV/AIDS community beginning in September 2006 to begin work on engaging in a policy dialogue to make PEPFAR more effective on the ground. I served as chair of the Global AIDS Roundtable and as chair I set up a process for identifying gaps between policy and practice and impact of policy on the ground. The Global AIDS Roundtable members went through the original legislation and convened working groups on prevention, treatment, gender, health workforce based on the original sections of the legislation. The working groups were tasked to review the original legislation and identified policy gaps that hindered programs to have a greater impact.

Concurrently, an HIV Implementers Roundtable, a roundtable that I also led, was established to help inform the policy recommendations based on actual field experience and knowledge. The HIV Implementers Roundtable identified programmatic gaps in implementing HIV/AIDS programs—what has worked, what has not worked and helped guide the specific policy recommendations. They helped determine what required a change in the actual law or legislation and what could be rectified through dialogue with US government agencies to make these programs more successful.

Together, the Global AIDS Roundtable and the HIV Implementers Roundtable came up with a specific set of areas in the original legislation that needed to be changed for more effective US assistance for addressing global HIV/AIDS. A few examples of items needed to be changed by law were: antiprostitution pledge, budgetary requirements (set funding allocations for treatment, prevention, care), ban on funding for safe needles, aligning with country's needs and situation, greater focus on gender equality, health systems strengthening including a specific focus on health workforce training.

As chair, I led the Global AIDS Roundtable in synthesizing the information gathered through the working groups and programmatic experience, helped develop specific recommendations, and used this information to engage in a dialogue with policy makers. I organized weekly roundtable meetings with key congressional staff who were writing the revised legislation, with the Administration, and with other stakeholders.

In these meetings, civil society presented policy makers (including staff) with suggested policy language to make aid more effective, using actual evidence from the field, changes to policy and technical guidances and also provided solutions on how to better execute the implementation of these programs at the country level.

To formulate these policy asks and ensure that the community was unified asks, I, on behalf of the Global AIDS Roundtable, convened numerous meetings—private meetings between the various working groups; between advocates and key congressional staff; large public meetings to arrive at a compromised set of recommendations. I also leveraged the programmatic experts found within its membership to make a solid case for a number of the requested legislative changes.

The efforts were not just limited to dialogue in Washington. Advocates mobilized American citizens across the country to write to their Member of Congress and urge them to take action and support key legislative changes and increase the funding for global HIV/AIDS programs. Hundreds of citizens took action through phone calls and letters and meetings with their policy maker. This includes faith based communities, students, and grasstops or influential leaders.

The end result was a revised law that included less strict budgetary requirements for HIV prevention, treatment, and care, establishment of partnership frameworks which were a joint collaborative strategy between the countries and US government, lifting of the ban on safe needles, a greater focus on reaching the most vulnerable populations, stronger indicators for more effective monitoring and evaluation, a specific target for training, equipping, and deploying health workers, and changes in technical guidances. The end result was more effective US assistance for addressing global HIV/AIDS.

Conclusion

Civil society played a critical role in making US programs on global HIV/AIDS much more effective and in having a greater impact on the ground. In the cycle of influencing policy, there was a great deal of dialogue between representatives of the US government and global HIV/AIDS advocates and other civil society actors such as faith-based groups.

The Global AIDS Roundtable was able to use the evidence to identify the policy gaps to make sound recommendations for more effective programming. This type of effective advocacy led to effective aid.

The 2008 legislative process on reauthorizing PEPFAR is an excellent case study on the role that advocacy plays in shaping donor global assistance programs. It is an illustration of the role of civil society advocates in fostering more effective aid.

Aid effectiveness is not just about donor harmonization or less duplication of resources and efforts on the ground, it is also about creating effective policies to have the desired impact. These effective policies are often informed by effective advocates who are able to identify the positive and negative aspects of programs and policies and engage in a dialogue at the national and global level. The 2008 PEPFAR legislation taught us that citizen action is critical to improving policies and for ensuring that the assistance indeed reaches those who need it the most and that this assistance is accountable to the people they serve.

I am grateful to be continuing to work to improve policies that impact the people we are trying to serve. Often we as advocates are speaking on behalf of those without a voice. And this is very true for the work that we do at Save the Children. Children cannot vote and often are not heard. Their voices are too small or distant. And newborns have no voices at all. It has been extra special working on behalf of these children, who are more vulnerable than even the most vulnerable adults. And to know at the end of the day, by calling on the US government to add more health workers to a community so that a pregnant mother can access the care that she needs or teaching health workers to counsel new mothers about newborn care and investing more for address malnutrition in children under five will make the world a better place for children is truly gratifying.

What You Can Do to Make Aid More Effective

All citizens can make sure that aid continues to be effective and has a positive impact on the people they are trying to serve. First, we must make sure that aid continues to flow to developing countries as it helps foster country ownership and increased country resources for human development issues, paves the way for diplomatic dialogue and partnership, as well as help build sustainable communities. Second, we must make sure that resources are being directed towards effective programs and address any barriers.

Your voice is extremely critical in making sure that governments, nongovernmental organizations, and other stakeholders are continuing to invest in programs that have the most impact.

Here are a few ways you can help in making aid more effective:

Ensure that the resources are there for effective aid. Every year, the US Congress evaluates and decides how much funding international assistance programs should get including poverty-focused programs. Congress needs to hear from you that you care about how much money goes to international programs focused on human development including addressing global health and humanitarian crises. You can help ensure that US assistance goes to programs helps communities in the developing world by going here: http://www.usglc.org/action-center/.

Help ensure that medicines, bednets, and other essential services and commodities reach the most hard to reach communities. Millions of people are living productive lives today because frontline health workers are there—to deliver vaccines, treat diarrhea or HIV, or provide bednets to prevent malaria. They are the ones who are providing health care in many of the hardest to reach areas, often traveling on foot with just a backpack of supplies. They include midwives, community health workers, physicians' assistants, peer counselors, nurses, and sometimes doctors serving in local clinics. The world needs one million more of these workers to ensure healthy lives and healthy communities and to make aid more effective. Take action now on www.everybeatmatters.org.

Ensure that the world continues to work towards ending preventable child deaths. In June 2012, the governments of the USA, Ethiopia, and India led a meeting on Child Survival: A Call to Action where governments, civil society organizations, faith-based organizations all pledged to end preventable child deaths within a generation. They pledged to ensure that resources helped improve children's lives, to use resources for programs that are most effective in helping children, and to design programs per country's needs and priorities.

You can help achieve the goal of ending preventable child deaths by signing a pledge: http://apr.nationbuilder.com/cso_pledge.

Suggested Readings

Aid Effectiveness. (2012, December). Retrieved from http://en.wikipedia.org/wiki/Aid_effectiveness

Baruah, S. (2012, April). *Making sure aid is effective.* Presentation to the summit on aid effectiveness in global health, Midego.

WHO. (2012). Global health and aid effectiveness. Global Health Observatory. Retrieved from http://www.who.int/gho/governance_aid:effectiveness/en/index.html

References

EveryOne Campaign. Retrieved from http://everyone.org/

P.L. 110-293 (2008, July). Tom Lantos & Henry Hyde U.S. Global Leadership against AIDS, Tuberculosis and Malaria Reauthorization Act of 2008. Retrieved from http://www.gpo.gov/fdsys/pkg/PLAW-110publ293/pdf/PLAW-110publ293.pdf

Chapter 23
Personalizing Health Communication

Gina M. Stracuzzi

> *People don't buy what you do; people buy why you do it*
> *(Sinek 2009).*
>
> *Simon Sinek, Author*

In his book and seminar series by the same name, *Start With Why*, Mr. Sinek explains how businesses that are built on, and marketed around their "why," i.e., the reason they exist, their driving motivation, are far more successful than those that only know "what" they do or "how" they do it. Companies immersed in their "why" are the leaders in their fields and have deeply loyal, committed clients. These companies inspire their customers to take action.

What is our "why?" What is the reason health communication exists? Most would likely argue that our purpose is to improve public health outcomes by conveying the impact and benefits of healthy behaviors. But isn't that what we do and in its simplest form how we do it, rather than the real "why" of our work? Is that enough however to inspire our "customers"—those on the receiving end of health communication messages—to make the kinds of changes we are promoting? Or should we be involving a more personal "why" to engender the kind of reaction needed to bring about lasting behavior change, the kind of inspiration that Mr. Sinek is referencing?

My goal in this chapter is to present the notion that by infusing health communication with the emotion and passion with have for our work—our personal "why"—we will improve our overall effectiveness. We will also at look how our personal motivation can be a powerful tool to illustrate our commitment to the communities we serve and to our counterparts who are learning to lead programs in their own countries.

G.M. Stracuzzi (✉)
Women International Mentoring Network, 8502 Rehoboth Ct, Vienna, VA 22182, USA
e-mail: ginastracuzzi@verizon.net

© Springer Science+Business Media New York 2015
E. Beracochea (ed.), *Improving Aid Effectiveness in Global Health*,
DOI 10.1007/978-1-4939-2721-0_23

Communicating in a Time of Change

Donor-driven development assistance is giving way to country-developed and implemented initiatives, which better serve developing countries and have the greatest chance of sustainability (Kharas et al. 2011). There must be similar modifications in our communication approaches. Over the last 50 years of development, a great deal of time, energy, and money has been assigned to development communication research, models, and strategies, such as *Behavior Change Communication*, *Communication for Social Change*, and *Participatory Communication*, which work on a macro-level (Waisbord 2008). While differing in approaches, the ultimate goal of each of the paradigms utilized today is to empower communities through discussion, training, and education programs (Bessette 2004). These models have their success and a place in our toolbox without question, but we can build upon their benefits and improve success moving forward.

All communication efforts have one inherent weak point: humans. Within all communication is the innately human dimension of what's heard (received) versus what is shared (sent). Most communication models are based on the notion of a balance or two-way flow of information (Bessette 2004). Almost anyone who has worked in communication or training can tell you that these two factors (sent/received and balance) can contrast widely depending on the message and the audience. Individuals in an audience (communities, health care workers, volunteers, etc.) receive and perceive messages through their own prism. Content aimed at large groups of people will have mixed results; interpretation can vary dramatically as can the acceptance or disregarding of that message (Chandler 1994). One macro-level communication theory, *Knowledge Gap Hypothesis* (Tichenor et al. 1970), highlights these disparities by suggesting that knowledge and information are not equally distributed across populations and that the kind of increased flow of information from major communication campaigns is more likely to benefit groups of higher socioeconomic status than those at lower income and education levels. The Knowledge Gap theory also states that large-scale public health campaigns would only perpetuate such inequities (Glanz et al. 2008).

If we acknowledge—or at least allow for the plausibility—that variances exist in the receiving and processing of communication messages across populations we can complement the data-driven, science-based communication models routinely employed in development communications with something more personal.

People-driven methods that harness the vision and personal missions of the thousands of dedicated professionals from around the world that comprise the field of development are an untapped resource. Each of us, whether a long-time international consultant from the north or a new local consultant from the south; a program officer or health official; or any other person working in development, has a story (maybe several) to share that illustrates our "why." In sharing our stories and personal missions, our driving motivation, we nurture one of the most effective communication tools we have to inspire change: human emotion (Ford 1992).

The Power of the Personal Story: Using Our "Why"

Emotion-driven communication, which is often the crux of a personal story, can tap into and build on the very individual nature of what development communication is trying to make happen, i.e., changes in behaviors. Whether as part of a large multi-region project or a small community-driven program, the vast majority of modifications being sought in change communication require changes at the personal level: the use of condoms, hand washing, sleeping under bednets, etc., all rely on individual action. For these changes to happen, however, individuals must act on the message, which means reaching them at the "gut level," where much of our decision-making takes place (Roller 2010).

So why is our "why" important in development aid communication? Reversing age-old, deeply ingrained "habits" or routines, as is needed to reach most development and behavior change goals, requires **an emotional "stirup"** (Lewin 1951). Sharing our passion and our belief in the message is one of the most influential ways to reach people at that gut, instinctual level, necessary for an "emotional stirup." This is where we can create excitement and build sustainable interest.

One of the best, emotion-based communication "stir-up" mechanisms we have is our own stories: our reasons for working in development and what inspires us to do the often difficult work of trying to save lives, improve living conditions, provide clean water, etc. In short, our "why." By leaning too heavily on communication models that rely on mass appeal for their success (Baran and Davis 2012) we overlook the impact of our individual "why" to create an emotional stirup.

Ultimately, communicating our inspiration can help others—especially our counterparts and colleagues in developing countries—begin to understand the power their own passion can have to create an emotional "stirup" in their work and communities.

> Long before the first formal business was established… the six most powerful words in any language were… "*Let me tell you a story.*"
> Ryan Matthews and Watts Wacker, "What's Your Story (Matthews and Wacker 2008)."

My Story, My "Why," My Defining Moment

After years of working in marketing communications in the commercial and non-profit sectors, I wanted something new, something that would allow me to use my education and experience in a way that truly benefited people. I was motivated to make this change after adopting our daughter, Talia, from Guatemala. The experience of picking her up in a country so rich in natural beauty, yet with such vast poverty and inequities, caused by decades of civil conflict and numerous natural disasters, left an indelible impression on me. These images helped guide me to the career change I was looking for and fueled my desire to someday help my daughter understand the hardships people in her birth country face. I started researching projects and efforts underway at that time to help Guatemala and its people. One of the lessons I learned is that like a lot of developing countries, Guatemala is a class-driven society in which marginalization, poverty, and chronic malnutrition are grimly interconnected. I also quickly began to understand that there was a lot I didn't know about development. To get a better appreciation of global efforts to help developing countries and build on my education and background in communication, I decided to pursue a career in Global Health Communications, which started with obtaining a graduate certificate in Global Health. I wasn't interested in implementing large communication campaigns as much as wanted to tell the stories of the people in developing countries—their hardships as well as their dreams—and the stories of the people, perhaps like yourself, from all over the world that have made bringing health and well-being to every corner of the world their personal missions.

Now, many years later, things have come full circle. I have had the opportunity to work on several development projects. I have had the humbling opportunity to coach dedicated health professionals from all over the world to help them improve their work and take their careers to new levels. I have traveled to Guatemala professionally, which gave me the chance to experience the country and its people more intimately, and I have started my own foundation, *e-Women*: *International Mentoring Network*, to connect women in the developed world with women in developing countries, like Guatemala, to mentor and coach them in areas such as health, family planning, education, and business. As Talia gets a bit older, I hope to involve her in e-Women so that she, too, can have the opportunity to support girls in her birth country. One day we will take her back to Guatemala so she can meet her country and experience its beauty for herself. Then my initial mission will be complete, but my story will continue.

I have told my story many times in my work and coaching, and each time I feel the emotions of carrying my new daughter in my arms for the first time. I remember how I cried both when we left Guatemala and as we brought her into her new home—the disparity between the two environments hitting me somewhere between immense gratitude for all that I had to share with her and sadness that she would not know her beautiful country, at least not for years to come. I share that emotion with my audience, whether it is one person or a crowded room. Many of those that I have shared my story with have told me that it has helped them find their own mission and they have begin sharing their stories.

Your Story, Your "Why"

That is my story, my reason for doing what I do. What is your reason? Why are you in the field of development? What is your personal story? Have you used your story to help others understand how much you care? Do you find and utilize opportunities to share your vision for development in your work. If not, I encourage you to begin thinking about your career and your knowledge in terms of its ability to motivate and inspire others. Start by thinking about your work; have you led a training session or implemented a program that required motivating people to take action? How do you feel about the experience? Were you able to share your experiences with enthusiasm and a sense of personal investment in the information you were imparting, or did you feel as though you were just pushing the material at people? Were you able to inspire them to apply what you taught or asked them to employ? Were you able to make them "feel" good about the changes you were asking them to make? Think about these ideas as you move forward in your work. How might a personal story—your story—be used to bolster interest and illustrate a genuine concern in helping others?

Perhaps you're thinking that you don't have a story to share, or maybe you do have something that drives you but you are not sure who to tell it to or how to begin. One easy way to start is with your coworkers. You may have worked alongside the same people for years, but have you ever shared what motivates you or your inspiration for the work you do? In fact, sharing stories in the workplace is a tool utilized by a growing number of corporations (Smith 2012) to communicate strengths and enthusiasm and to let others know that you are not afraid to take chances and show vulnerability. We can utilize this same thinking in development as a communication and training tool if we look at our stories as an opportunity to share our knowledge.

> A knowledge-sharing story offers a surrogate experience… when a story is recounted, the narrative form offers the listener an opportunity to experience in a surrogate fashion the situation that was experienced by the storyteller. The listener can acquire understanding of the situation's key concepts and their relationships in the same progressive or cumulative manner that the storyteller acquired that understanding. A key point of the surrogacy notion is that even though the listener did not directly experience the story situation, it must be possible, even probable, that the listener could experience a similar situation (Sole et al. 2012).

So How Do We Employ Our Most Effective Communication Tool?

Telling Your Story Effectively

Once you know what story you want to tell, the next step is to think about how you will tell your story. To motivate your audience, it is important to make your story compelling and to tie that excitement to an action you would like the person or people you are talking with to take (Mathews and Wacker 2008). Keeping these main ideas in mind will help you craft your story in an effective way:

- Start by thinking about what you want your audience to do (what action) and why?
- Next, think of a time in your career or life that compelled you **to take action**
  - Did you have a problem that needed solving? How did you solve it? What action did you take?
  - Did something unexpected happen? How did you deal with it?
  - Were you scared, confused, frustrated, or exhilarated?
  - Did someone or something take you in a completely different direction from your initial plan?

- Share how you felt at the time. What was going through your head? Include all the important details leaving out information that will detract from your overall point.
- Use humor, laugh at yourself; self-deprecation can be a great tool for breaking the ice and showing your vulnerability.
- Remember you are the most effective communicator of your own story—don't take yourself out of the equation. Keep this in mind as you are sharing your story. Tell the story in first person.
- After telling your story, start a discussion. Ask emotion-based questions:

  - Have you ever had something like that happen to you?
  - How did you handle it?
  - How did you feel when this happened?
  - What did you do about it?

The answers you receive can tell you a lot about a person or group and how best to reach them. With that information you can take communication to the next level.

Fostering Learning and Growth: Helping Others Cultivate Their Passion

Beyond improved acceptance of our training and communication messages, we should also be helping individuals and communities develop their dreams for a better life including better health. It will be their "why" for adapting healthy practices. We can aid this process by thinking about some of our own most memorable learning experiences. When considering your own memorable learning experience ask yourself, they involve someone just lecturing to share facts and information, or did they happen when someone took the time to share their passion about a topic and their enthusiasm was infectious? If we use our own stories of learning and growth as our guides we will make our messages and material more relevant, generate excitement, stimulate in-depth conversation, and earn the trust needed to make sustainable changes. There is a famous quote that has been attributed to both Theodore Roosevelt (The Examiner 2012) and John C. Maxwell (Good Reads 2012) that says, *"People don't care how much you know until they know how much you care."* Our personal missions show that we are emotionally invested in our work. Stories show we care by humanizing us, making us more approachable, and providing the opportunity to produce an atmosphere that allows for meaningful, grassroots communication. In turn, teaching this communication method can "help communities identify true problems and priorities and opens the door for making effective connections and encourages integration with a community's existing communication networks" (Mezzana 1996).

Sharing our passion and stories isn't just a communication tool that can inspire others and ignite change; it's also an opportunity. The field of development aid is rapidly changing as the mindset of "country-owned, country-led" aid grows stronger.

Our roles as development professionals are also changing, which, for many, is a frightening prospect. Rather than worry about what these changes mean for us, we can see this is as a unique opportunity to build relationships with colleagues and experts in developing economies who are working hard to improve their communities and their countries. Supporting their career growth and development through personal and emotion-based communication, such as mentoring and coaching, are just a few of the ways we can be more effective and help individuals and groups of health care professionals manage their new country leadership roles. Thanks to e-mail, Skype, social media, and other emerging technologies, developing these nurturing roles has never been easier. The rewards of building a network of support for these health professionals are limitless (Meyer 2001). From an effectiveness point of view such networks are great examples of what success could and should look like.

Make no mistake, these new roles—both for the experienced development professional and for the new professional in-country—won't always be easy. There are many very real differences in the way cultures communicate. Some things though are uniquely human, like the need to feel appreciated, the desire to do work that matters, to be recognized for that work, to have our opinions heard and respected. As Maslow's stated in his "hierarchy of needs," we all need to feel respected and valued and to know that we matter (Maslow 1954). This is true for all humans, not just those of us fortunate enough to be born in a rich and developed country.

In fact, we can learn a great deal from our colleagues in the developing world. Two great examples are within this book. I urge you to read Sam Daley-Harris' chapter on "Advocating for Aid Effectiveness," for his inspiring story, and the stories of the "everyday heroes" that motivated him to start RESULTS, a nonprofit, grassroots citizen's lobby group and the Microcredit Summit Campaign. Another chapter with powerful stories is that of Glenn J. Schwartz, the Executive Director of World Mission Associates. In his chapter Mr. Glenn shares some of the many stories that inspired and educated him throughout his missionary work. Like Mr. Daley-Harris and Mr. Glenn, as you begin using your story, remember to collect and share stories from your colleagues, people you encounter in your work, and especially the people you serve.

One amazing story of leadership that I often share is that of Sister Claudia Tukakuhebwa, Coordinator of the Rushoroza Community Based Health Care Programme. Sister Claudia looked at the high population of orphans and vulnerable children in the rural Kabale district of Uganda and immediately saw the need to support the hundreds of orphans and vulnerable children and families living in the area. She and her small but dedicated team set the goal of dramatically improving the lives and livelihoods of the more than 800 orphans and other vulnerable children (OVC) and 600 families in their community. Drawing inspiration, optimism, and enthusiasm from a *story* she read, *Health for All NOW*, (Beracochea 2005), about Amos, a district health officer facing seemingly insurmountable challenges to achieving better health to his district, Sister Claudia's team stated working with families in their homes and children from the OVC groups in educational environments. Through their hard work they have reached each of those 800 plus orphans and vulnerable children in less than a year, resulting in a huge reduction in the number of street children and those at risk of becoming one. They also brought about a greater awareness among community members of ways to assist orphans and vulnerable children, which has led to an overall reduction in the stigma for those with HIV and AIDS and has greatly reduced traumatic tensions and bereavement. Her team also noticed a much greater utilization of counseling and guidance, which has led to increased self-esteem among children and an on-going interest in health. I have shared Sister Claudia's remarkable story several times in my coaching to illustrate what one person can make happen when they put their mind to it. Sister Claudia was motivated to action after reading about Amos (the story of Amos is actually a composite of a number of people's stories presented together for even greater impact). One person has impacted the lives of more than 800 children and 600 families because of a story that compelled her. Another 700+ other health professionals from around the world have been moved to action through Amos and the *Health for All NOW story*, and now several hundred more through Sister Claudia's story. One story; many lives changed. Passion. Enthusiasm. Emotion. Powerful tools too often overlooked.

Women: The Ultimate Emotion-Based Communicators

Sister Claudia's story not only shows what one person can achieve but also highlights the important role women are playing in development. Involving ever greater number of women in development decisions will continue to be a priority for years to come. A 2008 report from The Development Assistance Committee of the OECD reported that in 2005–2006, approximately $8.5 billion was spent each year for gender equality and women's empowerment—almost 33 % of the $26 billion in overall aid spent by about 16 bilateral donors. This figure did not include the additional $27.8 billion in bilateral aid spent by seven other countries, including the USA (Selvaggio et al. 2008).

This investment in women is based on a single yet profound shift in global thinking: women are now seen as the economic engines of their communities and by extension their countries (Foroohar 2009). Moreover, it is quite often the sole responsibility of the woman, especially in rural areas, to raise and feed their families. However, the role of women working or engaged in development however is not equal to their level of responsibility. A 2000 report by the Food and Agricultural Organization of the United Nations (FAO) stated:

> Given the opportunity, women have shown themselves again and again to be highly responsive and responsible when helped to mobilize themselves, build upon available resources and produce sustainable results. Women need to learn additional technical and organizational skills and more women are needed at the center of decision-making. Specific challenges where communication is vital include helping women's groups to increase their self-determination and to broaden the dialogue between the sexes regarding rights, privileges and responsibilities (Colin and Villet 1994).

Working with women in developing countries as decision-makers is the perfect opportunity to utilize emotion-based communication. Women excel at open, horizontal, inclusive communication (Stillman 2005). Their stories inspire other women to take action, discover their own missions, and understand the impact they have on their families, communities, and country. Helping your counterparts in developing countries becomes more involved in development, and development communications is a logical step to harnessing their power to bring about change. Share your story or personal mission with them. Ask them to tell you a story about themselves; why are they working for change or pursuing a career or new livelihood? Collect their stories and share them yourself. You will discover the unique impact their stories can have. Given the opportunity to use these skills, women in resource poor settings can help lead their communities and countries especially in areas of development decisions. Helping women around the world find their voice through storytelling is a powerful and effective way we can help them be part of development process in their countries.

Stories Rarely Heard

The "last mile" is a term usually used in the telecommunications and technology industries to describe the technologies and processes used to connect the end customer to a communications network (http://www.investopedia.com/terms/l/lastmile.asp#ixzz2DjEguWlk). More recently the last mile has come to have a more profound meaning:

> Those living in the last mile comprise the majority of the world's poor. Most are disconnected from education and economic opportunities, and many more lack access to basic goods and services. Last mile work, therefore, implies a dedication to extending the benefits of development to everyone—even the hardest to serve (The Aspen Institute 2012).

We have accomplished a great deal in development, but we are not there yet. We still need to go that "last mile." Our communication efforts need to be evaluated and updated along the way. What if we apply "last mile" thinking to current development and behavior change communication methods? Are we getting there? Are we reaching the hardest to serve with models that mainly see communication as a "process of exchange, mutual influence, co-orientation, normative control, etc. of cognitive information processing (Bartsch and Hübner 2005)?" For communication and training efforts to be effective across all populations, we need to look beyond standard definitions and data and ask ourselves: Do our messages generate empathy while teaching new skills and encouraging individual participation in development activities such as hand washing and condom use? If not, then the likelihood is that we are not nearly as effective as we could be. Illustrating empathy shows we understand and care about a person's condition. Rather than just messages about the germs and disease associated with the lack of proper hand washing, for example, what if our efforts to teach communities the value of clean hands also included a vision for their "why." Instead of just the standard "hand washing saves lives (Center for Disease Control 2012)" message, if we begin talking about our desire to see people have a healthy life free from disease so they can watch their children grow, and help their families and communities improve, the message then moves from being about not getting sick and possibly dying to one of what a healthy future might look like for them. This is helping the person, group, or community define its "why," which is more powerful because the message is about them in a personal way. Starting with a story that illustrates your understanding of another human being's situation is a persuasive way to generate empathy and encourage greater response to your message.

> *What good is an idea if it remains an idea? Try. Experiment. Iterate. Fail. Try again. Change the world. Simon Sinek*

Improving Our Effectiveness

Evaluating aid effectiveness should not only look at what has worked in the past that we can build on; such evaluations should also consider how we can look at things differently. There is so much more to our work than how many people we have trained or how many communities received a behavior change message. Our work is, and must be, about getting the kinds of results that come from reaching people on a personal level. Sometimes, the most effective way to do to that is by reaching a few people, or even just one at a time, with a message that really resonates so they take action. Little else is as empowering, easily implemented, or constructive as personal, emotion-driven communication. We need not abandon current development communication models which are working at the community level to involve stakeholders in messaging and planning. However, passionately augmenting these efforts will make the message more personable, relevant, and powerful to exact a level of lasting change. Personal, emotion-based communication built around storytelling is one such model. Employing this approach will require that we step out of our comfort zone, to be sure. It won't always be easy; there will be naysayers, perhaps even harsh critics, but that often happens with new techniques. That doesn't mean we shouldn't use our "why"; it just means we need to show disbelievers that it can and will work. Our continued efforts will help us reach the level of consensus needed to bring about real, lasting change. Communicating our stories and our missions, with emotion, will help us reach our audiences more effectively and likely on a much more profound level.

As you start to integrate your story into your work, remember:

1. What is it you want to communicate and why? What do you want to have happen?
2. Adapt your story to be relevant to your audience. How can your story help them?
3. Don't just share knowledge; show how you feel about your work. Show your vulnerability which can be a powerful tool for supporting an environment for change.
4. Ask emotion-based questions to understand personal, social, and environmental factors.
5. Think about how you can use your story to coach others to take action.

6. Think about mentoring a colleague in a developing country. It could be a great new story for you and the beginning of your mentee's own personal story that she will be able to use to motivate and inspire others.
7. Never underestimate the power of reaching others on an emotional level: **aid effectiveness starts with each of us**.

References

Baran, S. J., & Davis, S. J., (2012). *Mass communication theory: Foundations, ferment, and future* (6th ed., p. 298). Belmont, CA: Wadsworth; Schlinger, M. J. (1976). The role of mass communications in promoting public health. *Advances in Consumer Research, 3*, 302–305.

Bartsch, A., & Hübner, S. (2005). *Towards a theory of emotional communication*. Retrieved from http://docs.lib.purdue.edu/clcweb/vol7/iss4/

Beracochea, E. (2005). *Health for All NOW!* Fairfax, VA: MIDEGO.

Bessette, G. (2004). *Involving the community: A guide to participatory development communication*. Penang, Malaysia: International Development Research Centre. Retrieved August 19, 2012, from International Development Research Centre: http://www.idrc.ca/openebooks/066-7.

Center for Disease Control. (2012). Retrieved November 20, 2012, from http://www.cdc.gov/handhygiene/resources.html

Chandler, D. (1994). The transmission model of communication. University of Western Australia. Retrieved June 11, 2011.

Colin, F., & Villet, J. (1994). *Communication: A key to human development*. Retrieved August, 19, 2012, from http://www.fao.org/docrep/t1815e/t1815e01.htm

Ford, M. E. (1992). *Motivating humans: Goals, emotions, and personal agency beliefs* (pp. 40–41). Newbury Park, CA: Sage.

Foroohar, R. (2009, September 11). The real emerging market. *Newsweek Magazine*. Retrieved September 25, 2012, from http://www.thedailybeast.com/newsweek/2009/09/11/the-real-emerging-market.html

Glanz, K., Rimer, B. K., & Viswanath, K. (2008). *Health behavior and health education: Theory, research, and practice*. San Francisco: Jossey-Bass. Retrieved November 20, 2012, from http://www.med.upenn.edu/hbhe4/part4-ch16-macro-level-theories.shtml.

Good Reads. (2012). Retrieved November 20, 2012, from http://www.goodreads.com/quotes/34690-people-don-t-care-how-much-you-know-until-they-know

http://www.investopedia.com/terms/l/lastmile.asp#ixzz2DjEguWlk

Kharas, H. J., Makino, K., & Jung, W. (2011). *Catalyzing development: A new vision for aid* (pp. 114–117). Washington, DC: Brookings Institution Press.

Lewin, K. (1951). *Field theory in social science*. London: Social Science Paperbacks.

Maslow, A. (1954). *Motivation and personality*. New York: Harper.

Mathews, R., & Wacker, W. (2008). *What's your story? Storytelling to move markets, audiences, people, and brands* (p. 135). Upper Saddle River, NJ: FT Press.

Matthews, R., & Wacker, W. (2008). *What's your story? Storytelling to move markets, audiences*. Upper Saddle River, NJ: Pearson Education.

Meyer, J.-B. (2001). Network approach versus brain drain: Lessons from the Diaspora. *International Migration, 39*, 91–110.

Mezzana, D. (1996). Grass-roots communication in West Africa. In J. Servaes, T. Jacobson, & S. White (Eds.), *Participatory communication for social change* (pp. 183–196). New Delhi, India: Sage.

Roller, C. (2010). Abundance of choice and its effect on decision making. Retrieved August 20, 2012, from http://www.uxmatters.com/mt/archives/2010/12/abundance-of-choice-and-its-effect-on-decision-making.php

Selvaggio, K., Mehra, R., Sharma Fox, R., & Rao Gupta, G. (2008). *Value added: Women and U.S. foreign assistance for the 21st century*. Washington, DC: International Center for Research on Women. Retrieved September 25, 2012.

Sinek, S. (2009). *Start with why*. New York: Penguin.

Smith, P. (2012). *Lead with a story: A guide to crafting business narratives that captivate, convince, and inspire* (p. 3). New York: Amacom.

Sole, D. W., & Daniel, G. Storytelling in organizations: The power and traps of using stories to share knowledge in organizations. Retrieved August 20, 2012, from http://www.providersedge. com/docs/km_articles/storytelling_in_organizations.pdf

Stillman, L. J., (2005). Culture and communication: A study of NGO woman-to-woman communication styles at the United Nations. Retrieved September 25, 2012, from http://hss.ulb.uni-bonn.de/2005/0527/0527.pdf

The Aspen Institute. (2012). Retrieved November 20, 2012, from http://www.aspeninstitute.org/policy-work/global-health-development/our-breakthrough-solutions/reaching-last-mile-geography

The Examiner. (2012). Retrieved November 20, 2012, from http://www.examiner.com/article/people-don-t-care-how-much-you-know-until-they-know-how-much-you-care

Tichenor, P. J., Donohue, G. A., & Olien, C. N. (1970). Mass media flow and differential growth in knowledge. *Public Opinion Quarterly, 34*, 159–170.

Waisbord, S. (2008). The institutional challenges of participatory communication in international aid. *Social Identities, 14*(4), 505–522.

Chapter 24
Asking Effective, Powerful Questions

Deanna M. Crouse

Conversation taking place in a clinic in a rural town in a Southern African country.

"Good morning. How can I help you today, Mrs. Wojoke?" the health provider asked while closing the door to the consultation room and inviting Mrs. Wojoke to sit down. The health provider smiled and waited until Mrs. Wojoke spoke.

"I came because I am worried about my baby. Precious is not eating well. I do not seem to have enough milk. I think she is too skinny."

"I would be worried, too, if my baby is not well. I am glad you came to get help, Ms. Wojoke. Your baby is 5 days old. You are still recovering from the delivery. I know it was not easy for you to get here, and I am glad you could today. I want to help you and Precious. What do you think is the problem with Precious?" said the health provider.

"I think my milk is not good, you know ... ." Mrs. Wojoke was so upset she could not finish her thought.

"I see you are worried, Mrs. Wojoke. It is good you care about your baby. Tell me more."

"Well, I am (HIV) positive, you know, and I worry a lot that my milk is bad. And that is why Precious looks skinny. I am afraid. Maybe my baby has HIV, too," as more tears run down Mrs. Wojoke's cheeks.

The health provider, holding Mrs. Wojoke's hands in hers, tells Mrs. Wojoke to take her time. Mrs. Wojoke calms down and continues her story. "I remember the maternity nurse told me because I am positive I should only breastfeed Precious.

D.M. Crouse, M.H.S., C.H.E.S. (✉)
Independent Consultant
e-mail: deannamcrouse@gmail.com

© Springer Science+Business Media New York 2015
E. Beracochea (ed.), *Improving Aid Effectiveness in Global Health*,
DOI 10.1007/978-1-4939-2721-0_24

She said not to give Precious formula, gripe water, or anything else. Only my breast milk. But I am afraid I don't make enough milk. Precious looks too skinny. I think I should give her formula so will grow as strong as the other babies in my village. My husband and his mother say the baby is too skinny and she must be fed formula, but… oh, I just don't know what to do," Mrs. Wojoke says while wiping her tears with her hand.

In this story, while the answers to Mrs. Wojoke's concerns about breastfeeding Precious can be answered with the surety of a medical protocol for the treatment and prevention of the transmission of HIV, of equal importance is helping Mrs. Wojoke better understand the social and cultural environment in which she lives. Through effective, powerful questioning, Mrs. Wojoke can learn about the "forces" that impact her choices and behaviors caring for Precious—and maybe even uncover how she wants to address them.

More than ever in today's global health environment, the basic principal of medical care—do no harm—must be broadened to include the social structures underlying causes of diseases and behavioral choices. The two go hand-in-hand. One way to help individuals and communities to broaden their understanding is for the global health workers to learn the power of questioning.

Why Asking Effective, Powerful Questions Is IMPORTANT in Global Health

The challenges global health workers face are many whether we are based in our home country in the industrialized world or in the field working hand-in-hand with our colleagues and those we serve. We work in countries ravaged with disease, epidemics, poverty, and food and political insecurities. We help deliver health prevention and curative services. We share our knowledge and experiences to strengthen health programs, policy, and service delivery systems. We collaborate on research activities. We work in rural areas where it can take days for the sick to get to a clinic and in overcrowded urban areas where hundreds of thousands of people migrate and may still find a shortage of health services.

All too often, our global health challenges are reduced to stories of dependency on international aid, greed, and corruption. At the same time, governments and their people often express the sentiment they have the know-how to fix their own problems. Still, for at least a half century, global health workers have been providing guidance and technical assistance for improving health. With the passing of each decade and each year we strive to do our work even better.

Today, we are bombarded with health data and instant information. *Everything* seems to be tracked and measured in our mobile and social media worlds. While we may see health improvements, we wonder whether the overabundance of information is the foundation for our success and whether it leads us to better decision making. Some have challenged that more information does not lead to making better decisions and suggest, rather, that it leads to thinking that is less clear and creative (Frank and Magnone 2011). Leaders across all disciplines recognize that to get meaningful answers we need to ask effective, powerful questions.

Global health programs are developed and planned based on clinically sound practices and research evidence. Often, cultural and behavioral objectives are part of the design. We know that funders—generally from Western cultures—develop interventions that tend to focus on individual risk factors. In many non-Western cultures, disease is a part of one's whole life (Azétop and Rennie 2010). That is, poor living conditions; inadequate health delivery systems; social inequality, myths and misconceptions about disease; or the expectation one's family has a say as to what should be done—taken together—are what make people vulnerable to disease. Under this paradigm individuals may feel they have little or no control over their health decisions and actions. Given these forces—the complexities of addressing the wider socioeconomic, cultural, and political barriers—make it more important than ever to ask effective, powerful questions in the search for meaningful answers for improving health conditions.

Is There a Difference Between a Question and an Effective, Powerful Question?

Yes, there is. A question asked with purpose—an effective, powerful question—opens a conversation to brainstorming an idea; discussing creative ways (thinking "outside the box") to solve a problem, resolving conflicts, negotiating. Effective, powerful questions are formulated for exploration, analyzing, evaluating, and inspiring action—indeed, for moving forward.

The literature on effective, powerful questions is prolific and found across many disciplines, such as education, business, marketing, and coaching. For example, the education sector has explored extensively the types of powerful questions that will engage students in the learning process. The most widely accepted framework is Benjamin Bloom's Taxonomy of the hierarchy of questions, which was first developed in the 1950s and is used today across disciplines (Canadian Education Association 2012; Hurley and Brown 2009). Dr. Bloom's hierarchy of questions is most frequently depicted in the pyramid in Box 25.1. At the bottom of the pyramid are knowledge-based facts and recall-type questions. Further up the pyramid are the questions asked for higher-level thinking skills and more complex responses—the ones for brainstorming, thinking outside the box, and problem solving (Box 25.1).

Box 24.1: Benjamin Bloom's Hierarchy of Questions

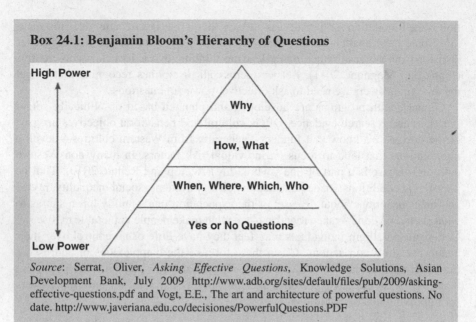

Source: Serrat, Oliver, *Asking Effective Questions*, Knowledge Solutions, Asian Development Bank, July 2009 http://www.adb.org/sites/default/files/pub/2009/asking-effective-questions.pdf and Vogt, E.E., The art and architecture of powerful questions. No date. http://www.javeriana.edu.co/decisiones/PowerfulQuestions.PDF

Researchers have put much thought into understanding what forms effective, powerful questions. From interviews conducted around the world the following themes emerged (Box 25.2):

Box 24.2: Themes of an Effective, Powerful Question

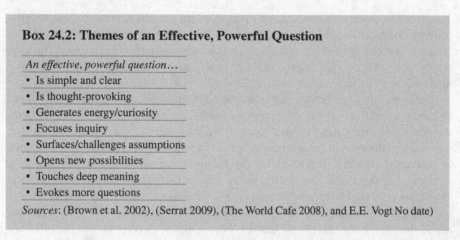

An effective, powerful question…
- Is simple and clear
- Is thought-provoking
- Generates energy/curiosity
- Focuses inquiry
- Surfaces/challenges assumptions
- Opens new possibilities
- Touches deep meaning
- Evokes more questions

Sources: (Brown et al. 2002), (Serrat 2009), (The World Cafe 2008), and E.E. Vogt No date)

Box 25.3 shows examples of questions that are powerful and not powerful. This instructional module was designed to help students learn to formulate effective, powerful questions. The "not powerful questions," are at the lower end of Bloom's taxonomy of hierarchal questions—that is, questions that are asked for facts or recall. The "powerful" questions are toward the top of the pyramid and ask for deeper thinking and complex responses (Box 25.3).

> ## Box 24.3: Examples of Powerful and Not Powerful Questions
>
> | Powerful questions | Not powerful questions |
> | --- | --- |
> | How did you decide that you wanted to do this job? | What is your job? |
> | What is the hardest part about your job? | What is your favorite hobby? |
> | What is the most interesting thing you do at work? | How long have you been working at your job? |
>
> *Source*: Excerpts from *Modelling the Tools*, Session 3, 2008. *LearnAlberta*, Department of Education, Alberta, Canada. http://www.learnalberta.ca/content/ssmt/html/docs/asking-powerfulquestions.pdf

One, Two, Three: The Basic Elements of Effective, Powerful Questions

One	Ask open-ended questions	Open-ended questions cannot be answered with a "yes" or "no." They bring energy and focus attention to the conversation. They elicit a wide range of possibilities. You can be sure that "yes/no" questions will cut short your conversation.
Two	No leading questions	Leading questions are asked in such a way that the questioner gets a desired response. It's a clever way to bring the listener around to the questioner's way of thinking. Rather, strive to help the listener uncover their own answers and solutions.
Three	No assumptions	Don't assume there is one right answer or one right way to do something. Keep asking questions. Suspend your own judgment and ways of thinking. Be assured common themes *will* emerge that will identify problems and ways to resolve them.

Examples

One	Open-ended questions	First, the close-ended (yes/no) question:
		Did you order the ART (antiretroviral therapy) drugs?
		Now, the open-ended question:
		Why did you order ART this week? (The answer should give an explanation for different situations, such as shortage of storage space, increased number of patients who screened HIV-positive over the past month/quarter, changes in revised ART guidelines, increased/decreased funds, etc.)
Two	No leading questions	First, the leading question:
		We can store our ART drugs in the second floor, don't you think? (The answer can only be a yes or no.)
		Now, the non-leading question:
		Where do you feel is the best and safest place to store our ART drugs? (The answer requires thought and an explanation as to why the place would be the best and safest.)

(continued)

Three	No assumptions	First, the assumption question
		How can we get the Igbo people in Gnifu Town to start their ART drugs? (This assumes only Igbo tested HIV-positive. People screened for HIV are identified by a number not by name or ethnic group. Those who tested HIV-positive in Gnifu Town would be Igbo and other groups living in Gnifu Town.)
		Now, the questions without assumption
		What do you think we can do to encourage Gnifu Town to help its citizens understand the importance of taking ARTs? (The answer shifts the "problem" from focusing on one group of people to opening a discussion for community education/action.)

Caution About "Why" Questions

Although the "why" question is powerful, be aware that to some asking "why" can make a person feel accused of something; that he or she has done something wrong. The person being asked the "why" question may expect the questioner has a specific ("right") answer that she does not know. A "why" question that has a negative connotation can become an effective, powerful. "How" question (see Box 25.4).

Box 24.4: A "Why" Question Becoming Even More Powerful

<u>Scene</u>: The mother, who is HIV positive, wanted to be sure her baby would not become infected with HIV and agreed she would breastfeed for 6 months as recommended by the PMTCT (Prevention of mother-to-child transmission of HIV) nurse at the maternity clinic (also the national guideline).

In month two after the delivery, the PMTCT community health worker arrived at the mother's village for her regularly scheduled visits. The community health worker was alarmed when she saw the mother bottle-feeding her baby and an empty box of formula setting on the table next to her.

Do not ask this *why* question	Rephrase the *why* question
Why did you bottle-feed your baby? You know your baby could get sick.	What is the most difficult thing for you about breastfeeding your baby?

The "do not" why question makes assumptions: the mother is feeding her baby formula because the PMTCT health worker sees the bottle and formula on the table when she arrives. The CHW also assumes the mother has not recalled correctly the information about exclusive breastfeeding for 6 months in her education session at the maternity ward.

The "rephrase" why question makes no assumptions. By asking more questions the PMTCT health worker will be able to learn more about the mother's experiences and, together identify the problems and solutions.

Culture and Language Matter in Asking Effective, Powerful Questions

Global health takes us to all continents where we work among diverse populations from a mix of cultures, ethnicities, and languages. Many global health workers speak local language and are very familiar with local cultures. This is very helpful, but we still need to be sensitive to a range of barriers (political, service delivery, health policies), and local traditions, attitudes, and values.

- **Do not assume common understanding of words**. Many of our country colleagues do speak English, but their English has been learned in different cultures and contexts than our own. Be sure everyone understands the words you use. If you sense the group is not getting what you say, it's probably true. Speak more slowly. Search for other words. Ask group members to repeat (in their own words) their understanding of what has been said. Be ready to say in different words what you have already said. Be patient. Be sure that all in the group are "on the same page."
- **Be aware that cultural "norms" do not apply to the behavior of a particular individual**. Each of us are shaped by our education, ethnicity, how and where we were raised, and the customs and values instilled in us. Simply put, respect others' opinions and how they are expressed. Do not assume one speaks for all.
- **Be aware of your body language and tone of voice**. Body language can be more powerful than the words we speak; let your body language and tone of voice "speak" to your authenticity and genuine caring.

Getting Ready for the Conversation

The following summarizes getting ready for a conversation (or meeting). Online sources that may be helpful include The World Cafe (www.theworldcafe.com/pdfs/cafetogo.pdf) and The Community Tool Box, Chap. 16 (http://ctb.ku.edu/en).

- Prepare the questions in advance. Know the purpose of the conversation (e.g., is it to explore ideas/finding insights; focus attention on a particular situation; launch a new initiative; or problem solving)
- Start with the big picture question and deepen the conversation to the "by using" prompts. For example:

General question	What do you believe are the two most important things we can do to improve care of new mothers and babies in our clinic?
Drill-down—Prompt #1	If you could improve one of these things, right now, what would it be?
Drill-down—Prompt #2	What are the 2–3 challenges you face to accomplish this?
Drill-down—Prompt #3	What changes do you think are needed to address these challenges?

- Decide who will participate, facilitate, and take notes (one-on-one or group)
- Keep the conversation group small: 5–6 people ideal
- Set a place, date, time

Starting the Conversation

(a) **Open to grace**
- **Explain why the conversation is important**. For example, tie the conversation to a health improvement identified by the community, a new initiative by the Ministry of Health, etc. When it makes sense explain the evidence/data that supports health improvement.
- **Put people at ease**. The group will most likely see you as the expert, the evaluator, a person of authority whether or not you are. Share something personal about yourself (see Box 25.5).

Box 24.5: Personal Sharing Tips
- Describe where you live in your home country. Find the common denominator to the lives of the people in your group. Do you also live in a rural area? An urban area? How similar or different is it compared to the community where you are now?
- Talk about your family in a general way. Family life is very important in most cultures. It makes no difference about your marital status or children status—people are interested in knowing something about your family life.
- Explain why you do the work you do and its importance to you.

- **Be curious and engaged**. You will find something you didn't know that could be important to the topic or an eye-opening story about the community/people in the group.
- **Be clear**. Not only should your questions be simply stated and easily understood, but state clearly it is each person's ideas, opinions, and experiences that are important. He or she is the expert, not you.
- **Believe in your group** (or individual). Most likely they have the answer to the challenges and problems under discussion. Your "job" is to help them uncover their own solutions and inspire to do things they never imagined.
- **Be respectful**. Participants may not be comfortable with or have the experience answering powerful questions. Give everyone the opportunity to speak.
- **Listen respectfully**. Be aware of taboo topics that you might have to talk about in the conversation. Be sure that each person in your group is comfortable giving their opinions.

(b) **Check assumptions**
    As global health workers our job is to elicit information, to learn from our counterparts, communities, and individuals and help them "learn" from their own words and ideas.
- **Verify what you hear**. Restate, follow-up, repeat, and ask more questions—"drill-down".

- **Check your own assumptions and biases**. We all have them. Our own opinions and beliefs must be set aside.
- **Respect silence**. Let people take the time needed to get their thoughts together to be said to the group. Do not assume "quiet" people have nothing to say. Sometimes you may need to encourage a participant to complete their thought. Give the "quiet" person the opportunity to talk (Box 25.6).

Box 24.6: A Note About Listening Skills and Asking Powerful Questions
Silence is one of four listening skills that are a part of asking powerful questions (Leonard et al. 2012). The three other skills are articulating, clarifying, and being curious—

Articulating. This is when we repeat back to a participant what we believe he means. This helps him feel "heard." For example, as a facilitator, we would say, "What I hear you saying is ..."

Clarifying. This is when we assist a participant who is vague or does not understand for herself. A facilitator makes a suggestion. For example, facilitator could say, "Here is what I hear you saying (say it). Is that right?" Clarifying and articulating may seem the same, but clarifying combines both articulation and clarification.

Being curious. This is about not making assumptions. Wait to hear what is actually being said. Do not assume you know what the participant(s) are going to tell you. Use your curiosity to explore the answers given and ask more questions to get more clarity.

Ending the Conversation

- Allow time to wrap up the conversation and, as necessary, state any follow-up steps. Engage the participants by asking if they want to add or clarify anything you have summarized.
- Write up the conversation notes and, as needed, share them with participants within 2–5 work days.

Summary

This chapter is a short guide about asking powerful and effective questions and explains their importance. Practice will help you find the effective questions that work best in your situation. Effective, powerful questions can be applied to any aspect of our global health work as we engage with our country counterparts, stakeholders, community leaders, individuals, and possibly, those we coach online.

Effective, powerful question can be applied one-on-one and with groups. We urge you to review the sources at the end of this chapter. Some of them offer toolkits with in-depth approaches to asking questions, managing conversation groups, and up-to-date information about working in a multicultural world.

Asking effective, powerful questions is a conscientious way to ask questions that will get meaningful answers. They are simple and clear; thought-provoking. Effective, powerful questions generate curiosity, focus the discussion, challenge assumptions, and lead to more questions to get to the heart of the matter. They inspire people to take action to do things they never imagined they could do.

Be clear about the purpose of the question you are planning to ask; thoughtful in preparing them; and be ready to "drill-down" for more detail. Powerful questions engage participants to think creatively, to express their ideas and opinions, to inspire fresh thinking, and to learn that one's own knowledge and wisdom will lead to the solutions that make a difference in improving health.

Powerful questioning leads to genuine and authentic collaboration, which will be successful when based on a sense of common purpose, trust, and respect.

Overcoming social and cultural barriers requires patience, practice, and determination. We need to be especially respectful and sensitive when we work in societies and cultures different from our own. The best approach to improving health resides within the societies and cultures in which we work.

Suggested Reading

University of Kansas, The Community Tool Box. (2012). The Community Tool Box is a global resource for free information on essential skills for building healthy communities. It offers more than 7,000 pages of practical guidance in creating change and improvement. Retrieved from http://ctb.ku.edu/en

References

Azétop, J., & Rennie, S. (2010). Principlism, medical individualism, and health promotion in resource–poor settings: Can autonomy-based bioethics promote social justice and population health? *Philosophy, Ethics, and Humanities in Medicine, 5*, 1. Retrieved from http://www.peh-med.com/content/5/1/1.

Brown, J., et al. (2002). Strategic questioning: Engaging people's best thinking. *The Systems Thinker, 13*(9), 2–6. Pegasus Communication. Retrieved from http://www.theworldcafe.com/articles/strategicquestion.pdf.

Canadian Education Association. (2012). Engaging students through effective questions, education Canada. *52*(5). Retrieved from http://www.cea-ace.ca/education-canada/article/engaging-students-through-effective-questions

Frank, C. J., & Magnone, P. F. (2011). *Drinking from the fire hose: Making smarter decisions without drowning in information*. New York: Portfolio/Penguin. Retrieved from http://www.firehosethebook.com/images/Drinking_from_the_Fire_Hose_Excerpt.pdf.

Hurley, T. J., & Brown, J. (2009). Conversational leadership: Thinking together for a change. *The Systems Thinker, 20*(90), 2–7. Pegasus Communication. Retrieved from http://www.theworld-cafe.com/articles/Conversational-Leadership.pdf.

Leonard, I. (n.d.). The art of effective questioning: Asking the right question for the desired result. Seattle, WA: Coaching for Change. Retrieved September 2012, from http://www.coachingfor-change.com/pub10.html

Serrat, O. (2009). *Asking effective questions, knowledge solutions*. Manila, Philippines: Asian Development Bank. Retrieved from http://www.adb.org/sites/default/files/pub/2009/asking-effective-questions.pdf.

The World Café. (2008). *A quick reference guide for putting conversations to work*. Retrieved from http://www.theworldcafe.com/pdfs/cafetogo.pdf

Vogt, E. E. (n.d.). The art and architecture of powerful questions. Retrieved from http://www.javeriana.edu.co/decisiones/PowerfulQuestions.PDF

Chapter 25
Lessons on Sustainability and Effectiveness

Barry Karlin

Numerous public health and development colleagues can readily present valid lists of factors associated with program success and failure, citing experiences throughout the world. Rather than going down that path or attempting to summarize such experiences, this chapter presents a program effectiveness framework by comparing experiences in two sharply contrasting countries, Thailand and Haiti, each with its own unique history, culture, and resources. We can begin with a few health statistics[1]:

Health-related factors	Thailand	Haiti
Potable water (%)	98	58
Improved sanitation (%)	96	17
Infant mortality	16.4 (2011)	54.0
Under-5 deaths/1,000 live births	21 (2011)	87 (1990)
Life expectancy at birth	73.6 years (2011)	61 years (1990)
Percent of routine vaccinations financed by government	90 %+	0 %

Why such startling differences? Haiti's soil and climate are no worse than Thailand's. Haitians certainly work as hard as Thais do. They love their children as much as Thais and all dream of better lives. Yet Haiti's infants die at over three times the rate as Thai infants do, and the average Thai lives almost 14 years longer than Haitians.

Here are a few key facts which help explain these differences:

---

[1] Data drawn from W.H.O. and UNICEF sources, and publications of Thailand's Ministry of Health.

B. Karlin (✉)
University of Colorado, Denver, CO 80203, USA
e-mail: vbkarlin@aol.com

© Springer Science+Business Media New York 2015
E. Beracochea (ed.), *Improving Aid Effectiveness in Global Health*,
DOI 10.1007/978-1-4939-2721-0_25

Haiti

(a) *Population origins and history*: Haiti was enslaved by France for decades. After the African slaves revolted in 1790 and, amazingly, in 1804, became the only slave nation to win its freedom, the young Haitian nation was forced to pay huge reparations to France, thus helping to keep it in poverty.

(b) *War and external occupation*: In 1919, during a period of unrest, the United States sent in the marines who occupied Haiti until 1935 (see "References" below). This history of occupations kept the Government of Haiti weak, limiting health and other social services, and hindering its ability to respond to emergencies such as earthquakes, hurricanes, and outbreaks of cholera and other diseases.

(c) *Economic exploitation*: France exploited Haiti for sugar and other crops, bringing in some 700,000 African slaves, many of whom were worked to death. Haiti, being a new black republic with a history of violence, was not attractive to outsiders, investors, educators, or other immigrants, in sharp contrast to the Dominican and other nearby nations.

(d) *Foreign relations*: Given its history of violent revolt, Haiti has been viewed by the United States and other governments as a place where communism might take hold and which could set an unwelcome example for other nations struggling for political and economic independence. Such viewpoints increased a willingness to accept ruthless Haitian governments which could suppress such influences and which were not interested in providing social services, including health. Rather than invest in human resources, rural infrastructure, or health facilities, investments in urban factories became dominant (see Rotberg 1971).

(e) *Natural disasters and disease outbreaks*: Following the 2010 earthquake, Haiti's extremely weak central government, further damaged by the quake, was unable to cope. As a result, the number of external nongovernmental organizations increased to an estimated 10,000–12,000, often working with little coordination, and with no guiding national health plan.

Thailand

(a) Thailand has never been colonized. Early contacts with foreigners included having American missionaries introduce smallpox immunizations and ether in 1838. One result has been a willingness to accept or reject foreign innovations on their perceived merit.

(b) The Thai royal family instigated building the first public hospital and a nursing school in 1895.

(c) Prince Mahidol, later King of Siam, graduated *cum laude* from Harvard in the early 1900s.

(d) With its concern for social conditions of rural Thais, as well as concern about revolutionary movements in Asia, the Government of Thailand signed an agreement with USAID in 1957 to initiate a Village Health and Sanitation Project (VHS). It began in the poorest region, the Northeast, and quickly expended to remaining rural areas.

(e) The VHS Project received guidance and support from American health advisors but the Thai Government remained fully in charge of the program.

(f) The VHS Project began with guidance from social scientists who studied rural Thai beliefs and practices related to health, as well as rural social organizational patterns. These insights were incorporated into training manuals developed by Thai health officials. Their content including ways of identifying respected local leaders, training villagers to map their communities, and to identify their own health-related priorities. Women played important roles, as did local teachers, children, and religious leaders.

(g) Thai Ministry of Health officials were strongly committed to improving health conditions in rural areas. Top Thai officials made regular visits to rural areas to identify existing needs and shortcomings, and to provide ongoing support.

(h) The VHS Project began by focusing on clean and conveniently located water. People preferred the taste of traditional pond water but they respected the advice of Thai health educators and sanitation workers. Such a willingness to change ancient practices was remarkable, keeping in mind that there was not even a common Thai word for "germs."

(i) The Project focused equally on safe disposal of human waste, coming up with a hand-flush squat-place water-seal latrine which the people greatly admired, not because of "germs" but because it was modern, odorless, and could be placed right next to their homes or under homes build on stilts. At the beginning of the Project, very few rural Thai families had access to potable water and sanitary latrines. Now, virtually every Thai family has such access.

(j) Once water and sanitation efforts gained ground, the Project went on to address MCH issues, nutrition, emergency care, immunizations, and so forth. Villagers felt pride and empowered in their efforts. At this moment, Thailand has over 800,000 trained Village Health Volunteers… the backbone of Thailand's health system. They are trained in skills such as identifying signs of high-risk pregnancies, keeping track of immunization status, and first aid. Every community is reported to have cell phones which can summon free and rapid ambulance services. The people's demand for decent health services eventually led to their government providing good quality free health care for all Thai citizens.

Should one ask Thai health officials about their rural sanitation staff, one is likely to get the reply: "What sanitation workers? That group worked their way out of their jobs long ago!" Present concerns have to do with chronic diseases, childhood obesity, traffic accidents, and the use of illegal drugs. HIV/AIDS and tobacco use remain problematic but Government policies and programs have been outstanding. As a result of early screening and drug treatment, almost no Thai infants are reported to be HIV-positive at birth. However, maternal mortality rates remain relatively high and mental health continues to be of concern.

Summary of factors which impact on health status

Factors	Haiti	Thailand
External exploitation	Yes	No
Significant history of violence	Yes	No
Being colonized	Yes	No
Significant despoiling of environment	Yes	No
Leaders with commitment to rural population	No	Yes
National control of health model	Limited	Yes
Strong public health leadership by nationals	No	Yes
Early emphasis on public health, disease prevention, water, and sanitation	No	Yes
Effective responses to epidemics, disasters	No	Yes
Strong national community development	No	Yes
Emphasis on sustainability and replication	No	Yes
Equitable distribution of wealth	No	Weakening
Democratic traditions	Weak	Relatively strong

The Government of Thailand and its Ministry of Health will continue to face challenges but are well prepared, as was demonstrated by their effective responses in the area of Phuket in the south following the great tsunami of 2005, in sharp contrast to post-earthquake events in Haiti only a few years ago.

This paper makes a number of references to program sustainability and replication. It suggests that these qualities are enhanced when a national government such that of Thailand has the ability to design and control its own health policies and system, while still being open to guidance from external donors. Problems associated with permitting external donors and experts to have major control of local projects is that, while their contributions may be quite effective on a relatively small scale, national leaders may have only limited knowledge and involvement in such projects. In addition, foreign workers from nations such as the United States may bring with them traditional suspicions of national models, preferring instead to design and test nongovernmental health systems. Replication on a national level becomes problematic, even when their concepts are quite sound. Publications of The Aga Khan Foundation offers such an example (Primary health care management advancement programme 2003).

Factors related to why health projects fail are similar to the broader question regarding why nations fail. For detailed discussions, see Acemoglu and Robinson (2012) as well as detailed reviews of their book by Diamond and others (Diamond n.d.). These authors examine institutional, political, social, cultural, and geographic factors associated with success and failure. These are complicated issues with which agents of change need to be familiar if they hope to achieve sustainability and replication.

Permit me to offer a small example of a cultural factor. When I arrived in Thailand in 1959 as a USAID advisor to the Ministry of Health, my first request to the Provincial Health Officer in Korat, Dr. Chek, was for an inventory of the contents of the warehouse so that I could begin requisitioning additional supplies. I asked if the inventory could be ready in 2 weeks. He smiled and assured me that it could. Two and then 3 weeks passed without the inventory. Had he forgotten my request? Was he ignoring it? Fortunately, I asked a Thai sanitarian rather than Dr. Chek directly and was told that such an inventory would take much longer but that it would have been impolite to tell me "no." I quickly learned that social and professional relationships are always more important than given tasks and deadlines!

References

(2003). *Primary health care management advancement programme*. Aga Khan Foundation.

Acemoglu, D., & Peterson, J. (2012). *Why nations fail*. New York: Crown Books.

Collapse, Jared Diamond, Penguin Group, USA. (2005). (See Chapter 11, "One Island, Two Peoples, Two Histories: The Dominican Republic and Haiti". Also see: *Questioning Collapse* by Patricia A. McNany and Norman Yofee, Cambridge University Press, 2010, Chapter 10.)

Danner, M. (2009). *Stripping bare the body*. New York: Nation Books.

Diamond, J. (n.d.). Why nations fail. *New York Review of Books*. 8/16/12.

Farmer, P. (2005). *Pathologies of power: Health, human rights, and the new war on the poor*. Berkeley, CA: University of California Press.

Haiti: Where did the money go? This excellent film is available from www.filmat11.com

Rotberg, R. I. (1971). *Haiti: The politics of squalor*. Boston: Houghton Mifflin.

Textor, R. B., et al. (1958). Manual for rural community health worker in Thailand. Thailand Department of Health. USAID: Thai-American Audiovisual Service.

Chapter 26
What Can Global Health Professionals Do to Improve Effectiveness

Elvira Beracochea and Aaron Pied

> We will have time to reach the Millennium Development Goals—worldwide and in most, or even all, individual countries—but only if we break with business as usual. (From the Address to St. Paul's Cathedral Event on the Millennium Development Goals, by Secretary General Kofi Annan, 2005 United Nations. Reprinted with Permission of the United Nations.) **United Nations Secretary General, Kofi Annan** G8 summit 2005.

Your Global Health Career

Let's start with me, Aaron Pied. I began my international development career as a Peace Corps Volunteer in Burkina Faso where I taught English and assisted with health campaigns to fight guinea worm and HIV/AIDS. I was later exposed to the economics of development while supporting research initiatives in Washington DC and later health financing programs. In between I spent years in Thailand, on the border with Myanmar, working at the national and local levels to assist refugees and migrants in their search to find a better life.

In my 14-year career, I was fortunate to get a perspective on development work from the field and policy levels. Like many in my cohort of young professionals in development, I have already encountered turning points in my career: deciding that teaching was not a good fit for me after returning from Burkina Faso, and more recently, transitioning from program management to a greater role in operations. I have been fortunate with my current employment at Realizing Global Health

E. Beracochea • A. Pied (✉)
Realizing Global Health Inc., Olley Lane 4710, Fairfax, VA 22032, USA
e-mail: aaron@realizingglobalhealth.com

© Springer Science+Business Media New York 2015
E. Beracochea (ed.), *Improving Aid Effectiveness in Global Health*,
DOI 10.1007/978-1-4939-2721-0_26

(RGH), a global health consulting company, to have the freedom and opportunity to combine my education and health interests and develop skills to improve my effectiveness and contribution in the advancement of the global health agenda.

Thirty years ago I (Elvira Beracochea) became a doctor because I wanted to save lives, and after a few years of practice, I got my Master's degree in public health because I wanted to save more lives. I later transitioned to work in global health because I wanted to make a bigger impact and help save even more lives. I have been involved in many global health projects and worked in academia, nonprofit sector as well as hospital manager and healthcare provider throughout my career.

There have been several turning points and roadblocks I have had to overcome. Let me tell you about my experience 12 years ago, when I had the honor of managing a project in Angola that expanded my mission in global health and led me to realize the importance and personal responsibility of improving my professional effectiveness. This project had a very effective expatriate director, whom I supervised, and who led an effective team consisting of more than 20 motivated and empowered young Angolan professionals, whose goal was to restore health services in one of the provinces most affected by the civil war. In just 12 months, where there had previously been no healthcare, there were 35 facilities delivering quality healthcare. Supplies were being delivered and staff were trained and motivated to overcome any challenge. They were enthusiastic and their enthusiasm was contagious at a time when hope and enthusiasm were much needed. The project team was also able to gather hundreds of people when they visited villages to promote healthy practices and timely use of the health facilities. In fact, when they went to every village, they were welcomed as close members of their communities. Many years later, I went back to some of the project villages and the communities still remembered the project and the enthusiasm of the team.

Unfortunately, this project ended after 12 months because the donor's priorities changed and they did not continue the funding. After a gap of about 2 years, the donor once again changed its priorities and started another project—from scratch and without building on the prior project's achievements or its lessons learned.

This experience of having a project end without ensuring the sustainability of the results achieved was very painful because we had to dismantle all the previous work and disband the team. However, my failure to convince the donor of the importance of sustaining the achievements made, and of the need for transferring the systems put in place in the 35 health centers to the Angolan health authorities so they could continue the work that the project had started, taught me some important lessons about effectiveness.

This experience led me to work for the last 12 years to find better ways to be effective, and expand my career mission to make sure this failure—of not strengthening the country's health system in a sustainable manner—did not happen again. This is the lesson I want to share with you so you do not have to go through it. Malcolm Gladwell in his book "Outliers" said it takes 10,000 h to become an expert in any field (Gladwell 2008). Well, I have more than that, and I am going to gift you my 10,000 h on effectiveness.

Professional Effectiveness

The way to improve your professional effectiveness is to develop and implement a career plan that delivers effective global health results and provides you with the satisfaction of a job well done. Before you begin to develop your career plan, you must figure out your strengths and weaknesses so you can build upon and lead with your strengths. More on strengths later. Having a written career plan will help you keep track of your progress to identify what is keeping you back so you can make changes where necessary.

The most important thing to remember is that you are not alone. In fact, you don't become effective on your own. You need to surround yourself with a team of peers, mentors and coaches, who help keep you moving forward through the various stages of your career. *My (Elvira) colleagues in Angola helped me realize my lack of effectiveness and to discover the Paris Declaration which I made my own and whose principles I apply every day.* There are always people along the way who can provide advice or suggestions and help you see your situation from a different perspective and find ways to make it better and you more effective. Do not disregard their support and views. Use them to become more effective.

Sometimes we choose our career because we have realized what our passion is and sometimes we fall into a career by necessity, by convenience, or just by accident (Karlin 2013). Most of us find ourselves somewhere between loving what we do and lacking satisfaction with our career and trying to find ways to motivate ourselves to deliver an effective performance. It is our job to make sure we truly love our career. If you do not truly love what you do, you won't get the results you want to achieve. In fact, if you do not love what you do, it is a sign it is time to change course because you are not being effective.

Sadly, we have all seen the results of not truly loving global health work— unsatisfied employees or coworkers who become negative and toxic to those around them. They typically have a bad attitude, poor performance below their potential, and no apparent motivation to achieve an effective sustainable result. Perhaps, they don't even know how to do a good job and do not care. They may not naturally be like this (though there will always be some that are negative and ineffective in all they do in life), but they are placed in the wrong job and the fact is that not everyone is right for every job. In any case, ineffectiveness cannot be accepted in our field of global health because it wastes valuable resources and costs lives.

To be effective you need to be satisfied and successful in your work, and to be satisfied and successful you must be effective. How can that be achieved? First, you need to remember your mission (Smith 2013) and why you chose a career in global health. Remind yourself of the reason you chose this career.

For me personally (Elvira), nothing gives me more satisfaction and inspires me to do my job more than helping my colleagues in developing countries improve how they work and become outstanding healthcare providers. You too might find inspiration in the work of others. We have all had an experience or met someone that inspired us to help others improve their health. You just need to remember that feeling of passion and keep it alive every day.

Another way to keep your career mission alive is to often ask yourself if in 30 or 40 years from now you will be proud of the career choices and the impact you've made. Is what you are doing now in line with what you wanted your career to be about? If not, figure out what you like, and do not like about your current work and start looking for your dream job or next assignment. If you do not have a job yet, figure out who has your "dream" job and what you like about it. Be clear about what you do not like and do not compromise. If you are still a student, start looking now for your dream job and start applying for volunteer work or summer internships in those organizations.

Second, get clear on what your strengths and weaknesses are. We all have strengths and weaknesses. Lead with your strengths. Your strengths are what make you unique and effective, work on making them even better and use them to explore different opportunities for what a successful career means to you. Use your strengths to choose the next career step that is right for you.

For example, in the Strength Finder test (Rath 2007), my main strength is "Relator." I am (Elvira) good at finding relations and patterns in apparently disconnected things, events or issues. This strength makes me a very effective problemsolver and good at explaining how things work in simple ways so people understand easily. So I focus my work on doing that instead of doing things I am not wired to do well. So, know your strengths and use them.

Knowing your weaknesses too will help you surround yourself with a team that is strong in those areas you are not (Rath 2007). Each person has a unique ability and you are doing a disservice to your organization and yourself if you are not making the best of it and waste your talent doing things you are not good at. It may seem scary at times because you may not have applied your strengths in this way before, but remember you do not have to do this alone. In global health, we must be effective team players and allow ourselves to focus and improve on what you are good at and enjoy doing.

Third, no matter where you are in your career, your performance and effectiveness is tied to your mindset and personal definitions of what it means to be successful. Therefore, you need to develop and maintain a flexible mindset and stay open to change (Dweck 2006). You may be afraid of change but we want to encourage you to see change as an opportunity to do more, and do it better. Don't stay in your comfort zone and let fear of change stop you. Keep your mind open to opportunities that present themselves for you to do things differently and more effectively because you don't always know how the potential change will affect your career, the organization you work for, and the lives you save.

For example, I (Aaron Pied) went to live in Burkina Faso as a volunteer with the United States Peace Corps 2 weeks after completing my undergraduate degree. I was excited to meet new people, learn a new language, and experience another part of the world. I had no idea how it would change me. I went with few expectations and a flexible mindset that I was simply exploring and seeking knowledge and experience. This way, the anger, fear, stress and other negative feelings that can arise when one is traveling somewhere foreign and unknown, that could have prevented me from being effective, were transformed into positive feelings. I embraced the excitement, mystery and intrigue that you experience only from something new, that you would normally never do, as well as the satisfaction of having improved someone else's life.

Living and travelling overseas with the desire to experience new things allowed me to learn different points of view and start lifelong friendships that changed my life. I came to understand that misunderstanding is usually not intentional, but comes from limited experience and knowledge, and often dictated by a fear grown from past negative life experiences. My Peace Corps service was a major turning point in my life but I had no idea that it would change the focus of my career—from a teacher in the United States to an international development professional. The simple act of leaving my own country and meeting hundreds of new people, motivated me to change and explore alternative careers.

Fourth, join professional organizations and attend their events not only to learn but also to network with your colleagues and peers. We suggest you join the Global Health Council (www.globalhealth.org), the International Health and Nutrition Group at the Society for International Development in Washington (www.sidw.org), and the International Health Section of the American Public Health Association (www.apha.org). Your enthusiasm for change and effectiveness will be renewed as you get involved in these organizations.

Fifth, keep a high level of motivation (Pink 2009) to do more and to do it better and use that to keep moving forward. We are all motivated by different things, and our definitions of success and what motivates us will likely change throughout the four main career stages: New Professional, Innovator, Expert, and Visionary. However, you must feel motivated to have the energy and enthusiasm to take effective action every day in global health.

As we develop in our careers, we encounter different challenges that may drain our motivation. We want you to be aware of that and see challenges as potential breakthroughs and opportunities to expand your effectiveness and make a bigger impact on those around you—both clients and colleagues. When frustrated or disappointed, tell yourself: "Ah, here is an opportunity to become better and more effective in my career." Your emotions will be the leading indicator telling you when you should start reflecting on your current challenges and potential opportunities. If you are not motivated and excited to get up and go to work every day, then it's time to reconsider whether or not you're in the right job. If you are not feeling satisfied with the results you are getting at work, it might even be a sign it is time to move to the next stage in your career.

In the next section, we will explore each of the four career stages of a global health professional and some of the most common roadblocks that limit our effectiveness at these different stages. Using our own experiences and anecdotal case studies, we aim to highlight what we see as some underlying issues that directly limit one's ability to become more effective, and then provide solutions to turn these roadblocks into opportunities for personal and professional growth.

Career Stages, Effective Performance, and Opportunities

New Professional

Your main career goal in this stage is to get your first professional job. You need and want to demonstrate you can do what your boss asks you to do and deliver an effective performance on time and on budget. You also need to surround yourself with colleagues who share their experience with you to help you grow and learn fast. To get a head start, you might want to start this stage while you are still an undergraduate through volunteer work or internships. If you have graduated already, you must start right away getting to know the people who will be your coworkers someday. Get appointments to have at least one "informational interview" every week with the people who have your "dream job" and ask questions to learn more about how the organization supports the development of new professionals.

If you are an undergraduate or are studying to get your Masters' Degree in Global Health or Public Health and are thinking about what you will do when you graduate, good for you! Most students do not do that until after graduation. You need to start thinking about what summer internships, part-time paid, and volunteer jobs you can get that will provide actual on-the-job skills and experience. Do not wait until you graduate to start gaining experience and looking for a job. Without experience and without knowing anyone working in global health (besides your teachers), it will be hard to get a job when you are competing against hundreds of other students who have also just graduated from the many other schools of public health. Give yourself an edge!

If you have already graduated and do not have any work experience, you can still do it. You can join the Peace Corps or you can volunteer to work in one of your target organizations. Yes, you need to find the organizations you would like to be part of and keep a list of the ones you need to interview with in the future. These will be your "target" organizations and you need to learn all you can about them. Visit their Web site every day, read their white papers, and like their Facebook pages. Watch their videos on YouTube and join their groups on LinkedIn. Remember you are a professional now, so make sure your Facebook and LinkedIn profiles are up-to-date and you use them to reflect the kind of professional you want to be and the kind of work you want to do.

Next, start to get to know the team in those organizations and arrange for several "informational interviews" in every one of your target organizations to find out what they like about their job and how the organization or company supports their growth and professional development. A report from the Dartmouth Atlas project highlights the need for students choosing their residency to not just focus on the curriculum but how the doctors treat patients to see the "hidden training curriculum" that exists (Arora and True 2012). This applies to target organizations too. You must be prepared to look not only at the job qualifications but the people who work there and how they approach their work. Informational interviews are important because they allow you to have a glimpse into the work environment you may be joining soon.

You will likely feel nervous and insecure at the first couple of interviews. That is fine and expected. Use that nervousness to your advantage by turning those nerves into energy and enthusiasm. Smile and make eye contact to show you are really interested. Do not beat yourself up if the first interviews did not go the way you expected or if you stammered, or failed to say something you wanted to say. You are learning. After a few more of these interviews, you will feel more comfortable and assertive and will be able to engage in productive conversation, ask the right questions, and be ready to answer in a calm, engaging, and confident manner. Remember, it's better to get the nerves out during these informational interviews than to do so during an actual job interview. No matter what the results of these interviews, reflect on what you learned and move on to the next interview and apply what you learned.

We suggest you start a "Career Journal" and write down your global health mission statement, keep track of professional goals, your short-term objectives, and lessons learned from these interviews, books, or articles you read and from people you meet at professional meetings and conferences. Looking back on the pages of your journal will help you get clear on what you want to do next and see what progress you are making.

Innovator

In the first years of your career, what we call the "Innovator" stage, your main goal is to fast-track your career, demonstrate that you can improve your performance, continuously strive for and deliver better results, grow in self-confidence and take on more responsibility. You need to focus on using best practices and systems that have proven results, so stay up to date on what is being published or new in global health so you can deliver effective results and build your experience. At this stage, you also need to demonstrate you can behave professionally and function as part of a team. You want to be able to work with, contribute, and take advice from colleagues who are much more knowledgeable than you.

Don't be intimidated by other experts around you! As an Innovator, you have something that is very unique to contribute to your team and your organization: you have a fresh perspective. There are many opportunities, gaps, mistakes, and problems that are only evident to the newcomer. You may not have all the answers that experienced professionals have, but you must tell it as you see it, speak up, and ask questions. You may not be an expert in your chosen field yet, but you must become an effective team player and ask questions that may point to problems that may have been overlooked and help your team take timely action. There are no stupid questions. People will take notice of you when you ask questions that make them think. They will recognize your value and acknowledge that you are thoughtful and valuable to the team, thereby fast-tracking your career and the impact you make. Alternatively, you can keep quiet and few people will notice you and you will not progress quickly in your career.

If you are currently working in a clinic or hospital and something does not work, or is dirty, broken and not used, ask about it. If the toilets in the health center are not clean, ask whose job description includes supervising the cleanliness of the patients' toilets and whose job is it to clean them. If a patient got a malaria medicine without lab confirmation, ask about the procedure the clinic or health center has for diagnosing and treating malaria cases. If a woman comes to the center with her sick child, ask about the procedure for checking the child's nutrition and vaccination status as well as the mother's own health and her use of family planning methods too. You may be the only one who perceived that these services were not offered. Trust yourself and speak up.

If you are currently working on a global health project with an organization, read Chap. 3 again. Ask yourself and your colleagues the "Three Questions" and determine how you can apply the global health principles described in that chapter. You will innovate and add more value to your organization by applying these principles. If a project does not a have an effective handover plan from day 1, ask what will happen when the project is over; who will continue delivering the medicines or do the training and supervision?

Some senior professionals do not realize it, but they often get comfortable and do not take risks attempting to change the status quo. You must take action and take risks to innovate and try something new to solve existing problems. These bold actions make you different from other professionals because you will be ahead of the pack in working to improve your own effectiveness as well as that of your team and your organization. In this stage, you must also hone your people skills and your public speaking skills because you will need to speak up and propose innovative solutions and make your point with clarity and confidence.

One way to do this is to take a page out of the playbook of many health entrepreneurs. They are encouraged to network with different groups within the project to gain different perspectives and develop relationships that can assist your communication and support for new ideas (Margolis 2013). Mert Iseri talks about the need for champions, that is, to develop relationships within different sectors of your institution so that you have advocates for your ideas who can promote your ideas on your behalf (Iseri 2013). This concept is important for all innovators looking to move forward. Remember; you want to be noticed, not to nurture your ego, but to influence more people to do effective work.

In this stage, you will also need to keep improving your writing skills because you will need to write effective reports and documents that share the work done concisely and effectively online and off-line. Look for and ask for opportunities to give presentations and coauthor papers and reports. Remember, if you are keeping your ideas to yourself, you are not innovating and making an impact!

This is the stage when you need to demonstrate that you are a good manager of people and resources. In addition to reading and self-teaching about management in global health, tell your supervisor you want opportunities to learn and improve your management skills, and ask about his or her management style and what techniques work for them. Also, identify who the best managers are in your organization and ask them to meet so you can ask questions and use them as a sounding board. It is very hard to think that anyone will turn you down.

Next, work on your coaching skills to work with others. Help others younger and older than you to succeed and you will develop lifelong partners among your peers in addition to uncovering the best solution for everyone. Learn global health coaching skills and practice coaching others every day because it is the best way to learn to ask the right questions, find innovative solutions to global health challenges, and become more effective and known as an Innovator in global health.

Do not get comfortable. In fact, at this stage we would like to encourage you to get comfortable with being uncomfortable because in this way you will strive for more effective solutions to global health challenges in your area of expertise throughout the rest of your career.

Expert

After a few years, you will transition from the Innovator stage to the Expert stage. By now, you will have identified your strengths and perfected your technical skills through substantive experience and gained demonstrated expertise in one or several technical areas: malaria prevention, HIV/AIDS, non-communicable disease, mental health, disease surveillance or health facility management, maternal or child health or training or hospital management, etc. At this stage, your global health effectiveness will be measured by the number of people you have been able to effectively help to do what you do.

It is at this stage when you realize that you must have a "platform" to convey your knowledge and share your experience. If you have not done it yet, you must write your own book, articles, LinkedIn discussions and blog, and speak about your topic or area of expertise. This is how you create a platform from where you will be able to influence how others practice global health. By now you are ready to lead others and create new solutions and training programs that benefit hundreds of health professionals so it is time to get your message out there in a bigger way to make a bigger impact. In this way, you will become better known, will be sought out as an expert in your field, and will be hired as a consultant or expert on various teams. At this stage, some global health professionals decide to freelance to have time to write books or choose the assignments that best suit their interests and area of expertise. Others work to get promoted to lead a project or a whole department in their organization. Remember to build your platform through writing and speaking at global health conferences and events so you can advance global health practice in your area of expertise.

You need to start thinking about transitioning to the Expert stage and what you want to do next while you are still in the Innovator stage. Find other experts. Who do you admire is 5, 10, or even 15 and 20 years ahead of you? What do these people do? How did they get there? Meet them and interview them; get together over lunch or coffee to chat informally. In these meetings, you will find the support and information that will help you get known as an expert. These meetings are the opportunity to find out how to best use your experience so you can make a bigger impact in global health.

It is important at the time of transition from Innovator to Expert that you keep working on and using what worked before in the Innovator stage. You must keep being a good team player and looking for the opportunity to be team leader while helping others and sharing your expertise. Other health professionals do not know what your hard earned experience has taught you. Therefore, you will need to train and coach others to help them discover the best ways to improve health programs and services. Most of the people you work with may have different perspectives and experience because their training may have been different; the structure of the health system, local cultural beliefs, and gender differences are also factors that will affect one's point of view. You must improve your coaching skills so you can transfer your knowledge and help others apply what you know even more at this stage; you must become effective at gathering evidence and become better at measuring and accounting for results. You will become a leader and this is a great responsibility and an exciting opportunity to influence other health professionals to save more lives.

Visionary

Still a few more years later, you may realize you are transitioning to a new stage in your career. You will grow dissatisfied with a certain challenge in global health because you will have developed a whole new vision of how global health must work. You will start feeling a bit frustrated because you want change to happen faster and more effectively and because your vision differs so much from the reality. Good! You are about to go through another career change. You will realize that while you still believe your mission and passion for global health, you have developed an intolerance for business as usual.

Your career mission will guide you more than ever to do something effective about it and significantly improve global health. You may even be wondering what else you can do and what the next stage in your career will be. If you only knew what! In any case, remember that a bit of frustration is good. It helps you come up with new ideas, not only to take action on what you do and how, but also how to lead others toward a new vision in global health. This is what people who gathered in Alma-Ata in 1978 did when they created the concept of Primary Health Care, or in 2000 when the Millennium Development Goals were created. You have arrived at what we call the Visionary stage. What you do at this stage moves the whole field of global health forward.

Those who reach the Visionary stage are the ones who will lead significant change and progress in global health. They will achieve the ultimate reward of a career and life well lived: no regrets. You will have become a game changer and someone who made a difference in the lives of millions. You will have made some mistakes along the way, but learned from them and made drastic changes in your work to achieve effective results. I hope everyone reading these pages will become a Visionary at some point and choose the road less traveled as Robert Frost said in his famous poem (Frost 1920).

You will train other experts and become known as an authority in your field. You will be training other experts, coaching other coaches, and advising other global health leaders who in turn will influence the lives of other health professionals serving hundreds of thousands of people. Your influence and the responsibility that comes with it are immense at this stage, but the professional rewards are immense as well. I am talking about the reward of having made a difference in the world, not excuses.

At this stage, it is very important to find and work along with other experts and visionaries who are taking their careers to a higher level. You should find the right advisors who help you take your impact to a C-level. This is the stage when you will be asked to be CEO of an organization or Dean of a school of public health, or feel the need to start your own organization to fulfill your new vision.

In this book, each author is a visionary in his/her own right. You have read what they have achieved and what they are doing to make sure their work is effective. I suggest you use their chapters not only as a source of information but also of inspiration to coach you when you face challenges. Contact them, and engage them, and share your ideas and the work that you are doing at whatever stage you are. At whatever stage, follow your unique global health mission and strive for effective results because if you don't, nobody else will do it for you.

Roadblocks

Main Roadblocks

It is important to understand in moving through the stages described above there will be roadblocks. We want you to be aware of the most common roadblocks to being an effective global health professional so you can quickly identify them and find a way around them. The first main roadblock is not having a Career Plan and not knowing at what stage you are and what you want to achieve in your global health career.

The second most common roadblock is not having a career "Think Tank" team of pacesetter colleagues you network with to help you find the answers you need. You also need them to find the opportunities to become more effective and deliver results that you may overlook because you are too close and you cannot see them although they usually are right in front of you. Find someone who is ahead of you in your career to be your guide and coach, or at least have a group of colleagues you trust and admire with whom you can bounce ideas and get clear on next steps.

The third roadblock is not keeping track of your ideas and progress, because it gives you the false impression that you are stuck and not moving forward or that you are making progress but that progress cannot be measured. Get a notebook and start a career journal and document what you do and the results you get. We know it seems strange if you have not done it before, but you will realize after the first few days how much you learn. If possible, use a notebook. (Handwriting is more effective than typing it because it helps you think. Don't ask why—it has something to do with how the brain is wired.).

Paralysis Problem

We have all felt this particular roadblock at one time or another and we will surely face it again throughout our career. It's the feeling of being overwhelmed and paralyzed from doing anything because the task seems so immense that you feel whatever you do makes no difference. At other times, your work has become more business as usual; routine and boring, and you feel stuck doing the same job over and over again. Avoiding the problem is not a solution. So when you realize you are not feeling excited and motivated about your work, you need to overcome this through working with others to help you check your progress and degree of satisfaction, and setting deadlines to implement changes.

One of our clients wanted to change jobs. He had grown tired of his job and did not want to be seen as new professional but as an innovator. But as the months went by and he was not getting the job he wanted, he wondered why he was stuck. The fact was that he was ready to assume more responsibility and had the skills to move on to a higher job in global health, and he knew it, but he was not communicating this in his CV and in job interviews. First of all, he needed to include his strengths and experience in a way that recruiters could identify him as a candidate for positions of higher responsibility than he had at that time. Having a resume or CV that effectively shows you have the qualifications and experience required for a job takes some work.

Sometimes it may be difficult for you to realize your own strengths and skills. So, take the Strengths Finder (Rath 2007) test and ask others what they think your three main strengths and skills are—basically what you are really, really good at. At our company we receive lots of CVs every week, but very few actually make it to our database because these professionals do not include the qualifications we require. If you are interested in a position, take the time to edit your CV to show you meet the requirements, and in those areas where you do not, offer other skills and expertise to complement or compensate. Nobody is perfect. However, you must show you are able to articulate your experience in a concise and clear way. The purpose of an effective CV is to get you an interview. You won't get the interview if you do not help the recruiters see you have what they need.

Once you get the interview, you must prepare for the interview. Really familiarize yourself with the organization's Web site and the job requirements. Lack of preparation makes you look unprofessional and not serious about wanting the job. You cannot wing it. You need to practice before you have job interviews, so have several informational interviews to make sure you are confident, make eye contact, and engage the recruiter and ask important relevant questions. A global health job requires that we work in teams and analyze evidence and information and articulate intelligent solutions. The interview is a way to demonstrate you can handle that.

Back to our client, we also showed him to set deadlines for his job hunt and to book at least two interviews every week with his target organizations. Also, he updated his LinkedIn profile, which was more than a year old, and we encouraged him to post in various LinkedIn discussions at least once a day to get his views and experience known. He also realized he was wasting his time attending conferences and meetings if he was not networking with colleagues, getting engaged in these meetings by asking questions and contributing to the discussions. In fact, it was at one of these meetings that he attracted the attention of a program manager who told him about a position open in her company. He had not thought of including this company in his target list but when he read the job description it was what he was looking for. He applied and got the job.

What is interesting about this story is that he was able to recognize he was paralyzed, stuck, and not doing what he had to do to get the job he wanted. He was telling himself that it was difficult in this economy to find the right job and that thought paralyzed him. He was not actively engaged in finding the right job. What's the lesson to overcoming this roadblock? In short, recognize paralysis, set a deadline, and take action weekly.

Experience vs. Education

Some see it as the chicken or the egg dilemma, but it's simpler than that. In global health, experience is key to landing a job. You can't keep going to school forever and depend on education without practical experience to get a job. That attitude is not as effective. While in school or when looking for work, utilize your downtime to get the experience you lack. Sometimes you just need to seek volunteer opportunities to get started.

This roadblock is very sad. It reminds us of a number of new professionals who called for advice because after getting their Master's degree they could not get experience because they could not get a job, and they could not get a job because they had no experience. Most people follow our advice to take action and start getting experience while still in school. However, there are a few people who, when we showed them what to do and what it takes to get a job, did not follow through. After a while, they decided to go back to school for a PhD instead. Getting more degrees is not going to get you a job unless you take action and actually get practical experience.

So start looking for jobs and contributing to global health in one way or another. If you go for more degrees, a job in academia might work for you, so while you get your degree do research and apply for grants so you can thrive in academia. Again, get a coach or a mentor if you are just starting to help you take action and do not invest in more education until you have gained experience. You do not need to choose between education and experience. You need both to work in global health!

Negative Fairy Tales

We all like to be comfortable, but comfort can lead to stagnation in your career. We often sell ourselves stories to justify our actions or inaction so that we stay in our comfort zone. We need to break away from this negative fairy tale and continue challenging ourselves to advance in our careers and make a difference. This road-block leads to ineffective action or inaction as the result of wrong interpretation or negative reaction to rejection, failure, or difficulties in your work.

Global health is not for the faint of heart. You need to write grant applications and proposals that get rejected 8 out of 10 times and you need to keep moving forward despite that. You need to help health workers in developing countries help communities that have been displaced or live in very poor conditions and you need to figure out how to help overcome these circumstances.

However, some global health professionals do not take action or do not challenge the status quo because they tell themselves all the reasons why things cannot work and why they cannot do one thing or another. We call these stories negative fairy tales because these professionals are stopped or guided to take a safe solution, not the right one, by negative self-talk that convinces them to stay in their comfort zone.

These "tales" most of the time are not based on any hard evidence so they need to be rebuked. Question yourself if you realize you are talking yourself out of doing something big, important or new that will make a difference. Then ask yourself: "How can I make this work, in spite of the difficulties and challenge?" Do not avoid risk. Instead, ask yourself, "How can I manage the risks?" Change is risky but not impossible if you take effective action and monitor and manage the process effectively.

Another solution is to prevent the fairy tales from taking over at the start by using checklists. You need to use checklists in your personal life and in your career to ensure that you have an effective way of doing things. In fact, using a checklist is the cornerstone of the health center delivery model in Dr. Beracochea book *Health for All NOW* (Beracochea 2008). A checklist ensures that every health provider delivers the same quality of care to every patient efficiently everywhere and every-day; thus preventing the fairytale of why he or she cannot deliver care in that way. A checklist also helps reduce preventable known errors in healthcare like forgetting to weigh a pregnant woman on every antenatal visit, or forgetting to wash your hands before giving a vaccine to a child—thus preventing the fairytale about why it is hard to remember to wash one's hands.

Another reason to use checklists is that they help maintain consistency and ensure all staff deliver the same quality of care, particularly when you must deal with staff turnover and have less experienced staff doing the job. Checklists assure that the job is being done correctly even at the beginning when new staff are just learning a new approach or process, and it helps the staff or team member to follow the correct way to do the job; no tales, no excuses.

A few years ago, I (Elvira) discovered "The Checklist Manifesto: How to Get Things Right" by Dr Atul Gawande (Gawande 2009) and it was like finding a soul mate. He also discovered the value and effectiveness of having checklists to imple-ment changes, or new solutions. In his book, he tells how people still resisted the use of his surgery checklists even when the results were clearly more effective. I guess the ones that resisted also were telling themselves a negative fairytale about why they could not change and use a simple checklist or implement changes that improve quality of care, efficiency and consistency.

Sticky Feet

You might have sticky feet when you can't let go of your job on a project and find a new job. Or when you don't know how to effectively handover your job to local health professionals and move on when it is time. To prevent "sticky feet," you need to ask yourself: "What will happen when my project ends? How will I transfer my skills and abilities to the local institutions, local schools of nursing, medical schools, authorities, or partners and get ready for a position that will give me the satisfaction of making a bigger impact and not more of the same?" You need to find innovative solutions to ensure the sustainability of any improvement (Tulenko and Preker 2013).

In fact, we see many clients whose staff get stuck in this roadblock because they failed to realize they need an exit strategy. You should start preparing for the end of a project at least a year in advance, preferably on day 1 when the project starts. You know the project will end and when, right? Handover and transfer of activities and responsibilities start at least 2 or 3 years before the actual end of the project. However, the actual planning of the exit strategy must start a lot sooner. Your plan needs to include the activities the project was funding into the local authorities' plans and budget so they are able to sustain the achievements and successes the project achieved. So why not start thinking how to do the handover and transfer effectively, and how you can effectively transition your career to your next assignment?

It is easy to give in to inertia and want things to stay the same, but in global health, nothing stays the same because we are always striving for more effectiveness and more impact. Project managers and technical experts need to overcome their sticky feet by preparing for the project's end from the first day. Please remember the "Three Questions" and focus on the third question about having an exit strategy from day one. Your project handover and sustainability strategy and the project staff phase-out need to be part of the project's overall strategy (Crye 2011). Do not wait until the last month of the project to make decisions about the future of the project's results and deliverables, and your own career and that of your team. In any case, it is never too late to recognize sticky feet and implement an effective exit strategy. Start right away.

Ego Traps

Although this roadblock is sadly more familiar and obvious to many, ego traps can also be quite subtle. In fact, we all fall victim of our egos sometimes in global health. Ego can play out as the money-driven competitive type that wants a promotion to director, or a chief position and the corner office. It can also be the person who doesn't know what to do and can't deal with failure because his or her ego got hurt. Ego, that is who we want other people to think we are can trap us all in ways that completely sidetrack us from our ultimate goals and mission in global health. Sometimes we fear what our colleagues will think if we do things differently. Or we get so excited about a recent achievement that we overlook the signs when things do not work as well. Be aware of this trap in yourself, your colleagues, and team and help everyone be aware so you do not fall into it. As the saying goes, be independent of the bad and good opinion of others.

In any profession and field there are people driven by their egos. In global health it manifests itself when people, who without realizing it, have become more interested in their project's interests than in the ultimate impact in the country's health system and the public good. It is the country's right to development (UN 1986) that must empower everyone in the country to collaborate and move forward. People with big egos are often more interested in being right or controlling others than doing what is right. They are "control freaks," become defensive and blunt, promote their organization at the expense of the country they are supposed to help. They can't admit an error or failure, because they are afraid it would reflect poorly upon them, find fault, and blame others. Personality and sometimes cultural characteristics fuel egos, but nevertheless we all have to learn how to deal with people's egos effectively.

First, think about your own motivations and what your ultimate goals are. What is really best for the project, or best for the team, best for the country, and the population? Empathize with those with big egos around you. However, keep reminding them to go back to the ultimate goal so you do not allow egos to compete and nothing getting accomplished. Focus on the task at hand and everyone around you will become more effective. Demonstrate your ego is not threatened; you are a confident responsible professional and know what you are doing. In this way, you will accomplish the goals you set for yourself.

We face this roadblock every day in global health as well as in other development fields. One of the good things about being a consultant is that you can say things that others are afraid to. I (Elvira) believe I am doing a disservice to my clients if I do not assess and address the effectiveness of their team to deliver sustainable results when I am asked to solve a problem or evaluate a project. The effectiveness of the professionals working in an organization or on a project determine the effectiveness of the overall organization. So when appropriate, I bring up these roadblocks to professional effectiveness and facilitate the identification of ego traps that may be affecting the projects or organization's results.

I have seen projects where partners from different organizations cannot get their egos out of the way and even scream and undermine each other's work. I have seen how members of a team insist on following a bureaucratic chain of command even when someone had to be medically evacuated. I have seen people invoke seniority to overrule the proposal of a junior staff that was clearly a more efficient solution. I have seen people losing their temper and finger pointing accusing and blaming others instead of using the time and energy to find a solution to the problem at hand. I have seen people avoid confrontations and others start them just to protect their egos. I have seen how personal rivalries spoil the opportunity to deliver important improvements. And I have seen people defensively use email to document all interactions and copy everyone to demonstrate they are right and the other party is at fault.

Human relationships and communication are complex and this is true among team members, supervisors, and subordinates in global health organizations and projects.

To be effective, global health professionals in any stage must prevent these ego roadblocks to personal and organizational effectiveness by setting rules at the start and setting the example by focusing on the work at hand and not letting egos get in the way. An outside consultant can facilitate communication and call on facts such as why only one person is doing all the talking and the others are just listening; or why only some people have access to resources or opportunities and not others; set guidelines for the use of e-mail; and practice and demonstrate team communication. In global health, people come from very different backgrounds and cultures so we need to make sure that we set guidelines to ensure we respect each other and communicate effectively to get job done and get effective results.

Conclusions

What Can One Global Health Professional Do to Improve Effectiveness?

Lots! This whole book has hundreds of suggestions for you to take action. So start now!

First, start by creating a career plan, and identify which stage you are in, and identify which steps you need to take to keep moving forward. Set one main objective to achieve every month and plan how to achieve it effectively using the lessons and ideas in this book. Stay focused on the objective. Ask yourself: "If I could only achieve one objective this month that will have the maximum impact on my project or the communities I serve, what would it be?" Of course, you can always strive for more than one, but only after you have met your most important objective.

Second, keep this book close so you can apply each chapter at the right time. Try to keep a flexible mindset about what you can do and what you can change. In fact, everything changes. We just need to figure out how to influence change for the better. When confronted by delays or roadblocks just remind yourself that some things might take more time and effort, or a change in mindset or strategy. Instead of simply asking, "Why does this not work?" remember to ask yourself, "How can I achieve my objective despite the challenges I face now?" Your brain will find answers to both questions. However, the second is more empowering and effective. So do not wallow in "why" things happened, instead ask, "How can I/we achieve our objective despite the challenges we face now?"

Third, be aware of the common roadblocks because they are real barriers to effectiveness for yourself and your colleagues. Keep in mind and apply in your everyday work the principles of the Paris Declaration (OECD 2005) and the "Three Questions" and the "Three Cs." (see Chap. 3). Remember that all you do must improve the country's health programs and lead to improve how the health system works and delivers services, and results must last after your work is done.

References

Arora, A., & True, A. (2012). *What kind of physician will you be? Variation in health care and its importance for residency training. The Dartmouth Atlas Project*. Lebanon, NH: The Dartmouth Institute for Health Policy and Clinical Practice.

Beracochea, E. (2008). *Health for All NOW!* Fairfax, VA: MIDEGO.

Crye, L. (2011). *Transition of management and leadership of HIV care and treatment programs to local partners: Critical element and lessons learned*. Arlington, VA: AIDSTAR-One. USAID's AIDS Support and Technical Assistance Resources, Task Order 1.

Dweck, C. S. (2006). *Mindset: The new psychology of success*. New York: Ballantine Books.

Frost, R. (1920). *Mountain interval*. New York: Henry Holt and Company.

Gawande, A. (2009). *The checklist manifesto: How to get things right*. New York: Picador.

Gladwell, M. (2008). *Outliers*. New York: Little, Brown.

Iseri, M. (2013). *Why healthcare entrepreneurs need multiple champions. Getting access: The paths for healthcare entrepreneurs*. Kansas City, MO: Kauffman Foundation.

Karlin, B. (2013). *Choosing a career in development: My five decades in international public health*. Fairfax, VA: MIDEGO.

Margolis, P. (2013). *A path to access: How one healthcare network integrates entrepreneurs into healthcare. Getting access: The paths for healthcare entrepreneurs*. Kansas City, MO: Kauffman Foundation.

OECD. (2005). *Paris declaration*.

Pink, D. H. (2009). *Drive: The surprising truth about what motivates us*. New York: Riverhead Books.

Rath, T. (2007). *Strengths finder 2.0*. New York: Gallup Press.

Smith, L. (2013, April 19). *Huffington post*.

Tulenko, K., & Preker, A. (2013). *Innovative financing options for the preservice education of health professionals* (Technical brief 8). Chapel Hill, NC: Intrahealth.

United Nations. (1986, December 4). *Declaration on the right to development*. New York: United Nations.

Further Reading

Alessandra, T. (n.d.). *The official site of Dr. Tony Alessandra. 1996-2013*. Retrieved February 24, 2013, from http://www.alessandra.com/abouttony/aboutpr.asp

ASPH. (2011). *Global health competency model*. DRAFT model version 1.0, Global health competency development project, Association of Schools of Public Health.

Duflo, E. (2011, April). *Policies, politics: Can evidence play a role in the fight against poverty?* The sixth annual Richard H. Sabot lecture. Washington, DC: Center for Global Development.

Lucier, C., Wheeler, S., & Habbel, R. (2007, June). The era of the inclusive leader. *Strategy + Business Magazine, 3*, 12.

Medhanyie, A., Spigt, M., Dinant, G., & Blanco, R. (2012). Knowledge and performance of Ethiopian health extension workers on antenatal and delivery care: A cross sectional study. *Human Resources for Health, 10*, 44.

United Nations. (1948, December 10). *Universal Declaration of Human Rights*. New York: The Commission on Human Rights.

United Nations. (2000, August 11). *The right to the highest attainable standard of health*. New York: Committee on Economic, Social and Cultural Rights.

Chapter 27
Conclusions on Improving the Effectiveness of Aid in Global Health

Elvira Beracochea

> *Until one is committed, there is hesitancy, the chance to draw back, always ineffectiveness. Concerning all acts of initiative (and creation) there is one elementary truth, the ignorance of which kills countless ideas and splendid plans: that the moment one definitely commits oneself, then Providence moves too. All sorts of things occur to help one that would never otherwise have occurred. A whole stream of events issues from the decision, raising in one's favor all manner of unforeseen incidents and meetings and material assistance, which no man could have dreamed would have come his way. Whatever you can do, or dream you can, begin it. Boldness has genius, power, and magic in it.*
>
> W.H. Murray, The Scottish Himalayan Expedition

This book was several years in the making. Great colleagues and visionary thinkers have shared their experience of many years striving for effectiveness in the hope that you, the reader, will benefit from this hard earned experience and the next generation of global health professionals will be more effective and achieves more tangible lasting results. One thing is common among all the authors of this book: we are committed to effectiveness. I believe it is that commitment that brought us together and turned the dream of having a book on effectiveness come true, and that commitment that will grow the Aid Effectiveness Movement.

I would like to finish this book by saying that after 30 years working to improve healthcare, I have realized that in fact, the key word is commitment. When I committed to achieve to do my share of achieving the Millennium Development Goals (MDGs) and to the principles of the Paris Declaration, I started to speak about them

E. Beracochea (✉)
Realizing Global Health Inc., Olley Lane 4710, Fairfax, VA 22032, USA
e-mail: elvira@realizingglobalhealth.com

© Springer Science+Business Media New York 2015

E. Beracochea (ed.), *Improving Aid Effectiveness in Global Health*,
DOI 10.1007/978-1-4939-2721-0_27

and write about them and started to attract like-minded professionals that also believed in the MDGs and in the need to increase the effectiveness of our work in global health and lots of "unforeseen, incidents and meetings and material assistance" came our way at a time when very few people thought that the MDGs mattered or that changing how global health worked was possible. There has been tremendous progress. However, we still have a lot to do to improve the quality of healthcare in developing countries and improve equity in developed ones. There really is power in boldness. We encourage you to also be bold and commit to achieving the right to health through effective global health programs that have organized and coordinated execution.

Here is THE question for you: do you commit to do effective work?

I believe that if you also commit, a whole stream of events will ensue from our joint decision. There is boldness in what we wrote in this book because we want others to be bold too and take the road less travelled, the road of effectiveness in global health, in which each country, donor, and organization working in global is accountable for and transparent in the results they achieve and that their results show that they have indeed progressively improved the country's health system, its health programs, and the performance of its facilities. The ultimate result is to impact the health of people globally and show we all increasingly make an effort to reach those that are vulnerable, marginalized, or at risk of disease or disability.

I believe it does not matter where you are in your career, you must commit to effectiveness and its "sister principle," that is, sustainability. You must not accept any less. You must not accept poor performance that cannot demonstrate that the health system of the country being helped is really improved as a result of the help provided. It is our hope that this book will raise the bar in global health, set a higher standard to practice and implement global health projects and start a new era of change, an era of intolerance for poor results that do not actually improve the results of the health programs of the countries where numerous governments and donors are pouring resources.

As you read in this book, Haiti is a clear example where we have failed to restore quality healthcare services after the earthquake in spite of the millions of dollars donated. Global health is about developing and reforming health systems, improving the effectiveness of health programs and improving the well-being of the people in each country and consequently, globally. We must act globally and ensure local impact. No excuses for not preventing preventable deaths, for not having medicines, for not having and accounting for an inventory of supplies and equipment in every health facility, for not having clean examination rooms and toilets, for not having screens on windows and mosquito nets over all hospital and labor room beds, for not having clean labor rooms and delivery kits, for not having a routine vaccination program that effectively immunizes children and all against vaccine preventable diseases, and for not mobilizing all resources available to make the required changes and make things work the way we know health services have to be delivered. The solution to all the problems above and more is to work in a different way from the usual way donors and governments and global health organizations have worked so far. We must create structures and procedures to effectively organize our work and communicate, collaborate, and coordinate (the 3 "Cs") to work together and ensure we make the best of all resources available. You have to be different to make a difference, follow the recommendations in the book, and be bold to go further.

At the time of this writing, we have been involved in the latest Ebola epidemic in West Africa. Concerts are taking place to fundraise for Ebola, and donors are pouring funding. However, like in Haiti, there is no clear joint and coordinated strategy to ensure that the epidemic will be, in fact, controlled and the countries will be strengthened so they can prevent future outbreaks and when they do occur that they are detected and controlled promptly. I encourage you to boldly ask the following questions:

1. Are the affected countries improving their health surveillance systems so they can monitor patterns of morbidity and mortality and improve their disease prevention and control programs better?
2. Have a number of facilities been upgraded to provide quality care to those affected but the epidemic and are these facilities able to continue and sustain the provision of care after the assistance ends?
3. Have healthcare delivery procedures, job routines and descriptions, and lines supervision and support been improved to ensure that the new healthcare delivery procedures are sustained?
4. Have the training institutions in the affected countries been helped to change their curricula so they can train future health professionals in the new healthcare delivery standards and procedures?
5. Are we making use of all the existing technology that can save lives?
6. Are public health programs, particularly, infection prevention and control programs, being sustainably improved and expanded to reach the most vulnerable, those in the risk regions and the underserved whose right to health is not being protected or fulfilled?
7. And finally, have infection control policies and plans and services included in the countries' next year's budgets been updated and include the contribution of various donors and international assistance projects and initiatives?

The need of a global strategy to finish the work started to achieve the MDGs and go further to ensure quality healthcare for all is now more clear than ever. We must have a concerted strategy and coordinated implementation programs of that strategy. And we must account for our progress. We all must contribute to the International Aid Transparency Initiative[1] to be accountable of effective work and correct ineffective unsustainable practices and global health interventions. We must implement reviews of effectiveness such as the European Court of Auditors did of the assistance to Haiti[2] and the Millennium Challenge Corporation did of its Threshold program.[3] These reviews must be carried by all donors and organizations and metrics for effectiveness must be used by all.

It is time we put effectiveness and sustainability in our code of practice and not just do things without clear strategy and outcomes and measures of success. It is frustrating and unprofessional for funding to go where it is not clear it will get the

---

[1] http://www.aidtransparency.net/

[2] https://www.devex.com/news/auditors-verdict-on-eu-aid-to-post-earthquake-haiti-not-effective-enough-84456

[3] http://www.mcc.gov/documents/press/factsheet-2010002048002-threshold-program-lessons-learned1.pdf

most results and highest return on the investment. In fact, as Glen Schwartz wrote, charity done like that destroys dignity and strengthens the sense and mindset of dependency and helplessness. On the contrary, our work must allow the strengthening of a "Can do" mindset, of ownership and proactiveness, of self-reliance and pride in the work health professionals do in their countries.

Dr. Binagwaho told us about the lack of respect and effectiveness of donations that are not managed by professionals that are really an insult. These practices must be stopped.

As Gina Stracuzzi and Sam Daley-Harris showed the power of the stories we create with our work and the legacy we build, I would like to finish with one last story:

I became a doctor over 30 years ago in Uruguay, then a developing country, now a middle income country in South America. About 25 years ago, I was fortunate to receive a scholarship to earn my Master's Degree in Public Health in Israel. It was a wonderful opportunity to advance public health in my country where such training did not exist at the time. I had Buddhist, Jewish, Christian and Moslem, Latin American, African, and Asian friends and studied among all of them. We all learned from each other too, shared our common goals of making an impact and advance global health, and were empowered to go back to our countries and apply what we learned. In fact, I helped create and teach a new Master's program in Epidemiology, applied and taught what I learned about research, and implemented new programs that improved the performance of my native country's teaching hospital.

Later, my experience and results allowed me work in other countries and I started to work internationally. I have now worked in over 40 countries to improve the effectiveness of various programs from family planning and MCH to logistics and rational management of medicines. Over the last 25 years or so, I have learned a lot about what works and what does not and have been sharing the lessons that I learned. I learned that we cannot just train people in a 3- or 5- or 11-day workshops and expect them to go back home and apply what they learned. There is need for coaching and support and effective supervision systems to help health professionals and all kinds of health workers to translate what they learned into new work routines and integrate the new knowledge with old knowledge into health service delivery. I learned that projects must be designed to contribute to improve the health system and not just show outputs to donors such as numbers of children immunized, children with acute malnutrition that are treated, or mothers that deliver with a trained attendant in a couple of states in the country. Global health projects must be designed to not just get children immunized but to ensure that the country's immunization program can continue immunizing children after the project if not in the whole country yet, at least in some part of it and keep expanding. Global health and nutrition projects must ensure that the country's nutrition program can continue preventing malnutrition and providing early detection and treatment and in this way the country can apply all the inputs from numerous donors; and that the country can continue upgrading its maternal and child health program in all facilities in all states in all countries.

About 10 years ago, my passion for results and to share all I had learned inspired me to commit and do all I could to achieve the health goals of the Millennium Development Goals and started, Realizing Global Health, Inc., a global health consulting company. That was a big step, a big personal and financial commitment to what I believed was right. I have learned a lot in the last 10 years about what works in our global health business sector, how the nonprofit sector works, and how philanthropy and development assistance works. Many things work well and some not so. Philanthropy needs to improve and conflicts of interest need to be systematically addressed.[4] This book was designed to help build on what works and help correct what does not work well. Global health IS a business that supports thousands of professionals to do their work and the overhead of the organizations they work for. We must ensure the global health business is effective, efficient, and accountable. Nonprofit does not mean organizations are efficient and for-profit does not mean they waste funds. What matters is to show effectiveness and progress.

As the targets of 2015 approach and a new set of sustainable development goals are being set, we must also change not only goals but how we work to achieve global health goals. We cannot continue business as usual. We know that many countries will not meet the 2015 targets and still have a lot to do to catch up. These countries cannot develop their health systems and deliver quality healthcare and succeed without everyone's commitment to changing the global health business so they have the knowledge global health professionals like the ones in this book have. We must commit to communicate and be transparent in our results, and share the good and the bad. We must commit to coordinate and collaborate so that multiple donors working in nutrition or HIV/AIDS or any other program do complement each other and keep things simple and thus make it easier for the government to sustain the improvements. Effective partnership models between the Public, Private, and Civil Society sectors are emerging[5] that will allow us to advance the sound normative foundation we have in the international human rights legislation and law; this is the mandate[6] for the global health business to embrace. The right to health, the right to development, the rights of child, and other international legislation must be the foundation of international development and global health practice. Good intentions are not enough; we must demonstrate effectiveness and sustainability in all we do.

The global health business must account and document progress in a continuous and transparent manner. The MDG annual reports have been a great improvement. Started in 2005, 5 years after the Millennium Declaration, these reports show the gaps in progress and the lack of urgency and concerted action placed on achieving the goals. We must not repeat this mistake with the 2030 agenda of sustainable development and particularly the health agenda because not meeting the 2030 goals will cost millions of lives. Just not reducing smoking is estimated to lead to over a billion tobacco-related deaths in the next 10 years.[7] We must have better monitoring

---

[4] http://www.plosmedicine.org/article/info%3Adoi%2F10.1371%2Fjournal.pmed.1001020

[5] http://www.google.com/url?sa=t&rct=j&q=&esrc=s&source=web&cd=1&ved=0CCAQ FjAA&url=http%3A%2F%2Fwww.brookings.edu%2F~%2Fmedia%2FPrograms%2Fglobal %2Fbbr2014%2FSession%25204%2520%2520Partnerships%2520%2520Herscowitz_FINAL. pdf&ei=NspoVPzTM5H3yQT-tYHoBQ&usg=AFQjCNEn00n8VmDodWx4EttpwoUQHv7CO w&sig2=q2djL54wSrzbMRekRW1new&bvm=bv.79142246,d.aWw

[6] http://papers.ssrn.com/sol3/papers.cfm?abstract_id=1024781

[7] http://www.who.int/mediacentre/factsheets/fs339/en/

tools and build global systems that allow global health organizations and countries to measure results such as monitoring mortality trends.[8]

Final message....

Improving global health, which is ensuring health for all on this planet, is a personal and professional journey. A new phase in your own journey starts today. Commit to see it through.

Commit to simplicity and commit to fulfilling your role in history. We all have a historical mandate to do our best in this life and leave the planet a bit better than we found it for our children's children. Learn from the past. Do not make my mistakes. Make your own and make it better.

In 2015, the global health business will start a new era guided by the 2030 sustainable development goals. It is time we all commit to practice effectiveness, realize human rights legislation, and apply the principles of the Paris Declaration. Just commit. Let's meet again in 2030 and celebrate the most significant achievement of human race, the elimination of preventable death, and of inequality of access to highest attainable standard of healthcare. I expect you, the reader, to be one of the main authors of the next edition of this book...

Further Reading

Brautigam, D. (2009). *The dragon's gift: The real story of China in Africa*. New York: Oxford University Press.

Farmer, P. (2013). *To repair the world*. Los Angeles: University of California Press.

---

[8] http://www.thelancet.com/journals/lancet/article/PIIS0140-6736%2814%2961591-9/abstract

Glossary

Aid effectiveness Aid effectiveness is the effectiveness of development aid in achieving economic or human development (or development targets).

Approved annual budget for the health sector It is the annual budget as it was originally approved by the legislature. In order to support discipline and credibility of the budget preparation process, subsequent revisions to the original annual budget—even when approved by the legislature—should NOT be recorded here. This is because it is the credibility of the original, approved budget that is important to measure and because revisions to the annual budget in many cases are retroactive.

Capacity development The process whereby people, organizations, and society as a whole unleash, strengthen, create, adapt, and maintain capacity over time.

Country procurement systems Donors use national procurement procedures when the funds they provide for the implementation of projects and programs are managed according to the national procurement procedures as they were established in the general legislation and implemented by government. The use of national procurement procedures means that donors do not make additional, or special, requirements on governments for the procurement of works, goods, and services.

Development partner Includes bilateral and multilateral donors, e.g., country aid agencies and international organizations.

Health aid reported on national health sector budget This should include all health sector aid recorded in the annual budget as grants, revenue, or loans.

Health sector aid ODA contributed to the health sector. ODA includes all transactions defined in OECD/DAC statistical directives paragraph 35, including official transactions that are administered with the promotion of economic development and welfare of developing countries as its main objective; concessional in character and convey a grant element of at least 25 %.

Health sector coordination mechanism Multi-stakeholder body that meets regularly (usually monthly or quarterly) to provide the main forum for dialogue on health sector policy and planning.

© Springer Science+Business Media New York 2015   343
E. Beracochea (ed.), *Improving Aid Effectiveness in Global Health*,
DOI 10.1007/978-1-4939-2721-0

IHP+ A global partnership that puts the Paris and Accra principles on aid effectiveness into practice, with the aim of improving health services and health outcomes, particularly for the poor and vulnerable.

IHP+ country compact The IHP+ is open to all countries and partners willing to sign up to the commitments of the Global Compact. IHP+ Global Compact defines commitments following Paris principles on national ownership, alignment with national systems, harmonization between agencies, managing for results, and mutual accountability.

Joint Assessments of National Strategies (JANS) Joint assessment is a shared approach to assessing the strengths and weaknesses of a national strategy. IHP+ partners have developed a process for the Joint Assessment of National Strategies (JANS) with the intention that a JANS assessment is accepted by multiple stakeholders, and can be used as the basis for technical and financial support. In this definition, a plan has been jointly assessed if the JANS process, or a similar joint assessment, has been completed (please provide details in the "Answers and additional information column of the survey tool).

Mutual accountability Two or more parties have shared development goals, in which each has legitimate claims the other is responsible for fulfilling and where each may be required to explain how they have discharged their responsibilities, and be sanctioned if they fail to deliver (DFID).

ODA Grants and concessional loans for development and welfare purposes from the government sector of a donor country to a developing country or multilateral agency active in development. ODA includes the costs to the donor of project or program aid, technical cooperation, debt forgiveness, food and emergency aid, and associated administration costs (OECD/DAC).

Parallel Project Implementation Unit (PIU) When providing development assistance in a country, some donors establish Project Implementation Units (they are also commonly referred to as project management units, project management consultants, project management offices, project coordination offices, etc.). These are designed to support the implementation and administration of projects or program.

Paris Declaration The Paris Declaration, endorsed on 2 March 2005, is an international agreement to which over 100 Ministers, Heads of Agencies, and other Senior Officials adhered and committed their countries and organizations to continue to increase efforts in harmonization, alignment, and managing aid for results with a set of monitorable actions and indicators (OECD).

Performance assessment framework The basis of a government's policy to make information about the quality and performance of healthcare services available to the public and partners. National Performance Assessment Frameworks should be comprehensive (i.e., cover all areas of health sector performance).

Pooled funding mechanism A funding mechanism which receives contributions from more than one donor which are then pooled and disbursed upon instructions from the Fund's decision-making structure by an Administrative Agent (or Fund Manager) to a number of recipients. Sometimes known as a Multi Donor Trust Fund. Taken from http://www.undg.org/index.cfm?P=152

Program-based approaches (PBAs)   PBAs are a way of engaging in development cooperation based on the principles of coordinated support for a locally owned program of development, such as a national development strategy, a sector program, a thematic program, or a program of a specific organization.

Public financial management systems (PFM)   Legislative frameworks normally provide for specific types of financial reports to be produced as well as periodicity of such reporting. The use of national financial reporting means that donors do not impose additional requirements on governments for financial reporting.

Sector budget support   Sector budget support is a sub-category of direct budget support. Sector budget support means that dialogue between donors and partner governments focuses on sector-specific concerns rather than on overall policy and budget priorities (OECD 2006).

Standard performance measures (SPMs)   Indicators developed and agreed by the IHP+ Working Group on Mutual Accountability. SPM were designed to track the implementation of development partners' and country governments' commitments as set out in the IHP+ Global Compact. They are based as closely as possible on the Paris Declaration indicators.

Technical cooperation (also referred to as technical assistance)   It is the provision of know-how in the form of personnel, training, research, and associated costs. Technical cooperation includes both free-standing technical cooperation and technical cooperation that is embedded in investment program (or included in program-based approaches).

About the Authors

Nana A. Mensah Abrampah is a global health professional with several years of experience in quality improvement (QI), systems thinking, and the spread of innovation across the African region. Prior to joining the World Health Organization in 2015, Ms. Mensah Abrampah worked as a consultant for the USAID Tibu Homa project in Tanzania. During this time, she worked with the team to develop a sustainable exit strategy by reducing direct donor support to in-country teams and promoting scale up. In Malawi, she worked at a tertiary referral hospital in Lilongwe, where she analyzed health system barriers for rational use of antibiotics. For 5 years, she worked in numerous capacities under the auspices of the USAID Health Care Improvement project, a global mechanism for applying improvement approaches that enhance healthcare in more than 30 countries within Africa, Asia, Europe, and Latin America. Ms. Mensah Abrampah serves as an Associate Faculty Member for Health Systems & Services Research for F1000 Research. She has published extensively in peer-reviewed journals and holds a B.Sc. Econ and an M.Sc. in International Health.

Laura C. Altobelli is a global health practitioner serving for over 35 years in 12 countries on research, evaluation, and program planning to improve health in resource-poor populations through community participation. Her work in Peru has been deeply involved with the community-based CLAS. Laura's doctoral degree is from The Johns Hopkins University School of Public Health with concentration in international maternal, neonatal, and child health. Since 2002, Laura has been Peru Country Director and more recently Professor of Equity and Empowerment in Health for Future Generations, an international nonprofit based in the USA that, in addition to programs in six countries, runs an accredited Master's program in sustainable development and community change with alumni from over 50 countries. Laura is a member of the Alpha Chapter of Delta Omega, the honorary public health society. Laura is Chair-Elect of the International Health Section of the American Public Health Association. She is author of numerous publications.

© Springer Science+Business Media New York 2015
E. Beracochea (ed.), *Improving Aid Effectiveness in Global Health*,
DOI 10.1007/978-1-4939-2721-0

Amy Ansehl, D.N.P., F.N.P.-B.C., is Assistant Dean and Associate Professor of Public Health Practice at New York Medical College in the School of Health Sciences and Practice. She is responsible for the Public Health practicum program and has placed more than 1500 students globally in projects. In addition, she has significant leadership experience in community-based organizations. She is the chairman of the board of directors of Visiting Nurse Services which serves the lower Hudson Valley of New York State and the Bronx.

Smita Baruah is Director of Global Health Policy & Advocacy at Save the Children where she leads policy and advocacy on global health issues related to maternal and child health including nutrition in health. She has over a decade of experience in the USA and global advocacy and policy analysis, most notably on HIV/AIDS and other US foreign assistance issues. Prior to joining Save the Children, Smita served as Director of Government Relations at Global Health Council, where she led the Global HIV/AIDS community in the reauthorization of PEPFAR. She has also worked at InterAction and RESULTS. She currently co-chairs the Policy and Advocacy subcommittee of the Frontline Health Workers Coalition, serves on the Executive Committee of 1000 Days Working Group on nutrition, and is co-leading a policy group on maternal, newborn, and child survival legislation.

Elvira Beracochea has more than 25 years of experience as a physician and a global health expert and has worked in over 40 countries. She is the founder and president of "Realizing Global Health" (RGH). RGH is a global health consulting company that assists donors, governments, and global health organizations to develop self-reliant sustainable health systems that deliver quality healthcare to everyone, everywhere, every day. Dr. Elvira has developed the "Health for All NOW" model to deliver integrated quality healthcare, The RGH100, a system for improving healthcare delivery in 100 days, the ABM system to strengthen health system performance, and numerous other solutions and training and coaching programs that improve the delivery of quality health services worldwide. She is an active advocate for the right to health through her participation in various professional organizations. She is chair of the Community-Based Primary Health Care work group of the International Health Section of the American Public Health Association (APHA), and co-chair of the International Health and Nutrition Work Group at the Society for International Development in Washington (SIDW). Elvira's recent books include: "Health for All NOW: How to transform the delivery of health services in developing countries," "Medicines for All," and "Rights-Based Approaches to Public Health" (co-editor). Dr. Beracochea received her M.D. from the University of the Republic of Uruguay and her M.P.H from Hadassah Hebrew University in Israel.

Agnes Binagwaho is the Minister of Health of the Republic of Rwanda. After practicing as a pediatrician for over 15 years, Dr. Binagwaho led the National AIDS Control Commission between 2002 and 2008. She then served as Permanent Secretary in the Ministry of Health until 2011.

Dr. Binagwaho serves on many academic boards academic. Her engagements include research on health equity, HIV/AIDS, information and communication technologies (ICT) in e-health, and pediatric care delivery systems. She has published over 100 peer-reviewed articles, serves on the International Advisory Board of *Lancet Global Health*, the Editorial Board of *PLoS Medicine* and of *Health and Human Rights*: *An International Journal*, and contributed to multiple books. She chairs the Rwanda Pediatric Society and is a member of the Global Task Force on Expanded Access to Cancer Care and Control in Developing Countries. Dr. Binagwaho is currently a Senior Lecturer in the Department of Global Health and Social Medicine at Harvard Medical School, and Clinical Professor of Pediatrics at the Geisel School of Medicine at Dartmouth. She also serves on the International Strategic Advisory Board for the Institute of Global Health Innovation at Imperial College London.

Dr. Binagwaho received an Honorary Doctor of Science degree from Dartmouth College in 2010. In 2014, she received her Ph.D. from the University of Rwanda. She is active in advocacy and political mobilization on behalf of women and children in Rwanda and worldwide.

Richard N. Blue, **Ph.D.**, for 30 years as a Senior Foreign Service Officer, a foundation executive, independent consultant, and Vice President of Social Impact, Inc., Dr. Richard Blue has developed and managed evaluation systems as well as conducted over 30 evaluations and other analytic services relevant to improving the results, impact, and sustainability of development programs. While with USAID, he created and supervised the USAID Impact Evaluation Program which broke new ground in the application of mixed method, participatory rapid appraisal approaches to determining ex-post effects of completed USAID programs. He was instrumental in the formation of USAID Center for Development Information and Evaluation. He also served as Director of the Office of Egypt Affairs, and later as Deputy Director of the USAID India Mission. He was seconded by USAID to assist the U.S. House of Representatives Foreign Affairs Committee in a rewrite of the Foreign Assistance Authorization legislation. With The Asia Foundation, Dr. Blue managed programs in Thailand, Laos, and Vietnam, and won USAID support for a major program in Cambodia. Dr. Blue has conducted complex, mixed method evaluations in 25 countries covering all regions except Latin America.... As an independent consultant, he was called on to conduct extensive program level evaluations of highly visible programs, including evaluations of Eurasia Foundation, ABA/CEELI, and the USAID-UNDP/UNOPS long-term program in Cyprus. He has extensive experience evaluating programs in SE Asia. Joining Social Impact, Inc., as Vice President for Evaluation Services in 2009, he led the Dept. of State's year long evaluation of US commitment to the Paris Declaration, involving case studies of seven Federal Departments and Agencies. He retired from Social Impact December, 2013.

Shaun Conway is a smart, creative physician who with more than 20 years of experience working in global health and international development. He has pioneered innovative development projects and founded ambitious social ventures that have improved access to essential healthcare in Africa. Through his direct involvement in service delivery, research projects, complex evaluations, and interests in digital health, he has had the opportunity advise government and international agencies, multinational corporations, and civic organizations on a range of policy and programmatic decisions relating to HIV/AIDS, TB, Health Systems, Human Resources for Health, Medicines Regulation, AID Effectiveness, and Health Innovation. He is a strong advocate for agencies to be more accountable for how they design and implement systemic responses to complex social and health problems. He founded the IHP+Results Consortium and led this accountability initiative for 4 years. He is currently working on new ways of delivering and accounting for health benefits, using blockchain technology.

Deanna Crouse, M.H.S., C.H.E.S., is a public health specialist program manager and educator with 35 years' experience in public and private sector agencies and organizations. Her career has been devoted to implementing projects involving chronic and infectious diseases with an emphasis on diverse populations and health disparities. In recent years, she has lived and worked in Sri Lanka and South Africa developing HIV/AIDS education programs for youth and mothers. She currently manages health research programs at Howard University in Washington, DC. Ms. Crouse is a graduate of the Bloomberg School of Public Health of the Johns Hopkins University.

Sam Daley-Harris founded the antipoverty lobby RESULTS in 1980, co-founded the Microcredit Summit Campaign in 1995, and founded the Center for Citizen Empowerment and Transformation (CCET) in 2012. CCET helps nonprofit organizations train their members to create champions in Congress and the media for their cause. The 20th anniversary edition of his book Reclaiming Our Democracy: Healing the Break between People and Government was published in 2013. Ashoka founder Bill Drayton called Daley-Harris "One of the certified great social entrepreneurs of recent decades."

Tom Davis is the Chief Program Officer for Feed the Children and the Director of the Center for Children and Social Engagement. Tom has 30 years of domestic and international field experience in planning, implementing, and evaluating maternal, child health and nutrition (MCHN) programs, and social and behavioral change activities in food security, child survival and nutrition, HIV/AIDS, and primary healthcare projects in 25 countries. He was the 2012 recipient of the APHA Gordon Wyan Award for Excellence in Community-Oriented Public Health, Epidemiology, and Practice. He has co-led the Food Security and Nutrition Network's Social & Behavioral Change (SBC) Task Force, and served as Chairman of the Board for the CORE Group and as a member of CORE's SBC Working Group. Tom developed the Barrier Analysis methodology for discovering determinants of behaviors in 1990, which has been used domestically and internationally. Tom has been a champion, pioneer, and regular author of papers on the volunteer peer educator Care Group model, which has significantly reduced malnutrition and child deaths in many countries, and co-authored the Local Determinants of Malnutrition Study methodology.

Dr. John Eriksson is President of Global Peace Services, USA, a nonprofit organization established in Washington, DC in 1998 that promotes the peaceful resolution of violent conflict. He held various positions in the US Agency for International Development, including Deputy Director of USAID, Sri Lanka; Director of USAID, Thailand; and Director, Center for Development Information and Evaluation, Washington. He has consulted for the African Development Bank: Danish Agency for International Development; Inter-American Development Bank; UK Department of International Development; US Agency for International Development and the Independent Evaluation Group of the World Bank. He has a Ph.D. in Economics from the University of California at Berkeley.

James N. Gribble is a senior fellow with the Palladium Group (previously GRM/ Futures Group), with more than 25 years of experience to the field of international population and family planning. His areas of expertise are policy, research, and synthesizing data and research findings for nontechnical groups, including policy-makers. He is deputy director for family planning and reproductive health of the USAID-supported Health Policy Project, where he provides oversight of the project's broad portfolio that includes costed implementation plans for family planning, development, and applications of policy models to generate support for family planning, and developing a better understanding of the linkages between population growth, family planning, and other health and development issues. Dr. Gribble has also authored a variety of publications on issues related to family planning, including contraceptive security, youth, and the demographic dividend. At the time of authoring this chapter, he was vice president of International Programs at the Population Reference Bureau. He holds his masters and doctoral degrees from the Harvard School of Public Health and undergraduate degrees from the University of Texas at Austin.

George F. Grob is President, Center for Public Program Evaluation, an evaluation company focusing on public policy, strategic planning, and communications. Prior to forming this independent evaluation consultancy, George was Director of Planning and Policy Coordination and later Deputy Inspector General for evaluation and inspections at the U.S. Department of Health and Human Services. Immediately prior to retiring from federal service, he was Executive Director of the Citizens' Healthcare Working Group, a congressionally established commission charged with developing options for health care reform based on citizen input. His work has centered on policy development and program effectiveness, largely in the fields of health, human services, and the environment as well as international evaluation capacity building. He received his M.A. in mathematics at Georgetown University.

Ruth Hope, As the Director of RGH's Center for Reproductive Health, HIV/AIDS and Gender Equality, Dr. Hope addresses critical public health issues in resource poor settings. She believes in order to realize global health individuals, families, and communities must be empowered to meet their reproductive health and development needs and governments must commit to strengthen health systems delivering quality health services. She focuses on the needs of the poorest and most vulnerable, providing technical support to sustainable approaches that enhance local and national capacity. Dr. Hope also designed RGH's 7-Day HIV/AIDS Program Manager Online Coaching Program that trains and coaches individuals in developing countries to become leaders in the fight against HIV/AIDS. Dr. Hope is a physician with postgraduate clinical qualifications in pediatrics, obstetrics and gynecology, and family planning. She has a Master of Science degree in Mother and Child Health from the University of London, Institute of Child Health, and a Master of Arts degree in Education from the UK Open University. She speaks Nepali and has worked in Eastern Europe, Central Asia, Latin America, the Caribbean, Africa, and Asia.

Sarah Kalloch is currently at MIT pursuing a graduate degree. Prior to that, she served as the Campaign Alliances Manager at Oxfam America, where she advocated for international development legislation and improved corporate practices to fight poverty, hunger, and injustice. Prior to joining Oxfam, Sarah worked at Physicians for Human Rights as Director of Outreach and Organizing, leading advocacy on HIV/AIDS, colleagues at risk, and more. Sarah is a Truman National Security Fellow, a member of the Food Tank Advisory Board, and was just elected secretary-elect of the APHA International Health Section.

Barry Karlin, Dr.P.H., served as USAID Public Health Adviser in Thailand from 1959 to 1966. He later worked for many years in Pakistan and Papua New Guinea with World Health Organization (WHO), and in numerous other nations, including Haiti. Dr. Karlin was in APHA's International Health Division for 8 years, and has taken numerous graduate classes to developing nations to study their health care systems. He is author of Choosing a Career in Development: My 5 Decades in International Public Health, published by Realizing Global Health in 2013. He currently leads efforts to reform Colorado's health care system.

Eckhard Kleinau is an experienced manager and technical leader committed to advancing global public health, strengthening health systems, and improving people's livelihoods through cross-sector approaches, social innovation, and reliance on evidence from implementation science. He is Vice President and Director of Evaluation Practice a AMEX International, and previously held similar positions at GRM Futures Group overseeing a large portfolio of international development projects funded by USAID, DfID, and DFAT with over 120 staff. Dr. Kleinau directed the monitoring of program performance, impact evaluations, creative but rigorous data analysis, flagship publications, and effective communication of agency achievements. He coordinated the standardization and harmonization of indicators in water supply, sanitation, and hygiene with NGOs, USAID, WHO, and UNICEF. He also developed and led an innovative and award-winning project integrating health, population, environmental management, and food security in Madagascar. Early in his career Dr. Kleinau led infectious disease control programs for malaria, tuberculosis, and leprosy as well as integrated the delivery of primary healthcare services in West Africa. Dr. Kleinau holds a Dr.P.H. in Health Policy and Management (Program Evaluation) from Harvard University; M.S. in Epidemiology and M.S. in

Health Services Administration from Harvard University; M.D. from Eberhard-Karls University, Tübingen, Germany.

Carl Mabbs-Zeno retired in 2014 as Senior Advisor for Economic Growth in the State Department's Office of Foreign Assistance Resources. He was formerly Senior Advisor for Global Health and a Division Director in the Bureau for Global Health at USAID. He began his career with the Economic Research Service of USDA and has worked in about 50 countries.

M. Rashad Massoud, M.D., M.P.H., F.A.C.P., is a physician and public health specialist internationally recognized for his leadership in global healthcare improvement. He is the Director of the USAID Applying Science to Strengthen and Improve Systems (ASSIST) Project. He is Senior Vice President of the Quality and Performance Institute at University Research Co., LLC (URC), leading URC's quality improvement efforts in over 40 countries applying improvement (aka implementation, delivery, execution) science to deliver better results in global health priority areas. He has a proven record of strong leadership and management. Previously, he was Senior Vice President at the Institute for Healthcare Improvement (IHI) in Cambridge, MA, responsible for its Strategic Partners—IHI's key customers working on innovation, transformation, and large-scale spread, such as HRSA's Health Disparities Collaborative, Kaiser Permanente, The NHS Institute for Innovation and Improvement in the UK and the DHHS Indian Health Service. Dr. Massoud previously served as Associate Director of the USAID Quality Assurance and Workforce Development Project (QAP 2 and 3) responsible for the Project's activities in Europe and Eurasia/Asia and the Middle East. Dr. Massoud pioneered the application of collaborative improvement methodology in several middle- and low-income countries. He helped develop the WHO strategy for design and scale up of antiretroviral therapy to meet the 3×5 target; large-scale improvement in the Russian Federation; improving rehabilitation care in Vietnam; developing the Policy and Regulatory Framework for the Agency for Accreditation and Quality Improvement in the Republic of Srpska; and developing plans for the rationalization of health services in Uzbekistan. He founded and for several years led the Palestinian healthcare quality improvement effort. He was a founding member of, and Chairman of the Quality Management Program for Health Care Organizations in the Middle East and North Africa, which helped improve healthcare in five participating Middle East countries. He has worked on healthcare quality improvement for the Harvard Institute for International Development and the Palestine Council of Health. He also served as a Medical Officer with the United Nations Relief and Works Agency, and he has consulted for and collaborated with several NGOs, KPMG, UNICEF, the World Bank, and WHO. Dr. Massoud is a regularly invited speaker at international conferences and chaired the April 2012 Salzburg Seminar: "Making Health Care Better in Low and Middle Income Economies: What are the next steps and how do we get there?" Dr. Massoud speaks English, Arabic, Russian, and basic French.

Pedro Mendoza-Arana is a physician and Surgeon (M.D.), holding an M.Sc. in Health Planning and Financing from the University of London, UK, and a Doctoral Degree (Ph.D.) by Universidad Nacional Mayor de San Marcos, Lima, Peru.

Previous experience includes top positions at the Ministry of Health, Ministry of Education, and Non-Governmental Organizations, as well as consultancies for UNAIDS, PAHO, IADB, JICA, GTZ, and Ministry of Health.

Currently devoted to the academia, at the Universidad Nacional Mayor de San Marcos, and consultant services. Author of three university textbooks: "Strategic Planning in Management: Applied for Health Facilities" (2000), "Economic Evaluation in Health" (2002), and "Strategic planning for health management" (2009).

Eric Muñoz is a Senior Policy Advisor with Oxfam America. His portfolio includes donor assistance for food security, domestic agriculture, and emergency food aid and food security policy. His advocacy experience ranges from influencing US policies to supporting global advocacy in multilateral fora including the Committee on World Food Security. He has more than a decade of experience working on hunger and human rights policy issues having previously worked as a Senior Policy Advisor with Bread for the World and as a paralegal with the Lawyers Committee for Civil Rights Under Law. He has co-authored research and policy papers along with five *Hunger Reports* on variety of global agriculture and food security issues. Eric studied English Literature at Rice University and International Relations at the Korbel School for International Studies at the University of Denver.

Padmini (Mini) Murthy is a physician (a trained obstetrician and gynecologist) and an activist who did her residency in Obstetrics and Gynecology. She has practiced medicine and public health for the past 28 years in various countries. She has been working in various arenas of the health care industry. She has a Masters in Public Health and a Masters in Management from New York University (NYU). Murthy has been on the Dean's list at NYU Steinhart School of Education and named Public service scholar at the Robert F. Wagner Graduate School at New York University.

She is also a Certified Health Education Specialist. Murthy is the NGO Representative of Medical Women International Association to the United Nations. She has served as a consultant to the United Nations and is on faculty at New York Medical College as Director of Global Health and Associate Professor; currently, Murthy also serves as member of the Executive Council of the NGO CSW Committee of NY at the United Nations. In this role, she has met United Nations Ambassadors, high-level UN personnel to discuss women's health challenges. She has been at the forefront of organizing workshops and seminars internationally on women's health and the challenges faced.

Murthy has been working on CEDAW and CSW issues namely women's health (throughout the life span) and human rights from a global perspective since 1998 as an NGO representative and later as a consultant to the United Nations Population Fund. In this role, she has organized conferences and workshops and has been an invited speaker every year at the CSW since 1998 to the present. In her role as

Executive member of the NGO committee of NY, she has been a team member working on the Beijing Plus 20 website and content for 2015.

Murthy is widely published and is the author and editor of *Women's Global Health and Human Rights* (*Jones and Bartlett publisher*) which is used as a text-book worldwide, and she serves as a peer reviewer for several publications. Her poetry book *Mini's Musings* was published in 2012. She has made over 100 presentations on women's and children's health nationally and internationally in scientific conferences and in the United Nations and countries where she has been invited. In April 2015, Murthy was inducted as inaugural fellow of the American Medical Women's Association. In June 2015, she received "Millennium Milestone Maker Awardee" at the 9th Annual Women's Symposium at Sias University China.

Aishwarya Narasimhadevara is an individual wishing to make a difference in society like others. Her background is International Development. She has completed her M.A. in International development from the School of International Studies at the University of Kent. She has been involved with different organizations that work with regard to international affairs. She is interested in Education in International Development. Travelling is a passion of hers, and she enjoys seeing new places and is widely travelled. She also enjoys learning, taking photos, and practicing karate.

Juan Carlos Negrette has more than 25 years of extensive international experience in health programs design, implementation, and management. He has successfully directed health service delivery programs and commercial healthcare activities, and has structured and developed productive partnerships of strategic importance with relevant private sector companies and government entities, resulting in tangible improvement of the health and social conditions of communities and populations served. Mr. Negrette has effectively adopted and adapted commercial tools, techniques, and approaches to primary care programs in different parts of the world. He has also designed and implemented effective strategic health marketing and communication interventions in challenging environments in Asia, Africa, and Latin America. Mr. Negrette is currently the Director of Global Health at the University of Utah.

Cristina de Nicolás, For over 15 years of overall experience in health systems strengthening, program management, strategic planning, monitoring, and evaluation, Cristina has brought growth and maintaining high profiles for organizations, as well as managing external communications and acting as the principal contact point for donors, local partners, and government representatives. Cristina has also provided strategic support to regional and international NGOs in the areas of organizational development, leadership, program and financial management of funds, Monitoring, Evaluation and Reporting, proposal development, as well as procurement and supply management. She also has a strong background in Global Fund-related initiatives (Governance and Leadership and Monitoring & Evaluation). As an organizational development consultant, she has worked in programs for a cross-section of development agencies and donors, including the Spanish Cooperation Agency (AECID), the European Commission Humanitarian Aid Office (ECHO),

USAID, and the Global Fund. Her work with bilateral donors has involved regular work with the NGOs receiving their funding. INGOs such as ACFI, MSF, and others. Her work for these agencies includes country representation, program management, training development tools in Project Cycle Management, and development of governance tools such as Manuals of Monitoring and Evaluation. Currently, as a technical adviser to countries recipient of Global Fund grants, she diagnoses, designs, and monitors Country Coordinating Mechanisms (CCM) to manage the funds supporting the establishment of governance tools and developing the capacity of various actors (mainly civil society) for improving performance. She is fluent in Spanish, English, and French and can work in Russian.

Henry B. Perry, III, is a Senior Scientist in the Health Systems Program of the Department of International Health at the Johns Hopkins Bloomberg School of Public Health. His primary research interest is on community-based primary health-care programs. He has a broad interest in primary healthcare and community-oriented public health, community participation, and equity and empowerment. He is the author of more than 125 scientific articles and other publications, many of which focus on child health and community-based approaches to improving maternal and child health. He teaches a popular massive open online course (MOOC) sponsored by Coursera entitled Health for All through Primary Health Care that has been taken by 50,000 people so far. He has worked as a consultant with UNICEF, the US Agency for International Development, the Gates Foundation, and many other organizations. Dr. Perry is a graduate of Duke and Johns Hopkins Universities with training in general surgery, public health, as well as sociology and anthropology. He lived in Bolivia, Bangladesh, and Haiti, where he provided leadership for health programs. He has a special interest in community health workers and their capacity to improve access to health services and improve the health of underserved populations.

Aaron Pied, For more than 15 years, Aaron has worked in Africa, Asia, and the USA as a teacher and administrative professional. After completing service as an English Teacher and health educator with the Peace Corps in Burkina Faso, Aaron returned to the USA and worked as a teacher before deciding to return to international development. He began by working to support international health research at the Center for Global Development. Aaron later relocated to Thailand where he was a consultant for local health and education organizations, a caseworker for refugees wishing to resettle to the USA, and an education coordinator for an NGO providing skills and opportunity to Thai and Burmese youth interested in vocational work. He is currently the Director of Operations for Realizing Global Health where he focuses on managing the finance, communications, human resource, and marketing activities for RGH while providing support to select projects.

Elisabeth Sandor is an international consultant in development with more than 20 years of professional experience in the areas of global health, health policies, public policies, governance, aid policies, and financing for development. Before becoming independent consultant, she has worked at the OECD and at the World

Bank as senior advisor in health aid and in the French public service as advisor in health (Palais de l'Elysée, French Ministry of health). Her article is based on her experience in managing a 4-year senior-level work stream on health and aid effectiveness at the OECD (2007–2011).

Glenn Schwartz served as a missionary with the Brethren in Christ Church in Zambia and Zimbabwe during the 1960s. He then served for 6 years during the 1970s as an administrator in the School of World Mission at Fuller Theological Seminary. From 1983 until 2014, he served as Executive Director of World Mission Associates (WMA) and has been researching, writing, and speaking about issues of unhealthy dependency and self-reliance in the Christian movement. He currently holds the position WMA Executive Director Emeritus. He and his wife, Verna, currently live in Lancaster, Pennsylvania, and have two adult children and six grandchildren.

Tim Shorten is an evaluation specialist with over 13 years of experience in international development primarily focused on Monitoring & Evaluation, Impact, and Accountability. He is experienced in coordinating high-profile, multi-stakeholder, multi-country processes, and effectively managing a wide range of stakeholder relationships to senior level. He has led and played key roles in high-profile evaluations including for DFID, the World Health Organization, Girl Hub, CHAI, and UNITAID. His areas of technical focus and experience include Aid Effectiveness, HIV and AIDS, Reproductive and Maternal Health, Health Systems, Education, and Governance. He is experienced in development and implementation of international and national level policy, working closely with developing country governments, bilateral and multilateral institutions, civil society and private sector, as well as with parliamentarians. His specific experience includes managing the consortium to provide four annual independent assessments of the implementation of the International Health Partnership (IHP+) with a primary focus of strengthening mutual accountability in the health sector. He has worked within the G8 to increase accountability, including through strengthening the Africa Partnership Forum and working with Parliamentarians and Civil Society to support their oversight and scrutiny of health sector interventions and results both in the UK and internationally.

Kelly Skeith is an international development M&E Specialist with expertise in the design, implementation, and management of performance monitoring and evaluation projects worldwide. She is currently the Senior Design, Monitoring and Evaluation (DM&E) Specialist at Freedom House, an NGO focused on human rights and democracy promotion. From 2010 to 2015, as Deputy Director for Social Impact's Performance Evaluation practice, she provided management and technical oversight and support for all evaluation, assessment, and performance monitoring contracts for USAID and the Department of State. Her technical work at Social Impact focused on the utilization of both qualitative and quantitative approaches to capture output, outcome, and impact level data to improve program and policy design and effectiveness in transitional, fragile, and conflict-affected areas. Ms. Skeith is also a certified trainer for USAID and DOS and helped to develop and facilitate

USAID's Evaluation for Program Managers (EPM), Evaluation for Evaluation Specialists (EES), and Managing for Results courses in DC and around the world. She is also a lead trainer for the US Department of State's Evaluation Design and Management courses. Prior to Social Impact, Ms. Skeith worked at USAID's Office of Conflict Management and Mitigation (CMM) and was a team leader in the AmeriCorps National Civilian Community Corps. She holds a Master's degree in Economic and Political Development from Columbia University.

Gina Stracuzzi is a communications specialist with more than 20 years experience helping organizations in the USA, Europe, and in developing economies build messaging strategies that capitalize on their strengths and tell their unique stories. Working across many industries including the nonprofit and global public health sectors, Gina joins her desire to advance social issues with her passion for storytelling to help clients learn how to tell their individual and organizational stories in ways that inspire action. As founder and Executive Director of eWomen International Coaching and Mentoring Network, Gina helps women in emerging economies and also helps them learn to share their unique stories as a tool for realizing their goals of starting businesses or venturing into their first career.

Gina has a Bachelors in Communication from American University, a Master's degree in Culture and Communication from New York University, a Graduate Certificate in Global Health from George Mason University. Professional development courses include Leading Change through Communication (The Johns Hopkins University) and Storytelling for Change (NovoEd).

Index

© Springer Science+Business Media New York 2015
E. Beracochea (ed.), *Improving Aid Effectiveness in Global Health*,
DOI 10.1007/978-1-4939-2721-0

Printed in the United States
By Bookmasters